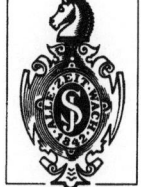

Nasser Javadpour (Editor)

Principles and Management of Adrenal Cancer

With 121 Figures

Springer-Verlag
London Berlin Heidelberg New York
Paris Tokyo

Nasser Javadpour, MD, Professor and Director,
Section of Urologic Oncology, Department of Surgery,
School of Medicine, University of Maryland,
University Hospital, Baltimore, Maryland 21201, USA

ISBN-13:978-1-4471-3136-6   e-ISBN-13:978-1-4471-3134-2
DOI: 10.1007/978-1-4471-3134-2

British Library Cataloguing in Publication Data
Principles and management of adrenal cancer.
1. Adrenal glands—Tumors
I. Javadpour, Nasser
616.99′445   RC280.A3
ISBN-13:978-1-4471-3136-6

Library of Congress Cataloging-in-Publication Data
Principles and management of adrenal cancer.
Includes bibliographies and index.
1. Adrenal gland—Cancer. I. Javadpour, Nasser, 1937–. [DNLM: 1. Adrenal Gland Neoplasms. WK 780 P957]
RC280.A3P75 1987 616.99′445 86-31443
ISBN-13:978-1-4471-3136-6

© Springer-Verlag Berlin Heidelberg 1987
Softcover reprint of the hardcover 1st edition 1987

The use of registered names, trademark etc. in this publication does not imply, even in the absence of a specific statement, that such names are exempt from the relevant protective laws and regulations and therefore free for general use.

Product Liability: The publisher can give no guarantee for information about drug dosage and application thereof contained in this book. In every individual case the respective user must check its accuracy by consulting other pharmaceutical literature.

2128/3916/543210

Preface

The vast amount of literature and rapid developments in the understanding and management of adrenal diseases have outpaced the ability of physicians to assimilate and utilize these advances in clinical settings. This book is designed to bring these developments to those interested in adrenal diseases and to assist clinicians in caring for patients with such diseases.

The recent advances in the understanding of steroids, catecholamines, and utilization of computed tomography and magnetic resonance imaging have rendered disease of the adrenal gland more rewarding in terms of early detection.

Although a number of basic and clinical improvements have been achieved in these diseases, there are still a number of unresolved problems, including the lack of effective cytotoxic agents for therapy of various disseminated adrenal malignancies.

The natural history of certain diseases of the adrenal glands and their proximity to the genitourinary system makes these essential organs very attractive to urologic surgeons. Furthermore, for a number of diseases such as adrenogenital syndrome, hypertension, and certain tumors of these glands it is obviously desirable that urologic surgeons are familiar with diseases of "the adrenal glands."

The first part of this book is an overview of the relevant embryology, anatomy, physiology, markers, pathology, imaging, and current progress. The second part covers specific diseases of the adrenal cortex and medulla. We hope that this volume will assist the physician in the diagnosis and management of patients with adrenal disease.

Baltimore, U.S.A.   Nasser Javadpour
February 1987

Contents

Contributors

D. R. Bodner, MD
Assistant Professor, Division of Urology, Case Western Reserve University, Cleveland, OH 4416, U.S.A.

S. A. Chalew, MD
Assistant Professor of Pediatrics, Division of Pediatric Endocrinology, Bressler Building, Rm 10-047, University of Maryland School of Medicine, Baltimore, MD 21201, U.S.A.

B. P. M. Hamilton, MD
Chief of Endocrinology and Metabolism, Veterans Administration Medical Center, Baltimore, MD 21218, U.S.A.

T. H. Hsu, MD
Assistant Professor, Department of Medicine, Johns Hopkins Hospital, 600 North Wolfe Street, Baltimore, MD 21205, U.S.A.

N. Javadpour, MD
Professor and Director, Section of Urologic Oncology, University of Maryland, University Hospital, Baltimore, MD 21201, U.S.A.

H. P. W. Kozakewich, MD
Assistant Professor of Pathology, Harvard Medical School, Children's Hospital, Boston, MA 02155, U.S.A.

E. E. Lack, MD
Chief of Surgical Pathology and Post-Mortem Section, National Cancer Institute, National Institutes Of Health, Bethesda, MD 20205, U.S.A.

P. A. Levin, MD
Assistant Professor of Medicine, Department of Pediatrics, University of Maryland School of Medicine, Baltimore, MD 21201, U.S.A.

B. López-Ibor, MD
Fulbright Fellow in Hematology and Oncology, University of Maryland School of Medicine,
Baltimore, MD 21201, U.S.A.

J. H. Mersey, MD
Assistant Professor, Division of Endocrinology, University of Maryland School of Medicine,
Baltimore, MD 21201, U.S.A.

J. E. Montie, MD
Professor and Chairman, The Department of Urology, The Cleveland Clinic Foundation,
9500 Euclid Avenue, Cleveland, OH 44106, U.S.A.

M. I. Resnick, MD
Professor and Chairman, Division of Urology, Case Western Reserve University, Cleveland,
OH 44106, U.S.A.

C. L. Schultz, MD
Assistant Professor, Division of Radiology, Case Western Reserve University, Cleveland, OH
4416, U.S.A.

A. D. Schwartz, MD
Chief of Pediatric Hematology/Oncology, University of Maryland School of Medicine,
Baltimore, MD 21201, U.S.A.

Chapter 1

Overview of Progress, Current Problems, and Future Perspectives

N. Javadpour

Recent advances in imaging and localization of adrenal tumors have had a remarkable impact on their surgical and medical management. Advances have also been made in the basic understanding of pituitary and adrenal function, and meaningful progress has been made in localization of tumors including venous sampling [8], computed tomography [9], magnetic resonance imaging, and brush biopsies of the intracaval tumor thrombi. A number of problems remain, the most immediate being a need for effective chemotherapeutic regimens in the management of local recurrences and disseminated adrenal tumors. In this chapter, I will review briefly the recent advances in the diagnosis and therapy of adrenal diseases with emphasis on surgical problems.

Adrenal Vein Sampling

The most definitive method of localizing adrenal aldosterone-producing adenomas has been selective adrenal vein catheterization with sampling of aldosterone concentrations [9]. Adrenal vein sampling is, in most cases, a safe and effective method of localizing an aldosterone-producing tumor. The technical adequacy of catheter placement in the adrenal vein, particularly on the right, is a critical factor in the accuracy of this test. On the left side,

a superior renal vein may occasionally be confused with the adrenal vein. Even when the adrenal vein is accurately catheterized, the concentration of aldosterone will depend on whether the sample is obtained proximal or distal to the entrance of the inferior phrenic vein (Fig. 1.1).

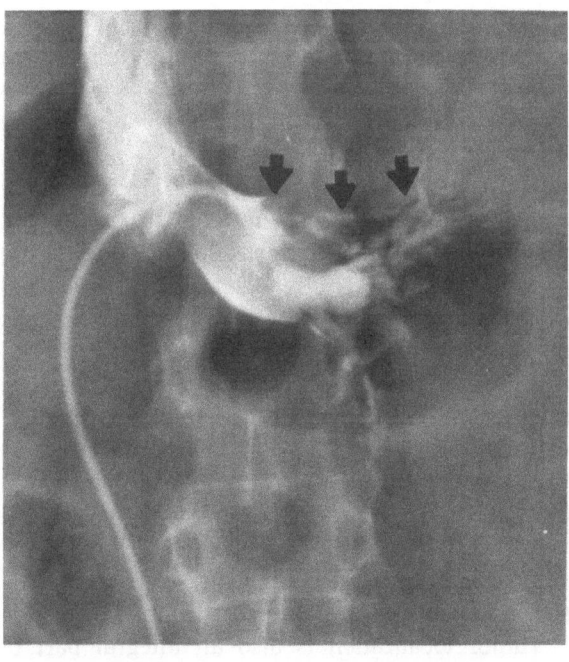

Fig. 1.1. Catheterization of the left renal vein with injection of contrast material.

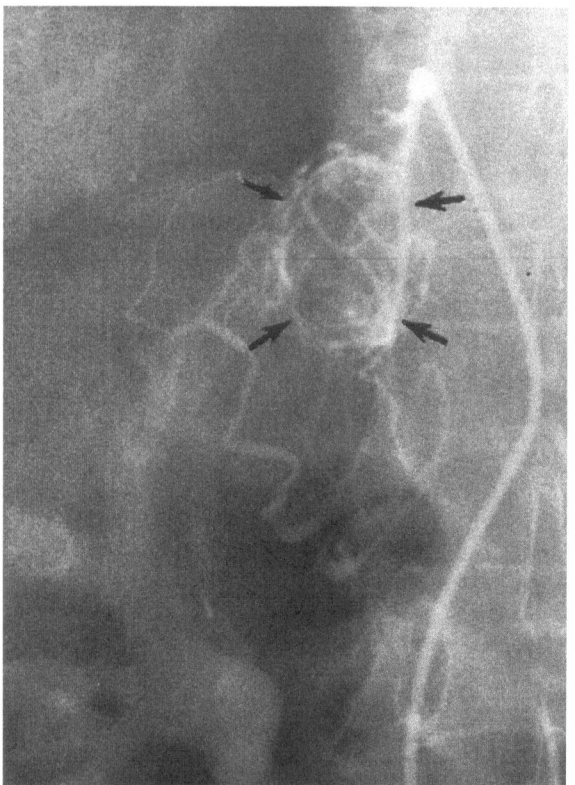

Fig. 1.2. A small aldosteronoma of the right adrenal gland with a moderately hypervascular adenoma.

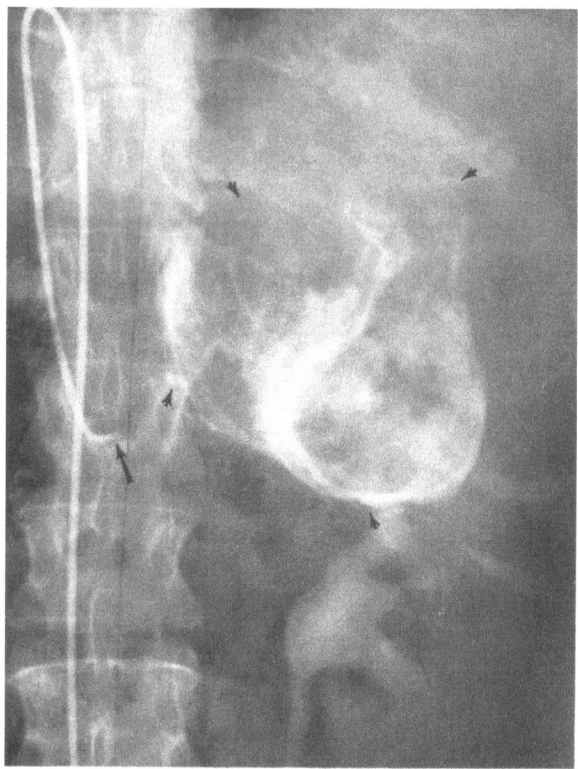

Fig. 1.3. Catheterization of the left adrenal vein with sampling and injection of the vein. Note a large hypervascular aldosteronoma of the right adrenal gland.

On the right side, the main problem is differentiation of the adrenal vein from the hepatic veins. Small hepatic veins may enter the inferior vena cava at the same level as the adrenal vein. Occasionally, the right adrenal vein drains into a hepatic or inferior phrenic vein (Figs. 1.2–1.4).

The use of the ratio of aldosterone to cortisol concentration in the adrenal vein to that in the inferior vena cava has been helpful in lateralizing adrenal adenoma [18]. By determining the level of cortisol in venous samples, a measure of the dilution of the adrenal efflux may also be gained. The aldosterone-cortisol ratio then reflects the aldosterone secretion corrected for the degree of selectivity of catheterization. Adrenal cortisol secretion is also unaffected by the aldosterone levels and provides a measure of the degree of accuracy of the adrenal vein sample. Thus, the ratio of aldosterone to cortisol affords a measure of the hypersecretion of aldosterone independent of the purity of the sample.

Tumor localization is also an integral part of the surgical management of pheochromocytoma. Although the diagnosis may be suspected from the

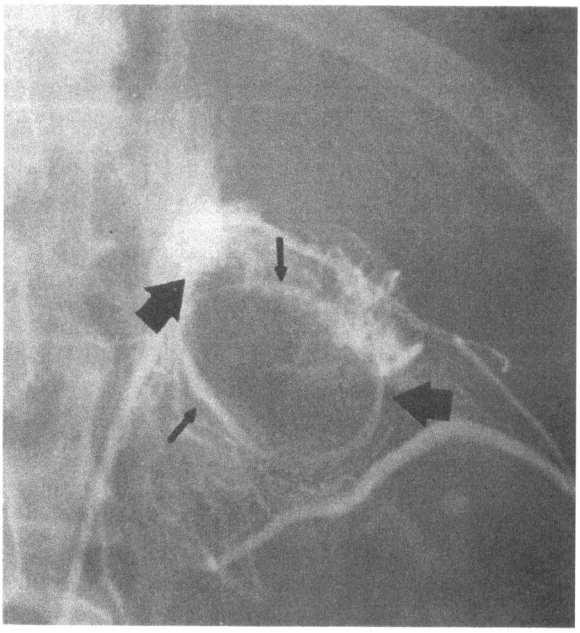

Fig. 1.4. A hypervascular tumor of the left adrenal gland.

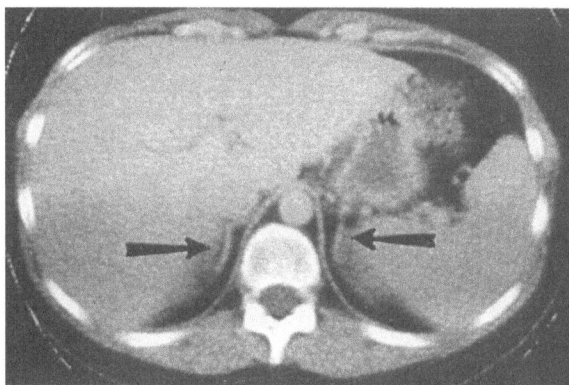

Fig. 1.5. Normal adrenal gland.

history and physical findings and confirmed by various pharmacologic studies, it is important for the surgeon to know the precise location and extent of the tumor when planning its safe and expeditious removal. Intravenous pyelography, even with laminagraphic views, may often fail to demonstrate these tumors. Selective arteriography may accurately demonstrate the blood supply and the extent of most pheochromocytomas, but it is an invasive technique with serious potential complications, including hypertensive crises. Adrenal vein and vena cava sampling of blood for catecholamines can help localize tumors in selected cases, although it, too, is an invasive procedure and is of little help in estimating size and extent of the disease.

Computed Tomography

The role of abdominal computed tomography (CT) in defining retroperitoneal anatomy and pathology is now well documented. Many reports have appeared in the literature emphasizing the usefulness of CT in identifying lymphomatous masses, renal tumors, retroperitoneal hemorrhage, and pelvic and presacral lesions [8,11,17].

The normal left adrenal gland can be visualized by CT in approximately 80% of patients; the right adrenal gland is visualized less frequently (50%). The left adrenal gland appears as a crescent- or triangular-shaped structure lying anterior and

medial to the upper pole of the left kidney posterior to the tail of the pancreas and lateral to the abdominal aorta. The normal right adrenal gland appears as a thin sliver of tissue lying above the upper pole of the right kidney and immediately posterior to the inferior vena cava.

Lesions of the adrenal glands as small as 1 cm in size can be identified since they distort the normal outline of the gland. The absorption coefficient values of these tumors are similar to those of normal surrounding organs, such as liver and kidney ($+32$ to $+40$ EMI units), and, depending on the vascularity of such lesions, absorption may be enhanced after intravenous infusion of contrast material. Hyperplasia, adenoma, carcinoma, and metastatic lesions of the adrenal glands may be demonstrated by computed tomograms (Figs. 1.5–1.8). Adrenal tumors appear as discrete masses in the adrenal gland. If the tumor is small, a portion of normal gland may also be identified. When the tumor is large, adrenal etiology may be suspected and CT may be the noninvasive evaluation that provides the best anatomic information of adrenal lesions. A number of adrenal tumors have low absorption coefficients even after injection of intravenous contrast material.

Our experience with CT shows that adrenal tumors whose total fat content is high will have absorption coefficient values approaching that of retroperitoneal fat. This constitutes a distinct pitfall in CT diagnosis, particularly when small adrenal lesions are sought. The normal adrenal glands, therefore, must be directly visualized before the presence of adrenal disease can be definitely excluded.

In 13 cases of adrenal cortical adenoma examined with CT at the National Institutes of Health, 11 of the 13 steroid-producing adrenal adenomas were correctly identified and there were no false-positive results. The smallest tumor identified was 1 cm in diameter. Two adenomas were missed: one was detected intraoperatively and measured as 0.5 cm in diameter, whereas the other was diagnosed by venous sampling. Tumors went undetected by CT in four patients with bilateral adrenal hyperplasia; we have not always been able to distinguish these glands from normal glands by CT scanning. However, a normal adrenal scan in the presence of Cushing's syndrome provides reliable, although indirect, evidence of adrenal hyperplasia.

In studying 26 adrenal neoplasms, we had an overall accuracy of 89% (23/26) with CT. In every

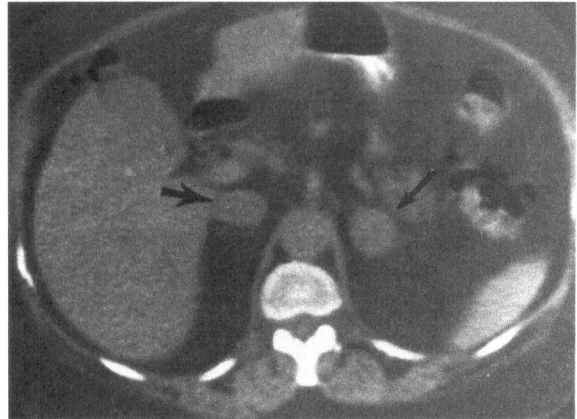

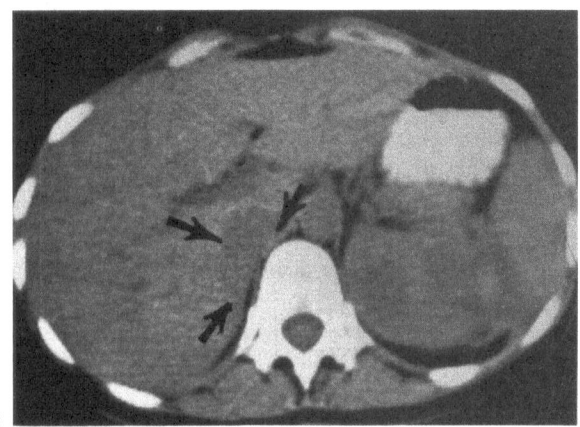

Fig. 1.6. a An abdominal CT of the bilateral adrenal carcinoma. **b** An abdominal CT of another patient with a right adrenal carcinoma (*bottom arrow*). Note the inferior vena cava also containing a tumor (*top two arrows*).

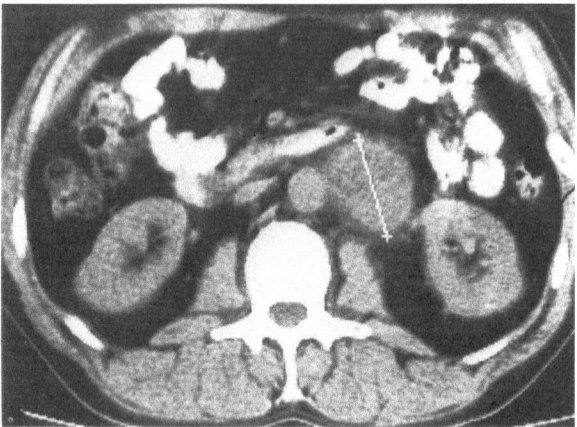

Fig. 1.7. An abdominal CT of a patient with a metastatic melanoma to the left adrenal gland (*linear mark*).

addition, one may detect extension of the tumor into the renal and adrenal veins and/or inferior vena cava without utilizing any contrast materials.

Furthermore, in certain cases, we have been able to differentiate a primary adrenal mass from the metastases to the adrenal gland, which is an important consideration in cancer patients with adrenal masses.

Currently, we are investigating the role of this imaging technique in various adrenal lesions and our preliminary experiences indicate its superiority to other conventional methods in the diagnosis and localization of these lesions.

case in which an adrenal lesion was detected by CT, the diagnosis was confirmed by operation.

Magnetic Resonance Imaging

This new imaging technique is based on magnetic resonance properties of certain elements. This magnetic property is found in elements with uneven protons and/or neutrons. In ordinary states, these magnetic fields are in different directions and are normally neutral. By introducing the human body into a magnetic field, and obtaining images from the various organs, one can differentiate normal and/or abnormal states of masses. Our experience with magnetic resonance imaging (MRI) in the past 3 years indicates more sensitivity and specificity than the other conventional techniques. In

Transcatheter Brush Biopsy of Intracaval Tumor Thrombi

Extension of tumor thrombus into major veins from neoplasms such as renal carcinoma, hepatoma, retroperitoneal sarcoma, glomus tumors, and pheochromocytoma has been demonstrated on venographic and arteriographic studies, but only rarely have these readily accessible glomus tumor masses been studied by biopsy to provide histologic confirmation for diagnostic or staging purposes [14]. Filling defects in the inferior vena cava (IVC) and iliac veins were encountered during the study of six recent patients with abdominal neoplasms at the NIH. Each underwent a brush biopsy via venous catheter, in one undiagnosed case in an attempt to obtain histologic material, and in the five patients with known primary tumors in an effort to distinguish neoplastic venous invasion from benign thrombus. In cases of renal carcinoma invading the IVC, biopsies have been performed by others by transcatheter aspiration by flexible gastroscopic forceps introduced through the catheter. There have been several reports of the radiographic manifestation of venous invasion by such tumors as renal carcinoma, hepatoma, pheochromocytoma, retroperitoneal soft tissue sarcoma, primary leiomyosarcoma of the IVC, and glomus tumors.

The technique of transvenous brush biopsy could easily be extended to smaller intrarenal and intrahepatic veins, in fact, into almost any tumor with accessible veins. Theoretical complications of this procedure include perforation of a vein or embolization of a benign or tumor thrombus. As in all diagnostic clinical procedures, the potential risks versus benefits need to be considered for each individual case.

Transvenous brush biopsy of filling defects in the abdominal veins seems useful in differentiating between benign and neoplastic thrombus. This not only confirms the extent of a known neoplasm, but may also provide the first histologic proof of the presence of a neoplastic process. Because of the easy accessibility via catheter of many abdominal veins, the potential utilization of transvenous brush biopsy is probably far greater than the limited experience indicates, and we are investigating this diagnostic approach in a wide spectrum of tumors.

After this overview of recent advances in imaging and localization I will briefly review the advances in pathophysiology and the treatment of the adrenal diseases.

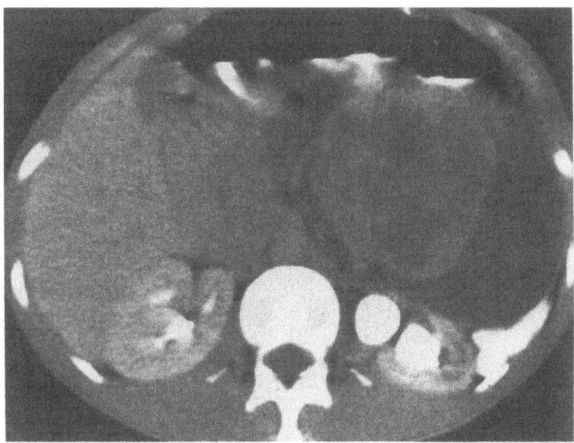

Fig. 1.8. A large pheochromocytoma of the left adrenal gland. Note necrotic and hemorrhagic areas in the left adrenal gland characteristic of a pheochromocytoma.

microadenomas, a long-term justification for these efforts at precise diagnosis can be expected.

Regardless of the etiology of the adrenal cortical excess, the symptoms are almost invariably the same and all are due to the increase in the levels of circulating functional corticosteroid. In addition, the characteristic diurnal variation of corticosteroid levels is lost.

Hydrocortical hyperfunction is characterized by the clinical syndrome of increased truncal obesity, the redistribution of truncal fat with a characteristic buffalo hump, and the development of rounded facies, abdominal striae, mild glucose intolerance, mild hypertension, and alterations in immune function. In any tests of suppression of the adrenal, the patient should not take estrogens as this produces high levels of plasma hydroxycorticosteroids.

Adrenocortical Excess

The surgeon faces the primary question: Is the cause of adrenocortical excess a hyperfunctioning pituitary, a syndrome of nonadrenal, nonpituitary adrenocorticotropic (ACTH) hormone production, or an intrinsic hydrocortical lesion? Only after this diagnosis has been made can appropriate therapeutic decisions be implemented. With the recent advent of precise assays for plasma ACTH and the burgeoning efforts with transsphenoidal microsurgery for

Cushing's Disease

Given the difficulties of making the diagnosis of a pituitary etiology of Cushing's syndrome [5] and, indeed, the variable criteria on which such a diagnosis is based, it is not surprising that the incidence of pituitary tumors causing adrenocortical hyperplasia (Cushing's disease) varies between 5% and 20% [19]. Most recently, emphasis on the existence of microadenomas has made previous estimates of the incidence of Cushing's disease erroneously low (Fig. 1.9).

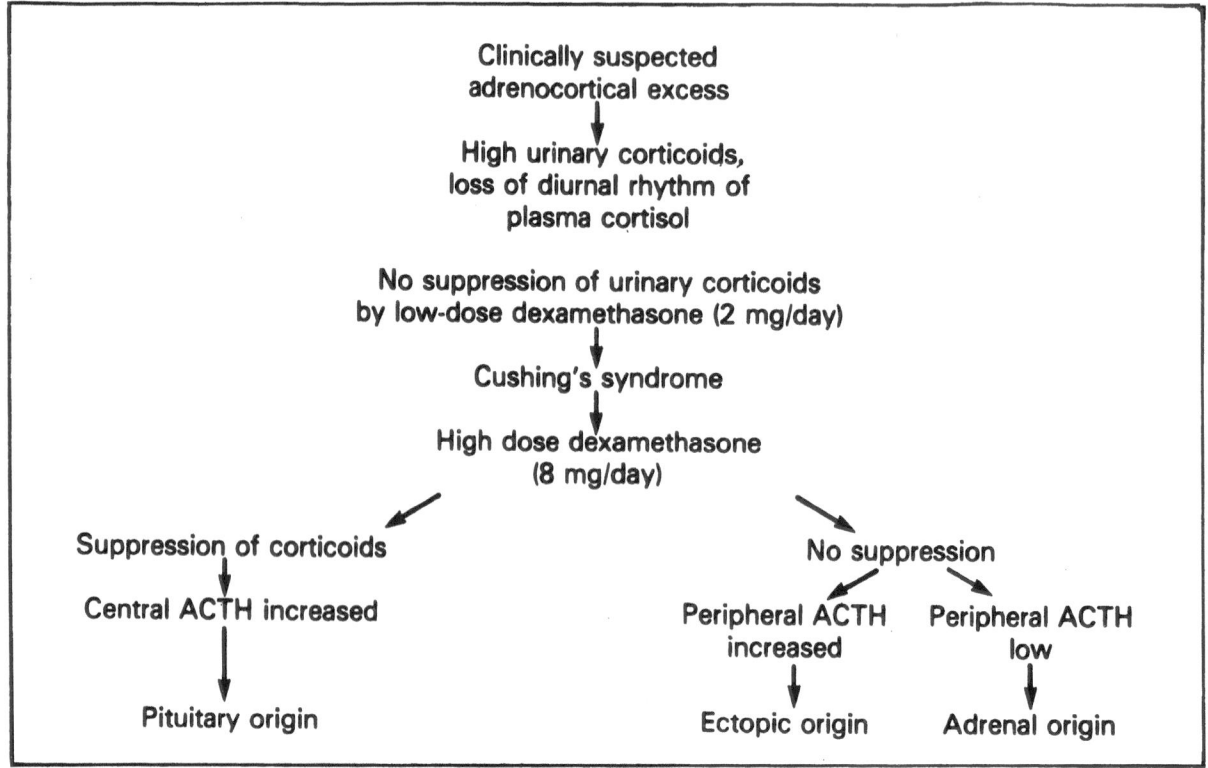

Fig. 1.9. Step-by-step elucidation of the etiology of Cushing's syndrome.

In a series of transsphenoidal microsurgical pituitary explorations for adrenocortical excess, pituitary adenomas were selectively resected, 14 of which were confirmed histologically. Of this total group of 20, normal cell tomography results were obtained in 8 (40%). Sixteen of the 17 undergoing selective tumor removal in this group had the hypercortisolism reversed. This incidence of pituitary adenomas is consistent with autopsy series.

"Normal" plasma ACTH levels can be found in patients with Cushing's disease, but they represent in reality an abnormal response in the presence of hypercortisolism. An elevated peripheral ACTH level does not elucidate a source and may be confused with the ectopic ACTH produced by some tumors. In the absence of an obvious neoplasm and with the availability of a reliable ACTH assay, selective venous catheterization of the jugular vein, sigmoid sinus, and petrosal sinus, as has been done for localization of other endocrine tumors, should be diagnostic.

Ectopic ACTH Syndrome

One of the findings that may be encountered in a hospital with a large number of cancer patients is the wide variety of tumors that can at some time in their course produce ACTH. The usual presentation is such that this syndrome is indistinguishable from Cushing's syndrome and can often be quite severe. The most common underlying lesion is carcinoma of the lung, and the inexorable progression of the primary disease results in a modification of the conventional Cushing's syndrome in that catabolic effects of the primary tumor are dominant.

In addition, difficulties remain in confirming the diagnosis as being secondary to truly ectopic ACTH production. Absolute diagnostic criteria require that the tumor be shown to have a high concentration of ACTH and that there be no evidence of a pituitary tumor. Presumptive evidence is obtained by the classical elevations of plasma cortisol and urinary 17-hydroxycorticosteroid excretion. The ability selectively to catheterize the draining veins of the cavernous sinus to identify the pituitary as a source of ACTH is a major advantage in the differentiation of those patients who have a nonpituitary neoplasm from those who have a pituitary neoplasm.

Oat cell carcinoma of the lung is the most common tumor responsible for the production of ectopic ACTH. Tumors in other sites, such as the pancreas, thymus, thyroid, and bronchus, and carcinoid tumors have all been reported to produce ACTH.

Therapy is aimed at the removal of the underlying primary neoplasm; however, the oat cell carcinomas are disseminated at the time of presentation and surgical ablation is not possible [3,11]. Conventional therapy for this tumor, i.e., irradiation and chemotherapy or chemotherapy alone, has resulted in some improvement in median survival (up to 36% 2-year survival for limited disease). Occasionally, the hypercortisolism responds to the chemotherapeutic agents given for the primary tumor. In rare cases in which prolonged survival in the primary neoplasm can be expected and there is poor response to metyrapone or o,p'-DDD (1, dichloro-2(O-chlorophenyl)-2-(p-chlorophenyl)-ethane), adrenalectomy can be considered.

Primary Aldosteronism

In 1952, Conn described a clinical syndrome induced by excessive production of aldosterone, which is accompanied by abnormally large amounts of serum aldosterone and urinary 17-hydroxycorticosteroids [1,4,6].

In primary aldosteronism, there is an increased secretion of aldosterone, which produces sodium retention, increased total plasma volume, increased renal artery pressure, and inhibition of renin secretion. In the secondary form of the disease, there is a primary decrease in the renal artery perfusion pressure, which stimulates the juxtaglomerular apparatus to secrete an increased amount of renin, thus leading to the production of angiotensin from angiotensinogen and stimulation of the adrenal to produce increased amounts of aldosterone. The two forms of aldosteronism can thus be differentiated by the determination of the plasma renin activity, renin being low in the primary and high in the secondary form.

Although children and young adults occasionally

have this syndrome, most patients are women in the age range of 30–50 years. The adenoma is rarely (5% or less) bilateral. Rare forms of the disease may be due to hyperplasia or adrenal corticocarcinoma.

Aldosteronomas are generally soft, yellow, and spherical and arise from the zona glomerulosa. They are usually single and circumscribed and can be clearly demarcated from a normal cortex. However, on occasion it is not possible to locate the lesion macroscopically and it is only on fine sectioning that the adenoma is found. The size of these adenomas has little correlation with rate of aldosterone production. The remainder of the adrenal cortex is not usually atrophic, but appears normal microscopically. The aldosterone-secreting cells may be a zona glomerulosa type but occasionally they do not appear to have components of either the zona glomerulosa or zona fasciculata. The normal zona glomerulosa is often hyperplastic and almost invariably present. Symptoms are often long standing. T-wave depression is noted with altered ST segments and left ventricular hypertrophy in a number of these patients.

Diagnosis

Differentiation between primary and secondary aldosteronism, which may be identical in signs and symptoms, is difficult without further studies such as angiography or venography, with careful evaluation of secretion rates and/or plasma renin activity. The diagnosis of primary hyperaldosteronism is established or at least suspected in patients with a low serum potassium level and high normal or elevated plasma sodium level. In secondary aldosteronism the serum potassium level is again low, but the sodium tends to be normal or low. Electrocardiographic changes of hypokalemia may be noted, including ST depression, invasion of T waves, prolonged ST, or the presence of U waves. In the differential diagnosis of primary hyperaldosteronism, it must be emphasized that secondary hyperaldosteronism may occur in cirrhosis of the liver nephrotic syndrome, congestive heart failure, and various hypertensive diseases.

In attempting to make the diagnosis, physicians should make sure that the patient receives no diuretic agents and has a normal sodium intake. The patient with hyperaldosteronism will have excessive urinary excretion of potassium and excessive retention of sodium. Differentiation of primary from secondary hyperaldosteronism is usually accomplished by the determination of plasma renin activity with the patient in the supine position.

The combination of high aldosterone and low plasma renin levels yields about 95% accuracy in the diagnosis of primary aldosteronism.

Adrenal Carcinoma

Adrenocortical carcinoma is a rare cancer arising in the adrenal cortex and it frequently retains the ability to synthesize steroids. Adrenocortical cancer is a slow-growing tumor with a relatively low propensity for metastasis [12,13]. The diagnosis of adrenal carcinoma is based on clinical, biochemical, and radiological findings. Functional adrenal tumors most commonly produce 17-ketosteroids (17-KS) or 17-hydroxycorticosteroid (17-OHCS). Rappaport and associates reported on 276 cases of adrenal tumors, including 188 cases of cancer. They found evidence of functional activity in 151 (80%) of these cases of proved adrenal cancer. The high proportion of functional tumors is no doubt explained by the fact that the detection rate is increasing. In the clinical setting, the majority of the tumors reported are functioning since they are more easily detected.

These tumors may manifest themselves as a palpable abdominal mass, Cushing's syndrome due to excessive production of glucocorticoids, or virilization due to excessive production of androgens. Less commonly, feminization due to estrogen secretion by the tumor of hypertension and hypokalemic alkalosis due to aldosterone production may be the main clinical feature in these patients.

The ACTH or dexamethasone tests may serve to differentiate between the benign and malignant adrenocortical tumors. The patients with cancer usually have a high urinary 17-KS or 17-OCHS level.

The main treatment of adrenal carcinoma is surgical excision. Since there is no other effective therapy available and the natural history of this tumor is that of a slow-growing one, the recurrences are also amenable to resection. The intracaval extension may also be resected with or without cardiopulmonary bypass in renal cell carcinoma [15,16].

Chemotherapy

The insecticide o,p'-DDD (1,1-dichloro-2-(O-chlorophenyl)-2-(p-chlorophenyl)ethane) has been shown to cause necrosis of the adrenal cortex in the dog and to produce regressions of adrenocortical cancer in man. Its mechanism of action is unknown [13]. The drug is not commercially available, but is supplied by the Cancer Chemotherapy National Service Center of the National Cancer Institute, Bethesda, MD, as 0.5-g tablets.

Any patient with metastatic adrenocortical carcinoma should have a therapeutic trial of o,p'-DDD. It is easier to anticipate the results of therapy in patients with functional tumors by monitoring urinary steroid excretion, but the final results in each patient category depend on decreasing the size of the tumor. Although we initially used a dosage regimen starting at 3.0–5.0 g daily and increased this to the maximum tolerated dose, we now begin therapy with 10 g daily. If the patient can tolerate this, then the dose may be increased in 2.0-g increments every few days until a total dose of 20 g daily is reached. The drug should be given in divided doses and is often tolerated better when given with meals. The dose in children should be reduced proportionately on a body weight basis.

The most troublesome side effects are those relating to the gastrointestinal tract. Almost every patient who continues on o,p'-DDD will develop anorexia and nausea. The CNS is affected by o,p'-DDD: somnolence and inability to concentrate are the dominant features of toxicity. Other infrequent manifestations of CNS toxicity are lateral nystagmus, blurring of vision, hypersialorrhea, and slurring of speech. Less frequently side effects have included diarrhea, vertigo, skin rash, urticaria, gynecomastia, and pigmentation. The side effects have usually subsided after cessation of therapy for a period of 2 weeks.

Bone marrow, liver, and kidney have not been affected by prolonged therapy. Hemoglobin and platelet levels remain unchanged and rarely there has been a mild leukopenia with extended therapy.

When regression has been achieved with o,p'-DDD, it is appropriate to measure urinary steroid excretion at regular intervals in those patients who have had a steroid-producing cancer. In a few instances, however, we have observed recurrence of disease without a proportionate increase in steroid production. Thus, the use of urinary steroid levels as the sole index of tumor growth may be deceiving and conventional measures against tumor recurrence should be instituted.

Pheochromocytoma

The optimal management of patients with pheochromocytoma demands a multidisciplinary approach [2]. Considerable progress has been made in the understanding of the physiology and management of chromaffin tumors particularly in preoperative, or operative, and postoperative management. Pheochromocytoma and pheochromoblastoma cannot always be classified separately because the tumor may include both types of cells. Although pheochromocytoma is usually benign, the histopathologic distinction between the benign and the malignant type is extremely difficult. The diagnosis of malignancy is reserved for those lesions that are locally aggressive or those that metastasize.

In the past several years, it has become clear that, although most pheochromocytomas are benign, they are functionally active and have clinical features such as headache, paroxysmal or sustained hypertension, excessive perspiration, angina, and cardiac arrythmias related to the secretory output of catecholamines by the tumor. In the normal person there are three naturally occurring catecholamines: dopamine, norepinephrine, and epinephrine. Each of these can be identified in adrenal medullary tissue, but at postganglionic sympathetic nerve endings apparently only dopamine and norepinephrine can be identified in other than the most minute concentration. In general, it appears that most of the extraadrenal pheochromocytomas are norepinephrine producers, whereas the tumors of the adrenal medulla produce both epinephrine and norepinephrine.

The clinical manifestations of pheochromocytoma are related to the concentration of catecholamines released into the circulation. If the tumors go untreated, a cerebrovascular accident (leading to death during one of the paroxysmal episodes), congestive heart failure with pulmonary edema, or ventricular fibrillation may result.

Typically, laboratory findings are those of elevated urinary vanillylmandelic acid (VMA) (normal, less than 6.8 mg/24 h), norepinephrine (normal, 100 ng/24 h), and epinephrine (normal,

25 ng/24 h). Abnormal glucose tolerance is common.

The radiologic studies recommended include IVP with nephrotomograms, abdominal arteriograms, selective venography, and CT of both adrenal glands (Figs. 1.8, 1.10, 1.11). These are useful tools not only in the diagnosis of the pheochromocytomas, but also in the localization of the tumor. This preoperative localization establishes the surgical approach for excision of these tumors. Although the histamine provocative tests, regitine-blocking test, and other indirect pharmacologic tests have been used in the past, the current consensus is more in favor of biochemical diagnosis and radiologic localization of these tumors. After the diagnosis and localization of the tumor has been made, the patient should be prepared for surgical removal of the tumor.

The alpha-adrenergic blocking agent phenoxybenzamine is given in a dose of 10–14 mg/day for 10 days to 2 weeks prior to operation and the dose is titrated to the individual patient's requirement. Efficacy of the regimen can be judged by the control of blood pressure, because in some patients other aspects of abnormal catecholamine excess, such as the glucose intolerance and the elevated lipolysis, will return to normal.

Beta-adrenergic blocking agents can be used, but are not essential in the preoperative management.

An alternative method that we prefer is the use of drugs that decrease catecholamine synthesis such as alpha-methyl-*para*-tyrosine (AMPT). This agent

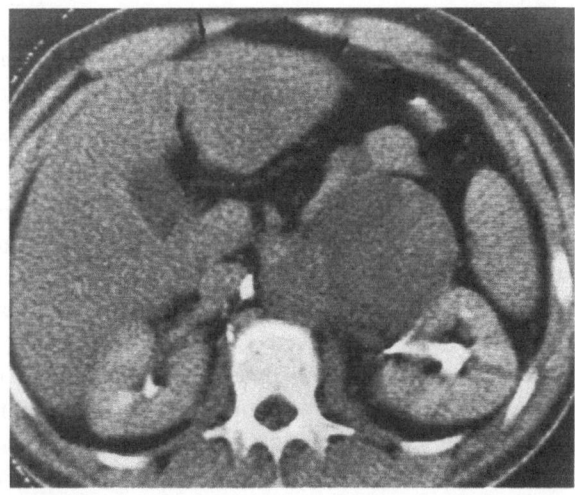

Fig. 1.10. Carcinoma of the left adrenal gland. Note the left lobe of the liver containing metastases (*arrows*).

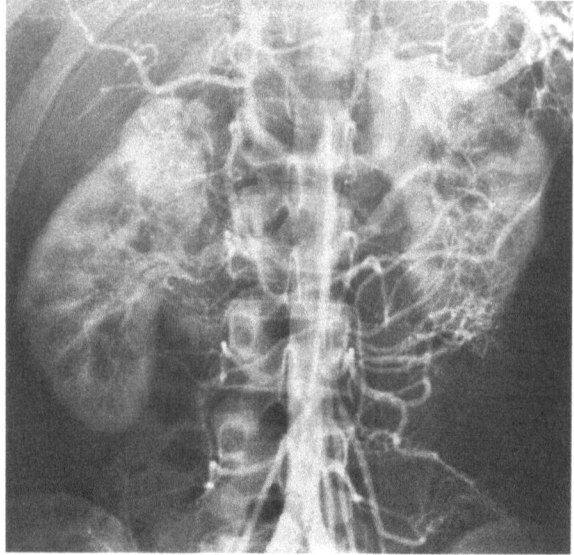

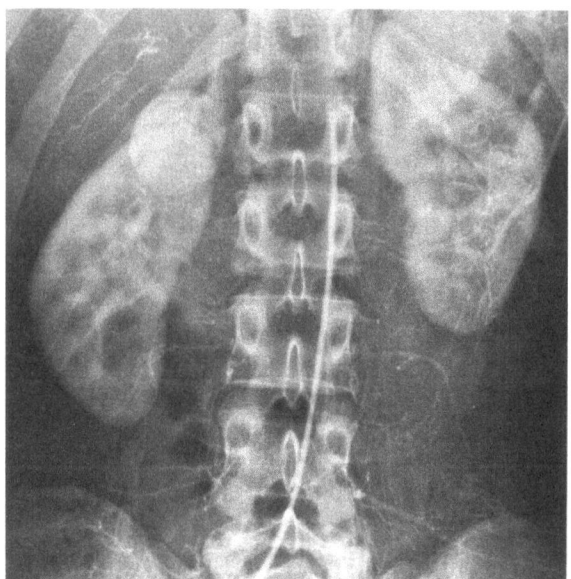

Fig. 1.11. **a** Aortogram for the left adrenal pheochromocytoma. Aortography is rarely used. **b** Tomographic phase of the same aortogram, demonstrating the tumor again (*bottom*).

controlled by the intraoperative use of an effective beta-blocking agent or lidocaine. Postoperative attention to the large fluid needs of these patients is mandatory.

At NIH incidence of surgically proved malignant pheochromocytoma in 22 of 68 (32%) is higher than that reported by Remine et al. or Scott et al., who found that only 5 of 44 (11%) and 18 of 138 (13%) patients, respectively, had malignant pheochromocytoma. This, however, reflects the referral nature to NIH rather than any variation in incidence of malignancy (Tables 1.1, 1.2).

Table 1.1. Malignant pheochromocytoma: symptoms. (NIH 1953–1977, 22 patients)

	No.	(%)
Primary site		
Adrenal	16	
Extraadrenal	6	
Major symptoms (%)		
Sweating	16	72
Episodic attack	14	63
Palpitations	13	59
Anxiety	11	50
Headache	10	45

Table 1.2. Therapy in 22 patients with malignant pheochromocytoma treated at the NIH from 1953 to 1972

Operation alone	6
a-Methyl-*para*-tyrosine (AMPT) alone	2
Surgery plus AMPT	4
Surgery plus propranolol (P)	1
Surgery plus dibenzamine (DBZ)	2
Surgery plus AMPT + P	1
Surgery plus AMPT + DBZ	2
Surgery plus AMPT + AMPP	1
Surgery plus AMPT + AMPP + P + DBZ	1
Surgery plus AMPT + AMPP + DBZ	1
Surgery plus chemotherapy + AMPT + DBZ	1

inhibits tyrosine hydroxylase and thus decreases catecholamine synthesis. AMPT (Merck Laboratories) is used in doses ranging from 500 mg to 2 g/day and the dose is titrated to individual tolerance.

The key to successful operative management is extremely careful intraoperative monitoring, particularly at the time of induction. We routinely use arterial pressure monitoring and usually induce a balanced anesthesia, occasionally with Ethrane. Catecholamine-induced arrythmias can be carefully

Surgically, the aim is to perform a radical adrenalectomy with removal of all surrounding adjacent fatty tissue and adjacent lymph nodes. On occasion, in the case of an extensive invasive tumor, a nephrectomy needs to be performed and most procedures are done through an abdominal approach with the option of entering the chest when appropriate.

Neuroblastoma

Neuroblastoma is the term applied to the malignant tumor arising from the embryonic sympathetic neuroblasts. The sympathetic ganglia are derived from primordial neural crest cells and neuroblasts [7,10]. Four types of tumors may arise from these cells; pheochromocytoma, ganglioneuroma, sympathogonioma, and neuroblastoma. Neuroblastoma is the most common extracranial malignant solid tumor in infancy and childhood comprising approximately 7%–14% of childhood, malignancies and 15%–50% of neonatal malignancies.

Sixty percent of neuroblastomas occur in children under 1 year of age, 26% in those between 1 and 2 years, and the remainder in those older than 2 years. There is a slightly greater frequency in males; the reported ratio varies in the range of 1.1:1.0 to 1.3:1.0.

Variations in the natural history of neuroblastoma are exceedingly common. Neuroblastoma has been reported to have the highest rate of spontaneous remission of any malignancy, and maturation into ganglioneuroma has been reported frequently. Despite advances in prolonging survival in other childhood malignancies, the prognosis for neuroblastoma has not changed appreciably in the past decade. The recommended evaluation of patients with neuroblastoma is shown in Table 1.3.

On gross examination, neuroblastomas are usually contained within a pseudocapsule, are nodular in appearance, and have a grayish surface when cut. There are frequent areas of necrosis, hemorrhage, and calcification within the tumor.

On microscopic examination, a typical neuroblastoma is a highly cellular neoplasm with cells arranged in broad sheets that in some areas form "rosette" patterns. Mitotic figures are often present in high numbers. The presence of rosette formations along with neurofibril formation is pathognomonic (Fig. 1.12a,b).

Staging

The most widely accepted staging method is that proposed by D'Angio, which is based on the extent of disease.

Stage I—Tumor is confined to the organ or structure of origin.

Stage II—Tumor extends in continuity beyond the organ or structure of origin but does not cross the midline.

Stage III—Tumor extends in continuity beyond the outline. Regional lymph nodes may be involved.

Stage IV—Remote disease involving skeleton, visceral organs, soft tissues, or distant lymph nodes.

Stage IV-S (special category)—Stage I or II, with remote disease confined to the liver, skin, or bone marrow (one or more of these sites) without radiologic evidence of bone metastasis on skeletal survey.

The treatment for neuroblastomas is surgery.

Prognosis

Most reports consider that a 2-year disease-free follow-up period separates survivors from nonsurvivors. Using this criterion, the single most important determinant of survival is age at the time of diagnosis, younger patients being associated with better survival rates. Other factors influencing survival include clinical stage, degree of cellular differentiation, the presence of skeletal or bone marrow involvement, and location of primary.

Overall 2-year disease-free survival rates of 86% for stage I, 63% for stage II, 37% for stage III, 6% for stage IV, and 78% for stage IV-S are reported, with an overall 2-year survival rate for all stages of 32%.

There is a generally more favorable prognosis for primary tumors of the neck, thorax, pelvis, and

Table 1.3. Recommended procedures for evaluation of patients with neuroblastoma

---

Complete blood count, including reticulocyte count and platelet count
Intravenous pyelography
Chest X-ray study, including tomography
Twenty-four hour urine concentrations of HVA[a], VMA[a], and cystathionine. If a 24-h urine collection is not possible, then HVA, VMA, and creatinine level determinations should be obtained from a single specimen
Bone marrow aspiration and biopsy
Skeletal bone survey
Liver, spleen, and bone scans
CT of the retroperitoneum

---

[a]VMA, vanillylmandelic acid; HVA, homovanillylmandelic acid

There appears to be an increased survival rate in girls. One large series shows this to be statistically significant, although this was a retrospective analysis that did not consider the possible effects of different treatments.

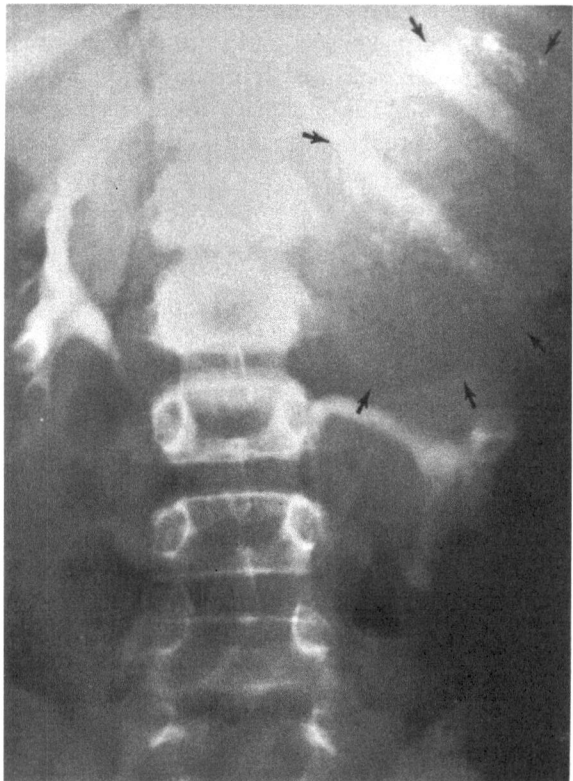

Fig. 1.12. A large calcified neuroblastoma of the left adrenal gland.

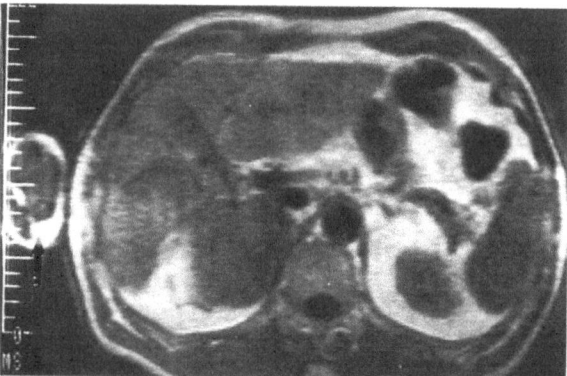

Fig. 1.14. Abdominal magnetic resonance imaging of patient with a large pheochromocytoma of the right adrenal gland.

midline than for tumors arising in the abdomen. The prognosis is particularly unfavorable when the primary tumor arises from the adrenal gland.

Although bone marrow involvement, when associated only with additional involvement of the liver and/or skin, comprises the more favorable stage IV-S, this should be distinguished from skeletal bone involvement, which predicts a significantly decreased survival rate.

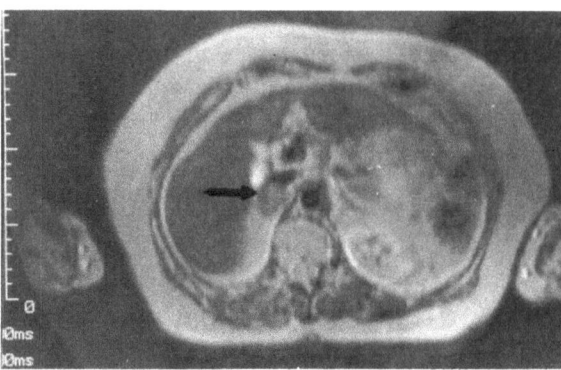

Fig. 1.13. Magnetic resonance imaging of a right adrenal adenoma (arrows).

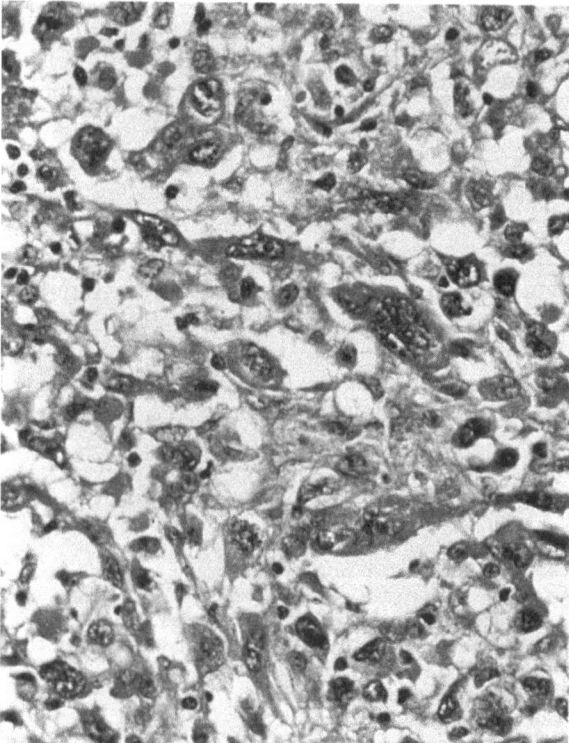

Fig. 1.15. Histologic appearance of a malignant pheochromocytoma. These histologic features may also be present in a benign pheochromocytoma.

Future Perspectives

There has been some progress in the field of adrenal diseases in terms of diagnosis, localization, and utilization of tumor markers. A number of problems remain unresolved, though, such as finding effective cytotoxic agents with minimal toxicity and maximal efficacy. However, current medical and surgical approaches are curative in a number of benign diseases of the adrenal glands.

In the area of basic research the role of the *N-myc* oncogene in neuroblastoma has produced a new dimension in the understanding and explanation of the mechanism of rapid growth of a subset of these tumors [20]. The association of multiple copies of the *N-myc* oncogene with rapid growth of these tumors has been observed. Currently the role of MRI in detecting the size and extent of adrenal tumours (Figs. 1.13, 1.14) and the use of newer immunocytochemical techniques to differentiate benign from malignant pheochromocytomas are under study (Fig. 1.15).

References

1. Auda SP, Brennan MF, Gill JR (1980) Evolution of the surgical management of primary aldosteronism. Ann Surg 191:1–7
2. Bergman SN, Sears HF, Javadpour N, Keiser HB (1978) Postoperative management of patients with pheochromocytoma. J Urol 120:109
3. Bigos ST, Robert F, Pelletier G (1977) Cure of Cushing's disease by transsphenoidal removal of a microadenoma from a pituitary gland despite a radiological normal sella turcica. J Clin Endocrinol Metab 45:1251
4. Conn JW (1955) Primary aldosteronism: a new clinical syndrome. J Lab Clin Med 45:6
5. Cushing H (1932) The basophil adenomas of the pituitary body and their clinical manipulations (pituitary basophilism). Bull Johns Hopkins Hosp 50:137
6. Danford DN Jr, Orlando MD, Bartter FC, Javadpour N (1977) Renal changes in primary aldosteronism. J Urology 117:140
7. D'Angio GJ, Evans AE, Koop CE (1971) Special pattern of widespread neuroblastoma with a favorable prognosis. Lancet 1:1046
8. Dunnick NR, Schaner EG, Doppman JL, Strott CA, Gill JR, Javadpour N (1979) Computed tomography in adrenal tumors. Am J Roetgenol 43
9. Dunnick NR, Doppman JL, Mills SR (1979) Preoperative diagnosis and localization of aldosteronoma by measurement of corticosteroid in adrenal venous blood. Radiology 133:331
10. Jaffe N (1976) Neuroblastoma: a review of the literature and an examination of factors contributing to its enigmatic character. Cancer Treat Rev 3:61
11. Javadpour N, Woltering EA, Brennan MF (1980) Adrenal neoplasms. Curr Probl Surgery 17:1–52
12. Huvos AG, Hajdu SE, Brasfield RD, Foote FW (1970) Adrenal cortical carcinoma—clinicopathologic study of 34 cases. Cancer 25
13. Lippsett MB (1966) Treatment of adrenal carcinoma. Mod Treatment 3:1377
14. Mills SR, Doppman JL, Head GL, Javadpour N, Brennan MF, Chu EW (1978) Transcatheter brush biopsy of intravenous tumor thrombi. Radiology 127:667
15. Paul JG, Rhodes MB, Skow JR (1975) Renal cell carcinoma presenting as right atrial tumor with successful removal using cardiopulmonary bypass. Ann Surg 181:47
16. Rote AR, Flint LD, Ellis FH (1977) Intracaval recurrence of pheochromocytoma extending into the right atrium. N Engl J Med 296:1269–1271
17. Schaner EG, Dunnick NR, Doppman JL, Strott CA, Gill JR, Javadpour N (1978) Adrenal cortical tumors with low attenuation coefficients, a pitfall in computed tomography diagnosis. J Comput Assist Tomogr 2:11
18. Scoggins, BA, Oddie CJ, Hare WSC, Coghlan JP (1972) Preoperative lateralization of aldosterone-producing tumors in primary aldosteronism. Ann Intern Med 76:891
19. Scott HW, Goster JH, Rhamy RK, Klatte EC, Liddle GW (1971) Surgical management of adrenocortical tumors with Cushing's syndrome. Ann Surg 173:892
20. Seeger RC, Brodeur GM, Sather H (1982) Association of multiple copies of the *N-myc* oncogene with rapid progression of neuroblastomas. N Eng J Med 313:111

Chapter 2

Embryology, Anatomy, Physiology, and Biologic Markers

N. Javadpour

Embryology

The adrenal gland develops from two distinct primitive embryonic layers. The adrenal cortex originates from the splanchnic mesoderm and the medulla originates from the neural crest, an ectodermal derivative. The primitive sympathetic cells, which are characterized by an affinity for chromium salts, have been designated as sympathogonia. These cells differentiate along two lines, as indicated in Fig. 2.1. Sympathogonia may differentiate into sympathoblasts and the tumors of these cells are often grouped together as neuroblastomas. The sympathoblast may further differentiate into the sympathetic ganglion cell and give rise to the often benign tumor called ganglioneuroma. The sympathogonia may also differentiate into pheo-

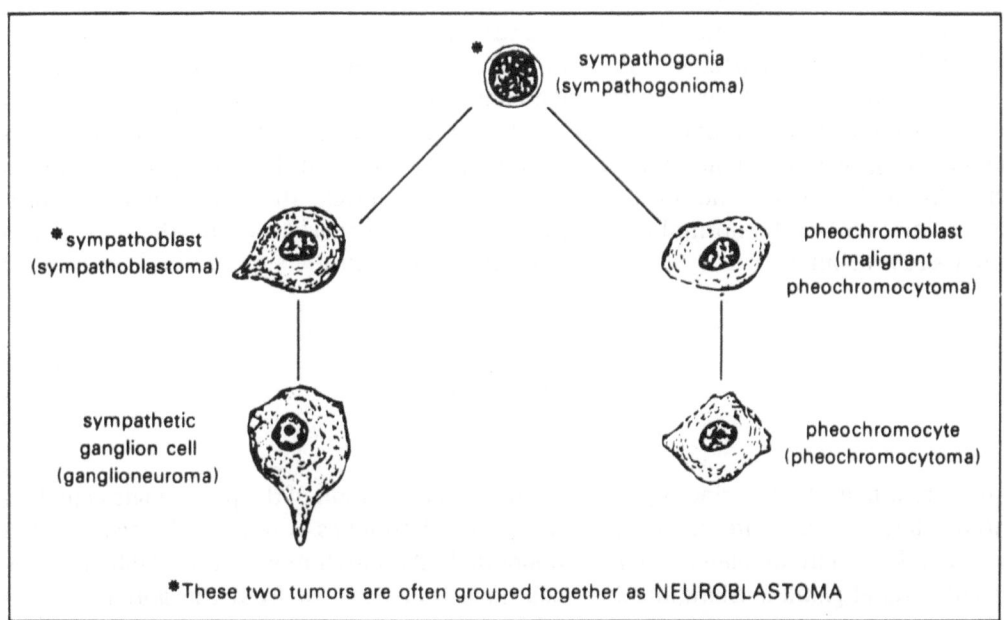

Fig. 2.1. Embryologic derivation of the cell origins of the adrenal medulla and their tumors.

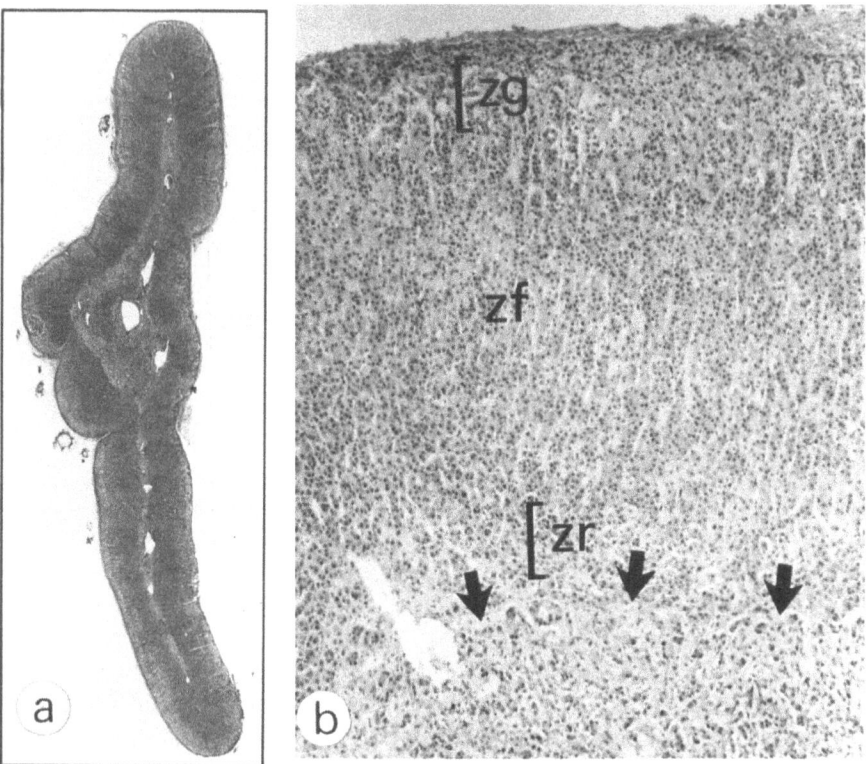

Fig. 2.2.a Gross anatomy of a normal adrenal gland. Note the medullary and cortical components. **b** Normal histologic components of the adrenal glands. Note the zona glumerulosa (*zg*), zona fasciculata (*zf*), and zona reticularis (*zr*). The adrenal medulla is shown by the *arrows*. [4]

chromoblasts, giving rise to a malignant pheochromocytoma. The pheochromoblast may also differentiate into pheochromocytes that are the cells of origin of a benign pheochromocytoma. During the 3rd and 4th months of fetal life, the adrenal glands are larger than the kidneys, mostly as a result of the rapid growth of the adrenal cortex. However, this initial rapid growth is not maintained and, at birth, the adrenals are about one-third as large as the kidneys. In adult life, the normal ratio of adrenal to kidney size is about 1:28.

vessel. The left adrenal is close to the aorta, pancreas, and spleen, with longer veins that empty into the left renal vein. Each adrenal has three arteries: one from the inferior phrenic artery, one from the aorta, and one from the renal artery. The lymphatics of both glands accompany the suprarenal veins and drain into the lumbar lymph nodes. Microscopically, three distinct zones are recognized in the adrenal cortex: the inner zona reticularis, the outer zona glomerulosa, and the middle zona fasciculata (Fig. 2.2b).

Anatomy

The adrenal glands are a pair of endocrine organs within the perirenal fascia located in the retroperitoneum (Fig. 2.2a). Each adrenal gland weighs about 5 g. The right adrenal gland is triangular in shape and close to the inferior vena cava, with several short veins that empty directly into this

Physiology

An in-depth discussion of the physiologic activity of the adrenal hormones is beyond the scope of this monograph. Although more than 50 different steroids have been isolated from the adrenal cortex, only a few are secreted into the bloodstream; the rest are intracellular intermediates. Recent studies of the biosynthetic pathways of adrenal steroids have shown that the main steroids synthesized by the adrenal cortex are hydrocortisone, corticosterone, aldosterone, and 11-hydroxyandrostenedione [1–3].

The adrenal cortical hormones are derivatives of cholesterol and are basically of two structural types: those with a 2-carbon chain at the 17 position of the D-ring and containing 21 carbon atoms, and those with a keto or hydroxyl group at position 17 and containing 19 carbon atoms. For practical purposes, the only steroids secreted in sufficient quantities to be physiologically active are aldosterone, cortisol, corticosterone, and dihydroepiandrosterone. Also secreted is deoxycorticosterone, a mineralocorticoid with only a very small physiologic effect compared with aldosterone.

Adrenocorticotropic hormone (ACTH) acts by stimulating adenyl cyclase and a protein kinase to increase the amounts of cholesterol that enter the mitochondria and by another mechanism stimulates conversion of cholesterol to pregnenolone, a precursor of cortisol and progesterone. The understanding of the enzyme systems involved in steroid biosynthesis allows production of the defects to be expected from congenital inborn errors of metabolism or those changes produced by selective use of chemical antagonists or agonists. Therapeutic gains can then be derived from this knowledge, e.g., metyrapone inhibits a conversion early in the formation of cortisol, whereas orthopara-DDD (o,p'-DDD) would be expected to block the secretion of all of the steroids. The effectiveness of o,p'-DDD in lowering cortisol production has been demonstrated. The major excretory end products of the androgens are the 17-ketosteroids; for practical purposes it can be assumed that approximately two-thirds of the ketosteroids of cortisol in the male urine are derived from the adrenal or are a consequence of breakdown of cortisol in the liver and about one-third is derived from the testes.

About 10% of cortisol is converted in the liver to the 17-ketosteroid derivates, but most of it is converted to cortisone and then to tetrahydrocortisone, which is fairly soluble and is rapidly excreted in the urine. Therefore, the major cortisol derivatives in the urine are glucuronides, 20-hydroxy derivatives of tetrahydroglucuronides (30%), and the tetrahydrocortisol (25%) and tetrahydrocortisone (15%) glucuronides.

The physiologic effects of corticosteroids are well known; they are also involved extensively in inter-mediary metabolism since they affect water and electrolyte balance as well as carbohydrate, protein, and fat metabolism. In addition, glucocorticoids play a permissive role in a number of intermediate metabolic events and participate in the response of vascular smooth muscles to norepinephrine and epinephrine. The surgeon most often encounters problems of glucocorticoid imbalance when the patient who is adrenally insufficient is exposed to any form of stress. The failure to increase available corticosteroids can result in sudden collapse and death.

The adrenal medulla excretes both epinephrine and norepinephrine. On average 80% of the adrenal catecholamine output is epinephrine and 20% norepinephrine. Secretion of catecholamines is initiated by the acetylcholine released from the neurons that embrace the secretory cell. It has been suggested that acetylcholine acts by increasing the permeability of the secretory cell and allows calcium to induce secretion of the catecholamines. Catecholamines in turn act for a short time in the circulation and are reduced after oxidation to 3-methoxy-4-hydroxy mandelic acid (VMA). These substances can be detected in the urine, where approximately one-third of the total secreted catecholamine appears as VMA and one-half is secreted as free or conjugated metanephrine.

For practical purposes, epinephrine and norepinephrine both simulate effects that are similar to adrenergic discharge although each has its own specific actions. These catecholamine effects are widespread and involve actions on the myocardium and vascular smooth muscle, as well as multiple intermediary metabolic effects, such as the mobilization of glycogen from the liver, induction of lipolysis, increases in metabolic rate, stimulation of glucagon release, inhibition of insulin secretion, and inhibition of peripheral insulin sensitivity.

Table 2.1. Normal range of urinary end products of adrenal hormones utilized as tumor markers

Urinary metabolites	Normal range (per 24 h)	
	Women	Men
Cortisol	78–365 μg	108–409 μg
17-OH corticosteroids	2–6 mg	3–10 mg
17-Ketosteroids	6–15 mg	9–22 mg
Catecholamines	>136 μg	>135 μg
VMA	0.7–6.8 mg	0.7–6.8 mg

Markers in Adrenal Disease

The adrenal cortex produces a number of hormones that are derivatives of cholesterol and either the hormones or their end products could be utilized as an index of the adrenal activities. There are a number of steroids that are synthesized in the adrenal cortex but only a few are excreted into the circulation and are biologically active. These compounds are hydrocortisone, corticosterone, and aldosterone. The adrenal medulla excretes epinephrine and norepinephrine; about 80% of the adrenal vein catecholamines is epinephrine. The measurement of catecholamines and VMA is utilized in the diagnosis and follow-up of these tumors. Currently, the diagnosis of pheochromatization is made by measuring the blood catecholamines and localizing the tumor by abdominal CT.

The role of various markers is demonstrated in Table 2.1 for malignant pheochromocytoma. Also, in pheochromocytoma originating from the adrenal generally there are elevated levels of epinephrine and norepinephrine, although in extra-adrenal pheochromocytoma the main catecholamine is norepinephrine.

In summary, the serum levels of cortisol, ACTH, aldosterone, epinephrine, and norepinephrine may be utilized in the diagnosis and/or monitoring of certain adrenal diseases. Furthermore, the urinary excretion of the metabolites of these markers may also be conveniently used for this purpose. These end products are shown in Tables 2.1 and 2.2 including 17-OH corticosteroids, 17-ketosteroids, metanephrine, and VMA. The frequency of elevated urinary catecholamines in malignant pheochromocytoma is shown in Table 2.2.

References

1. Javadpour N, Brennan MF, Woltering EA (1980) Recent advances in adrenal neoplasms. Curr Probl Surg 17: 1–52
2. Conn JW (1955) Primary aldosteronism: a new clinical syndrome. J Lab Clin Med 45: 6
3. Danforth DN Jr, Orlando MD, Bartter FC et al. (1977) Renal changes in primary aldosteronism. J Urol 117: 140

Table 2.2. Urinary catecholamine excretion in malignant pheochromocytoma[a]

	Normal value[b]	Abnormal test (%)
Catecholamines	<200 mg/day	100
Epinephrine	~40 pg/ml (0–20 µg/day)	70
Norepinephrine	~300 pg/ml (10–70 µg/day)	62
Normetanephrine	0.3–1.3 mg/day	80
Metanephrine	0.3–1.3 mg/day	100
VMA	1–9 mg/day	100

[a] From 15 patients operated on at the NIH from 1965 to 1977.
[b] Stressed.

Chapter 3

Pathology

E. E. Lack and H. P. W. Kozakewich

Introduction

The adrenal glands are two endocrine glands in one with cortex and medulla having disparate morphology, embryology, and physiologic function. These fundamental differences mandate separate consideration of pathologic processes affecting cortex and medulla. A useful and intuitive approach to the pathology of the adrenal cortex is based upon the clinical effects of endocrine hyper- or hypofunction. Simplistically, diseases affecting the cortex can be subdivided into those which are associated with excess or decreased steroid production and those which have no obvious effect on endocrine function. Using this functional approach, the pathology of the adrenal medulla is limited mainly to conditions causing excess catecholamine production since there is no well-defined endocrinopathy related to adrenal medullary insufficiency in humans. The intent herein is to illustrate various aspects of adrenal pathology in both adults and children utilizing material seen at the National Institutes of Health, Bethesda, Maryland, and the Children's Hospital, Boston, Massachusetts.

Normal Anatomy of the Adrenal Glands

Gross Anatomy

The paired adrenal glands are closely related to the superior poles of both kidneys and in the adult have been arbitrarily divided into three regions—the head and body, which are directed medially and contain almost all of the medullary tissue, and the tail, which is situated laterally. The gland on the right side has an approximately triangular shape, and the one on the left is more elongate. The anterior surface of each gland is relatively smooth, while the posterior aspect is convex with a prominent ridge or crista flanked by two lateral projections or alae (wings). On cross section the cortex in adults is normally golden-yellow with an inner, slightly pigmented zona reticularis and a central gray medulla. In elderly patients pigmentation of the zona reticularis may be accentuated. The fetal and neonatal adrenal cortex is paler because of the poorly lipidized provisional cortex. Due to the prominent vascularity of the provisional cortex, it may appear congested and give a spurious impression of hemorrhage.

It is not uncommon to see small spherical nodules of adrenal cortical tissue either attached to the capsule of the gland or free within periadrenal fat. With appropriate sectioning one can often demonstrate continuity of the nodule or its capsule with the underlying adrenal cortex or its investing connective tissue. Microscopically, there is no medullary tissue and they lack the normal zonation seen in the adrenal cortex. There may be minor variations in the shape of the adrenals. In cases of renal agenesis, for example, the ipsilateral adrenal is flattened anteroposteriorly and has a more rounded contour.

Normal Adrenal Weights

The individual and combined weights of adrenal glands vary with age and other factors, such as underlying disease state and whether the glands have been obtained surgically or at autopsy. The available data regarding adrenal weights in children are based solely upon postmortem studies. The maximum size of the adrenal gland relative to body weight is reached at about 16 weeks gestation. Stoner et al. [46], in an autopsy study of 184 children ranging in age from newborn to 15 years, found that the average combined weight at birth was 10 g (range, 2–17 g), and by 7 days of age it had decreased to an average value of 6 g (range, 3–12 g). The combined weight remained relatively

steady for 2 years then gradually increased to an average combined weight of 15 g at 12 years. In a more recent evaluation of adrenal weights in children and young adults, one of the authors (Kozakewich) has found a similar trend but lower mean values for combined weights (Fig. 3.1). In this study, individuals with multiple congenital anomalies were excluded. In the first year of life, most of the adrenals were obtained from victims of sudden infant death syndrome. The majority of older children and young adults had congenital heart disease or cystic fibrosis.

The marked decrease in adrenal weight in the first few weeks of life is due to regression of the fetal or provisional cortex, a process which is nearly complete by 3 months of age. In adults, much of the data regarding adrenal size is also derived from postmortem studies. Careful examination of adrenals from patients who died suddenly or from women undergoing bilateral adrenalectomy for breast cancer has shown that the average weight of each gland is between 4 and 4.5 g. The size of adrenal glands obtained postmortem under ordinary circumstances tends to be somewhat larger.

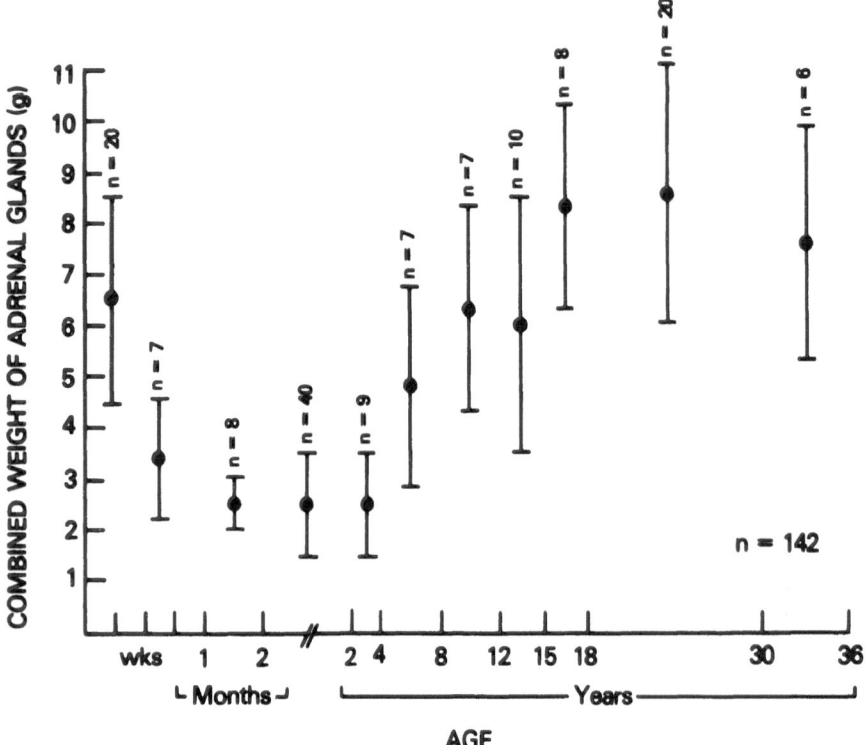

Fig. 3.1. Average combined weights of adrenal glands from 142 patients ranging in age from newborn to 35 years. *Vertical bars* represent one standard deviation. Note the marked decrease in weights during the first few weeks of life.

Adrenal Cortex

Microscopic Anatomy

The adrenal cortex is derived embryologically from coelomic mesoderm of the urogenital ridge. The first part to appear is the provisional or fetal cortex, which accounts for the bulk of the cortical mass in utero. This occurs during the 4th–6th week of intrauterine life. The fetal cortex produces a large quantity of dehydroepiandrosterone and also 16α-hydroxyepiandrosterone, which undergo aromatization in the placenta to form estriol that circulates in late pregnancy [31]. The provisional cortex is composed of large cells with compact, lightly eosinophilic cytoplasm and a prominent, well-stained nucleus (Fig. 3.2a, b). The definitive or adult cortex is formed during the 10th week of gestation and appears as a thin subcapsular band of cells immediately adjacent to the provisional cortex. It is composed of smaller cells with relatively scant vacuolated cytoplasm and less conspicuous vasculature (Fig. 3.2a, b).

In the adult gland, the adrenal cortex shows both structural and functional zonation (Fig. 3.3a, b). The three recognizable zones are (1) the zona glomerulosa with a discontinuous array of ball-like (glomeruloid) clusters of cells involved in the synthesis and secretion of mineralocorticoids; (2) the zona fasciculata, a thicker middle zone occupying about 80% of the cortical width with radially oriented columns of lipid-rich cells; and (3) the zona reticularis, a thin inner zone abutting upon the medulla with an anastomosing net-like arrangement of cells having compact cytoplasm. The zona fasciculata and zona reticularis elaborate and secrete glucocorticoids, as well as androgenic and estrogenic steroids.

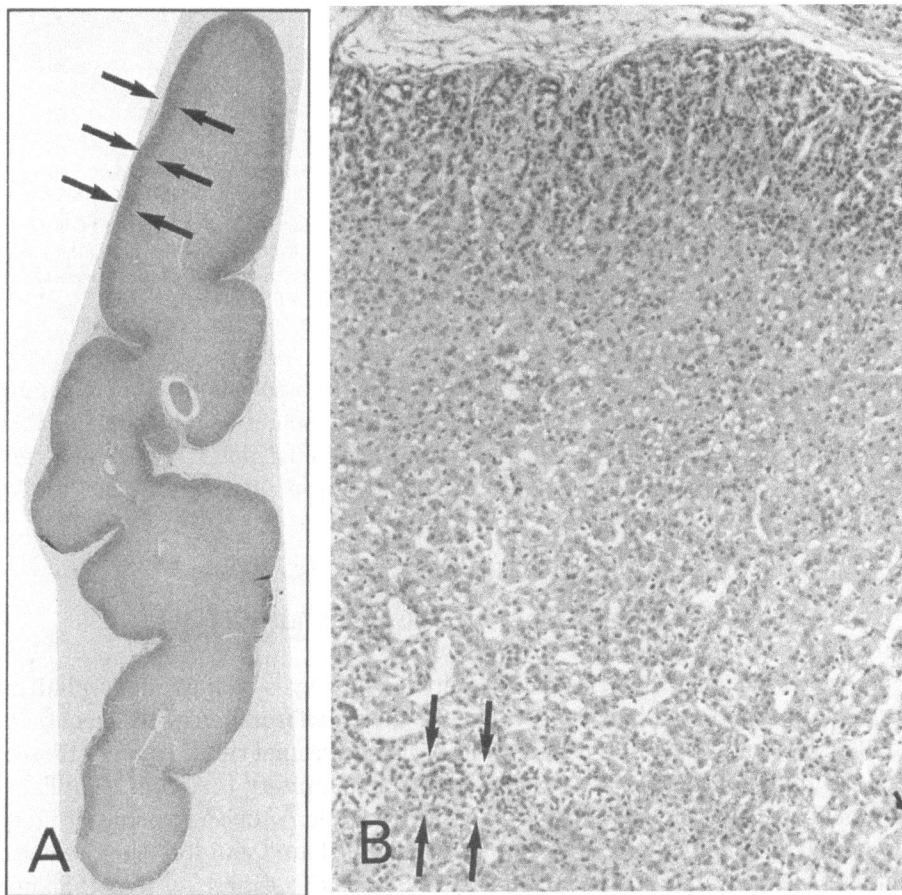

Fig. 3.2. a Cross-section of adrenal gland from a newborn shows dominant provisional (fetal) cortex and thin peripheral rim of definitive (adult) cortex (*arrows*). H & E, × 5. **b** Pale inner zone represents provisional cortex. Note prominent vascular sinusoids and sparse medullary tissue typical of the newborn gland (*arrows*). H & E, × 90

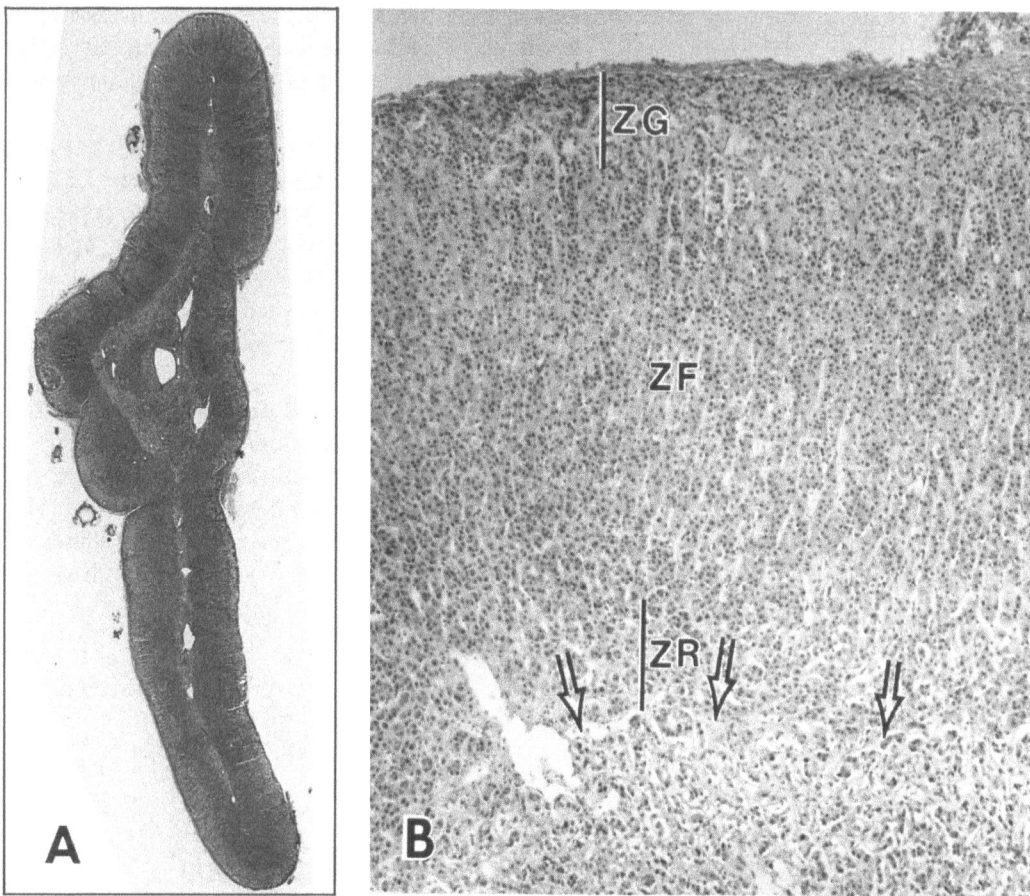

Fig. 3.3. a Cross-section of adult adrenal gland showing well-defined cortex and medulla. Section taken through the body of the gland where the ratio of cortex to medulla is approximately 15:1. H & E, × 4. **b** Adrenal gland from an 18-year-old patient with cystic fibrosis. There is mild lipid depletion. Note adrenal medulla at bottom (*arrows*). About 80% of cortical width is occupied by zona fasciculata (*ZF*). Zona glomerulosa (*ZG*) and zona reticularis (*ZR*) are also indicated. H & E, × 65

Pathology

Adrenal Heterotopia and Accessory Adrenals

Nodules of accessory adrenal cortical tissue (adrenal rests) are usually small encapsulated structures which can be found incidentally in a variety of sites—adjacent to the adrenals, in the retroperitoneum, beneath the capsule of the superior pole of the kidney or the undersurface of the liver. When visible grossly they usually measure less than 3 mm in diameter. In females, they may be found in the mesovarium close to the hilum of the ovary and in males on the spermatic cord or in close relation to the rete testis or epididymis (Fig. 3.4a, b). Medullary tissue is characteristically absent in accessory nodules. In children with congenital adrenal hyperplasia, accessory cortical tissue may also undergo enlargement. Rarely, adrenal glands may

be fused, sometimes in association with congenital midline defects such as spinal dysraphism (Fig. 3.5). True heterotopia of adrenal glands is extremely rare but has been reported in sites such as the cranial cavity and lung [1].

Adrenal Glands in Anencephaly

Bilateral adrenal atrophy is seen in anencephaly, a severe neural tube malformation with agenesis of most of the brain and cranial vault. The sella turcica is flattened and the pituitary is seldom identifiable by gross inspection. Microscopically, some pituitary tissue can usually be found, but it is often reduced in amount. Atrophy or agenesis of hypothalamic structures may also contribute to the adrenal atrophy. The combined weight of both adrenals is often less than 1 g. The provisional cortex is rudimentary

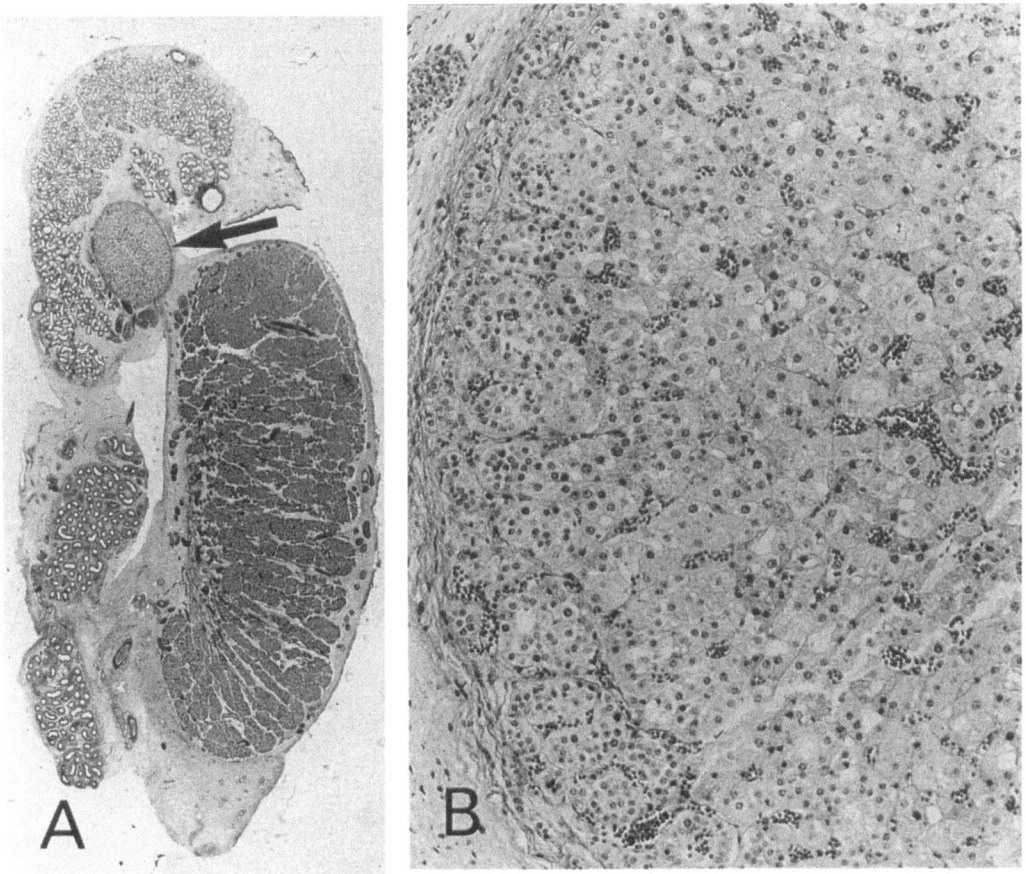

Fig. 3.4. a Sagittal section of testis and adnexa from a newborn. Note nodule of accessory adrenal cortical tissue adjacent to the head of the epididymis (*arrow*). H & E, × 6.5. b Cortical nodule is composed of small cells at periphery representing definitive (adult) cortex. Larger, more compact cells with congested sinusoids are provisional (fetal) cortical cells. H & E, × 130

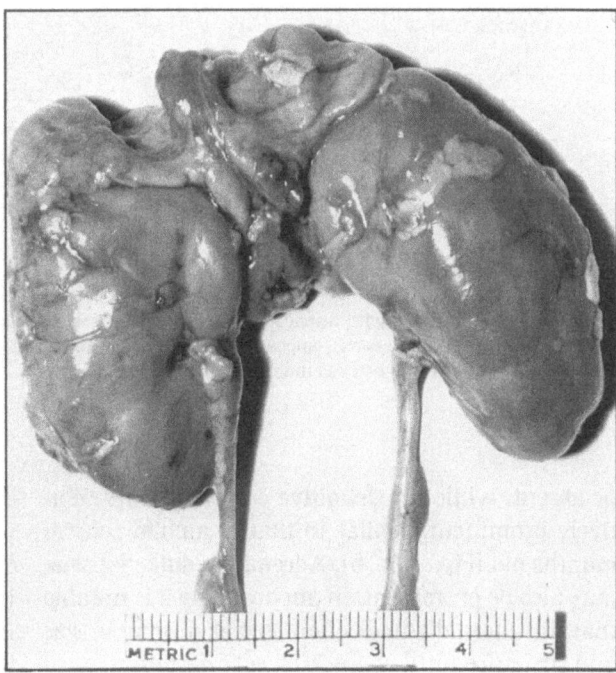

Fig. 3.5. One-month-old child with multiple congenital anomalies including spinal dysraphism. Kidneys were more medially placed than usual and note fusion of adrenal glands.

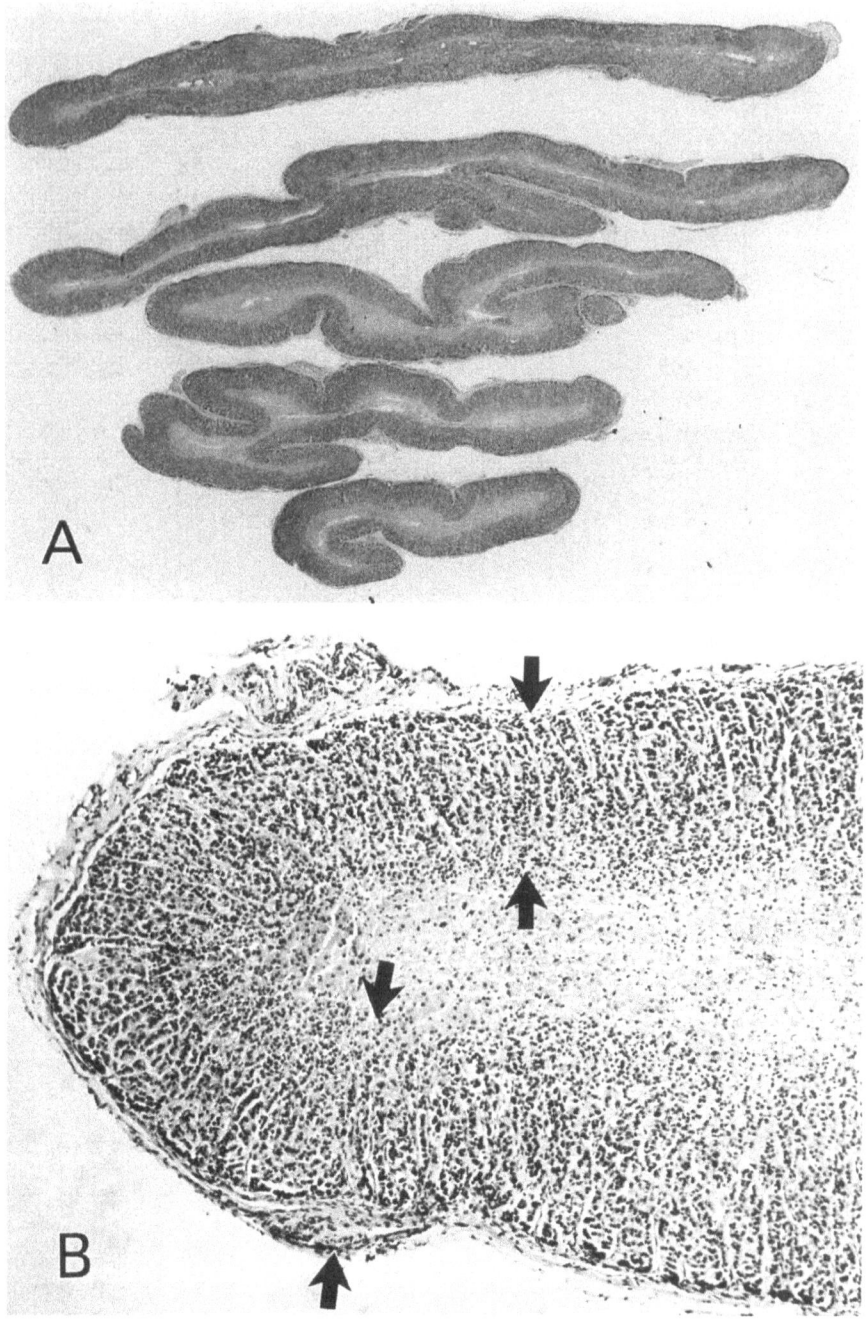

Fig. 3.6 a Newborn child with anencephaly. Note in comparison with Fig. 3.2a that the provisional cortex is markedly reduced in volume and the definitive cortex appears relatively prominent. H & E, × 7.7. **b** Provisional cortex is markedly reduced compared with Fig. 3.2b. Definitive cortex is indicated by *arrows*. H & E, × 58

or absent, while the definitive cortex appears relatively prominent, similar to that of a child several months old (Fig. 3.6a, b). Adrenal medullary tissue may also be prominent. In anencephaly it is notable that the adrenal glands often appear normal in size and structure until about 20 weeks gestation.

Reactions to "Stress"

The autopsy affords the major opportunity to examine the adrenal glands for the effects of "stress" imposed by terminal illnesses or systemic and debilitating diseases. The most common reaction to

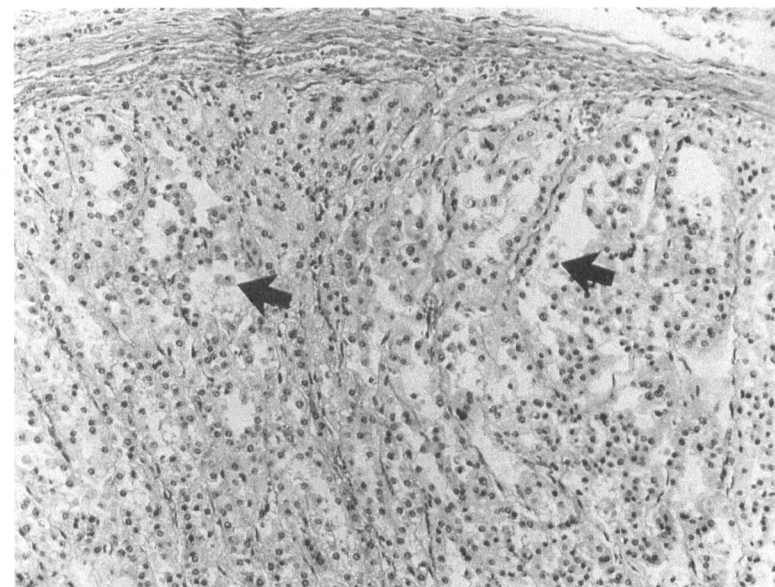

Fig. 3.7. Cords of outer zona fasciculata are widened with evidence of cytolysis (*arrows*) and secondary tubule formation. Many cortical cells have compact cytoplasm representing lipid depletion. H & E, × 120

stress is known as lipid depletion where cytoplasm of cells of the zona fasciculata becomes compact as opposed to the normally vacuolated lipid-rich or clear cells. There may be some degree of cellular enlargement. The zona fasciculata and zona reticularis may then appear as a unified zone of compact cells with inconspicuous zona glomerulosa.

Lipid depletion in the adult is often focal and may remain so for some time, but in children it is thought to become diffuse rather quickly. In some areas of lipid depletion, the outer part of the zona fasciculata may undergo degenerative change with cytolysis and formation of tubules as noted by Wilbur and Rich [50] (Fig. 3.7). It is presumably related to intense stimulation by adrenocorticotropic hormone (ACTH). In the earlier literature, tubular degeneration had been associated most commonly with fatal cases of diphtheria and meningococcemia.

Effects of Drugs and Cytotoxic Agents

Relatively little is known about cytotoxic effects of drugs on the adrenal cortex. Early investigation of the effects of the common insecticide dichlorodiphenyltrichloroethane (DDT) in dogs demonstrated selective destruction of the zona fasciculata [31]. The potent cytotoxic agent was found to be a derivative of DDT known as *o,p'*-DDD. This agent, marketed as Mitotane, has been used for palliative treatment of patients with adrenal cortical

carcinoma but with somewhat limited long-term success [19]. It appears to have an "adrenolytic" effect with specificity for adrenal cortical cells, both normal and neoplastic. Another group of chemicals causing selective necrosis of the adrenal cortex are derivatives of 12-methylbenz(α)anthracene. Polymers such as hexadimethrine also cause cortical necrosis and hemorrhage. Extraadrenal toxicity has limited their use in humans [31]. 5-Fluorouracil has also demonstrated cytotoxicity in vitro [30].

Secondary Aldosteronism

Secondary aldosteronism is associated with sodium retention and loss of potassium and is distinguished from primary aldosteronism by high renin output. Hyperplasia of the zona glomerulosa has been reported in some patients with secondary aldosteronism associated with hepatic cirrhosis and ascites, nephrotic syndrome, cystic fibrosis, and Bartter's syndrome. The latter is a rare disorder characterized by hyperplasia of juxtaglomerular cells in the kidney with elevated renin secretion and secondary stimulation of the zona glomerulosa. In secondary aldosteronism, the hyperplastic zona glomerulosa appears as a continuous cortical band usually greater than $100\,\mu$m wide. In patients receiving spironolactone (Aldactone), a competitive antagonist of aldosterone, glomerulosa cells may show characteristic cytoplasmic "inclusions" as early as 10 days following treatment for primary or

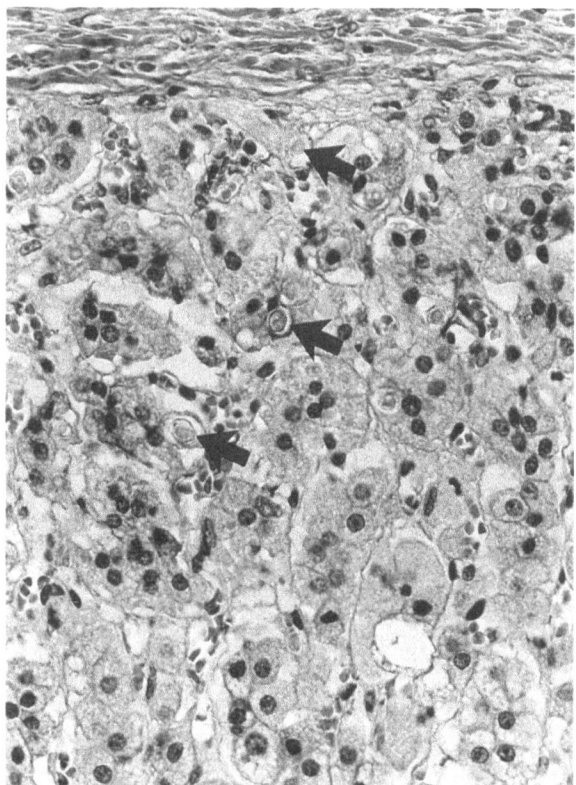

Fig. 3.8. Scroll-like cytoplasmic inclusions represent so-called spironolactone bodies. They are surrounded by a clear halo (*arrows*) and are largely confined to cells of zona glomerulosa. Inclusions vary in size from one-half to two times the size of a nucleus. H & E. × 300

secondary aldosteronism (Fig. 3.8). Ultrastructurally, they appear to be membranous structures in continuity with smooth endoplasmic reticulum, and a recent immunohistochemical study has demonstrated their capability of storing or binding aldosterone [18].

Systemic Infections Involving the Adrenal Glands

The adrenals can be involved by a variety of infectious agents, including viruses, bacteria, and fungi. A well-known example of "viral adrenalitis" is seen with disseminated herpes simplex in the newborn. The affected infant usually has cutaneous and other disseminated lesions, but there is a distinctive tropism for adrenal glands and liver resulting in hepatoadrenal necrosis. There are punctate sharply defined foci of necrosis with little or no host inflammatory response. The cortical necrosis can become extensive and confluent. A similar histo-

logic appearance can be seen with disseminated varicella and cytomegalovirus (CMV) infection (Fig. 3.9a, b). With the emergence of the deadly acquired immune deficiency syndrome (AIDS) in recent

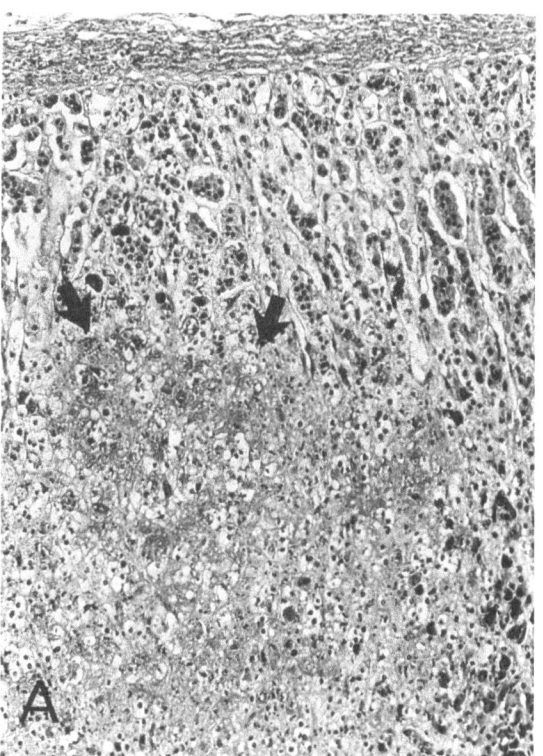

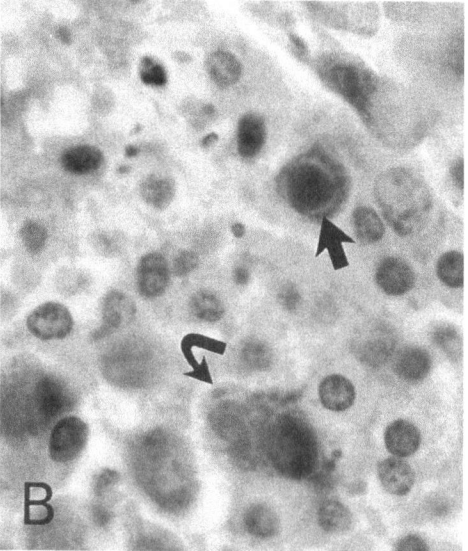

Fig. 3.9. a Adolescent with acute myelogenous leukemia and disseminated cytomegalovirus (*CMV*) infection. Note well-defined zone of necrosis in cortex (*arrows*). H & E, × 115. **b** Higher magnification showing characteristic nuclear inclusions, some of which are surrounded by a clear halo (*arrow*). Other cells contain cytoplasmic inclusions (*curved arrow*). H & E, × 570

years, CMV adrenalitis and necrosis may be extensive enough to cause adrenal insufficiency in some patients.

Tuberculosis may also involve the adrenal glands to such an extent that chronic adrenal insufficiency results. This is an unusual cause of Addison's disease in developed countries today. Both glands tend to be somewhat enlarged. Similar to disseminated herpes infection, there may also be involvement of accessory adrenal cortical tissue. The classic tuberculoid granulomatous reaction is usually not seen, but instead there is prominent caseation necrosis. The adrenals may also be involved in systemic mycotic infections such as histoplasmosis (Fig. 3.10) and blastomycosis. Similar to tuberculosis of the adrenals, a granulomatous or tuberculoid reaction is usually not seen.

Ovarian Thecal Metaplasia

This is an unusual microscopic finding of unknown functional significance which consists of wedge-

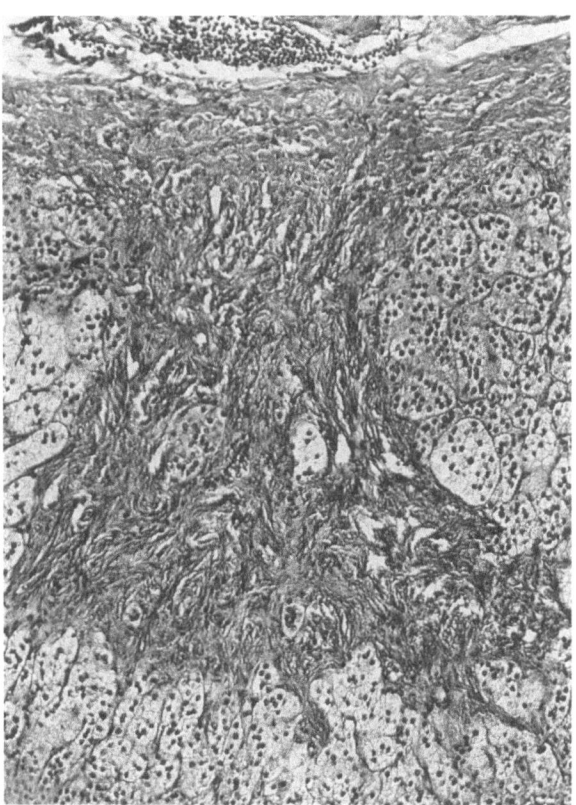

Fig. 3.11. Wedge-shaped area of thecal metaplasia contains bland spindle cells and much collagen. It is attached to adrenal capsule at top and contains small nests of cortical cells. H & E, × 120

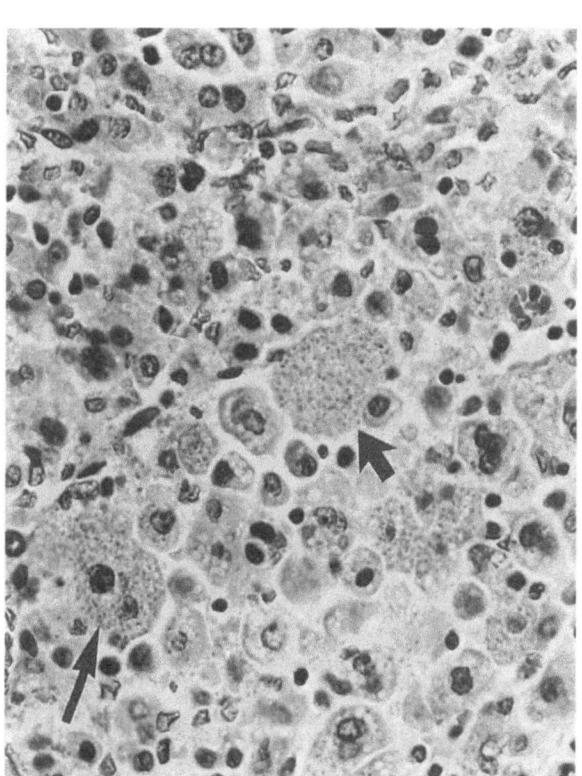

Fig. 3.10. Disseminated histoplasmosis involving adrenal gland. Many cells resembling histiocytes contain numerous organisms measuring about 2–3μm in diameter (*arrows*). Residual cortical cells are difficult to identify. H & E, × 460

shaped foci usually less than 2 mm in size (Fig. 3.11). They have been seen in about 4% of women undergoing bilateral adrenalectomy for metastatic breast cancer and are frequently multiple and bilateral just beneath the adrenal capsule [14]. Their occurrence may explain the rare examples of ovarian-type sex cord-stromal tumors reported in this location.

Amyloidosis of the Adrenal Glands

The adrenals are usually involved to some degree in secondary amyloidosis and may be enlarged. With advanced amyloid deposition, the inner zones of the cortex are virtually replaced by homogeneous eosinophilic material, which causes severe atrophy of the zona fasciculata and zona reticularis (Fig. 3.12). There is often a peripheral rim of clear (lipid-rich) or compact cells of residual zona fasciculata. Adrenal insufficiency is only rarely seen. In primary

28   Pathology

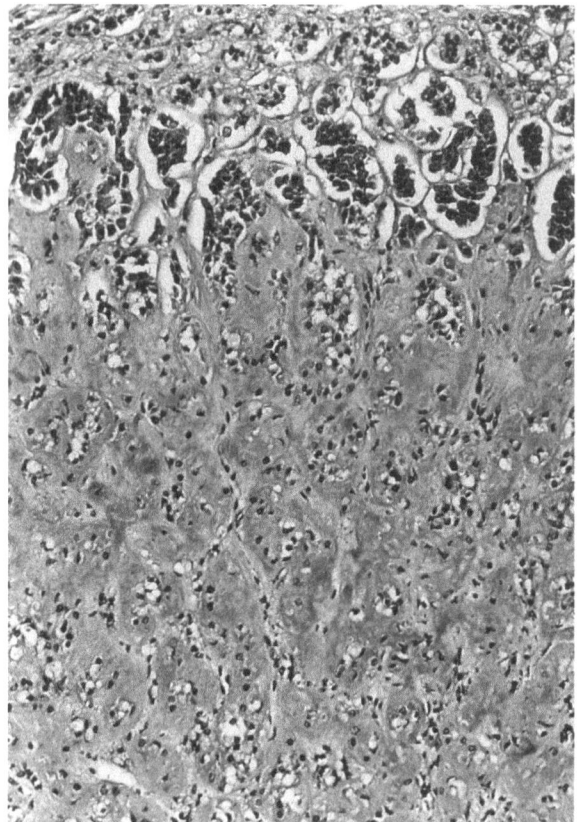

Fig. 3.12. Twenty-five-year-old man with cystic fibrosis and secondary amyloidosis. Amyloid deposits cause severe atrophy of inner zones of adrenal cortex. There are small collections of clear cells beneath capsule representing zona glomerulosa and an inner band of darker compact cells. H & E, × 125

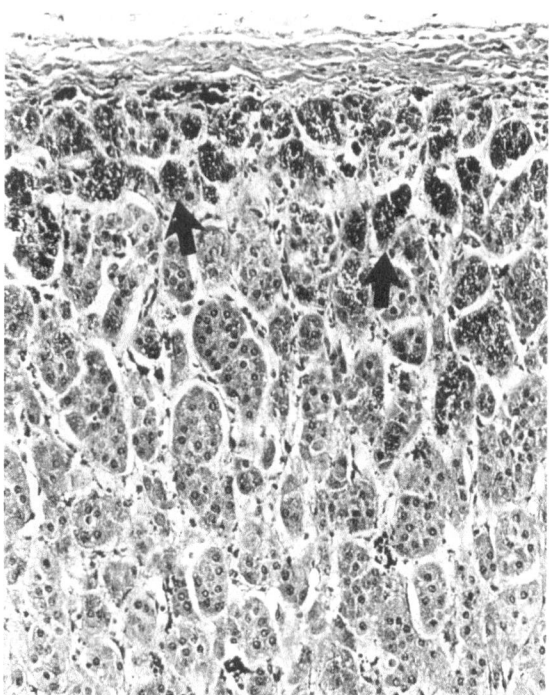

Fig. 3.13. Hemosiderosis of adrenal gland obtained at autopsy from a patient with beta thalassemia major. It shows darkly stained deposits of hemosiderin within cells of zona glomerulosa (*arrows*). Patient had hemosiderosis due to multiple transfusions. H & E, × 60

amyloidosis, there is preferential involvement of arterioles.

Hemosiderosis of the Adrenal Glands

Iron deposition in the form of hemosiderin can be seen in patients with hemosiderosis or primary hemochromatosis (Fig. 3.13). There is distinct predilection for the zona glomerulosa which can be dramatically accentuated in sections stained for iron. There may be deposition in adjacent cortical cells, but usually the zona fasciculata and zona reticularis are spared.

Congenital Adrenal Cytomegaly

This peculiar condition is usually an incidental microscopic finding in adrenals which are otherwise

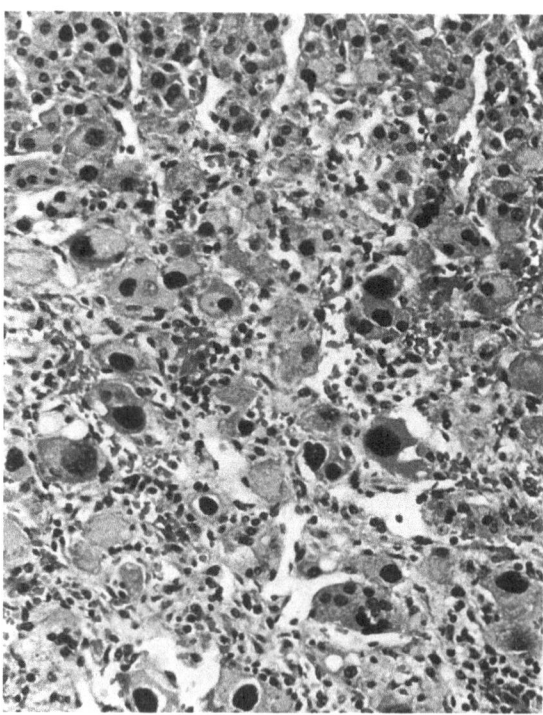

Fig. 3.14. Marked cytomegaly of cells of provisional cortex. There are numerous enlarged hyperchromatic nuclei. Child had Beckwith-Wiedemann syndrome. H & E, × 195

grossly normal. It is relatively uncommon, occurring in about 3% of stillborns and infants less than 2 months of age [9]. The cytomegaly may be focal or diffuse. Cells of the fetal cortex are enlarged with increased volume of both nucleus and cytoplasm (Fig. 3.14). Nuclei may be markedly pleomorphic. One may also see so-called pseudo inclusions due to intranuclear herniation of cell cytoplasm. Cytomegaly can also occur in accessory tissue elsewhere.

Adrenal cytomegaly is a characteristic feature of Beckwith-Wiedemann (exomphalos-macroglossia-gigantism) syndrome, which consists of macrosomia, macroglossia, omphalocele, and pancreatic islet cell hyperplasia with neonatal hypoglycemia. A number of other abnormalities may be present. The condition may be associated with childhood tumors such as nephroblastoma (Wilms' tumor), adrenal cortical carcinoma, or hepatoblastoma.

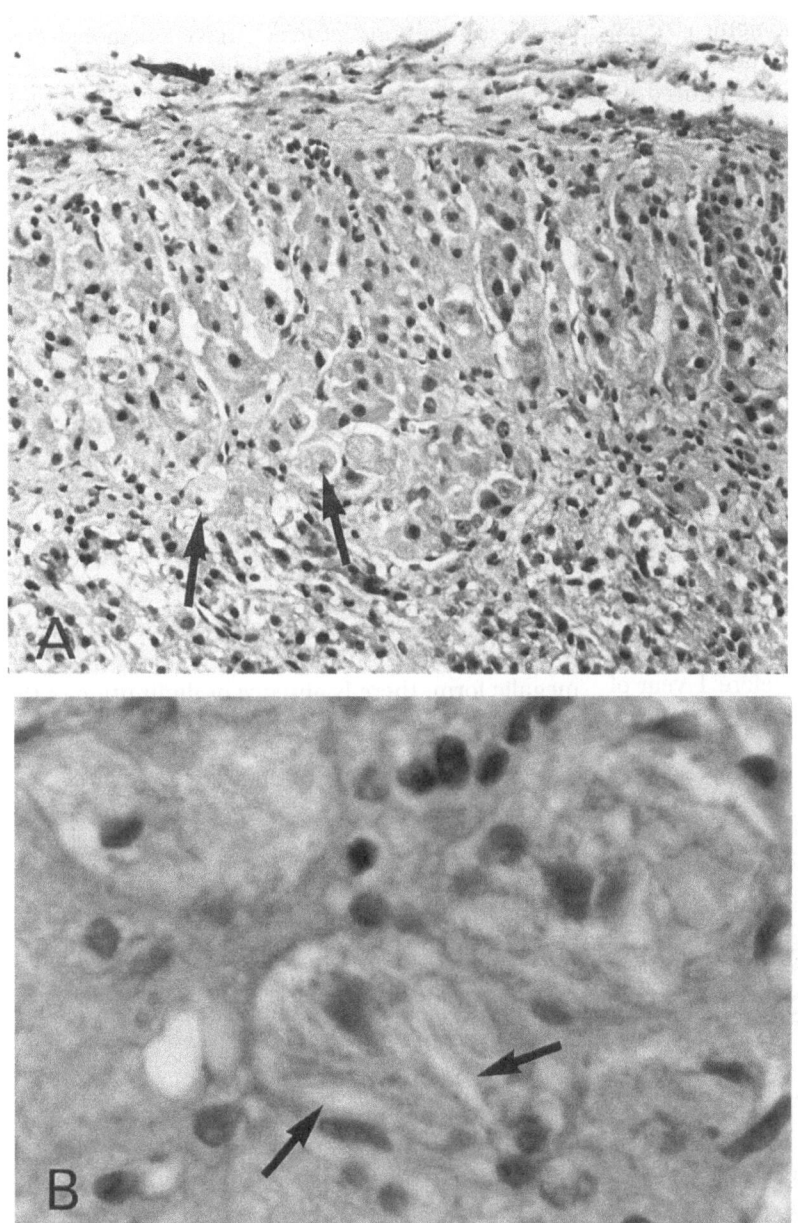

Fig. 3.15. a Nine-year-old child with adrenal leukodystrophy. Note marked atrophy of cortex and the large ballooned cells (*arrows*). Portion of adrenal medulla is present in lower half of field. H & E, × 255. b Some of the ballooned cortical cells contain striate clefts in cytoplasm (*arrows*). H & E, × 600

Storage Diseases Involving the Adrenal Glands

Adrenoleukodystrophy. This hereditary, sex-linked disorder affects mainly male patients toward the end of the first decade, but it can be seen in the neonatal period as well [36]. Occasionally, females may be affected. It is a metabolic disorder in which unbranched long chain saturated fatty acids of 24–30 carbon atoms (usually esterified to cholesterol) accumulate. Affected sites include central and peripheral nervous system, adrenal cortex, and testis. The basic defect appears to be a diminished capacity to oxidize these fatty acids. Pathognomonic striated inclusions are found in adrenal cortical, Leydig, microglial, and Schwann cells and are caused by accumulations of lamellar-lipid profiles and crystalloid clefts which contain long chain saturated fatty acids. Clinical and laboratory evidence of central nervous system and adrenal cortical dysfunction is prominent in the congenital, neonatal, juvenile, and adult forms [36]. The adrenal glands are usually small with thinning of the zona reticularis and inner zona fasciculata. The most typical cells are ballooned with striated lamellar material within the cytoplasm (Fig. 3.15a, b). These acicular clefts represent lipid which has been extracted during routine processing of tissue.

Wolman's Disease. This metabolic storage disease caused by deficiency of lysosomal acid lipase results in massive accumulation of cholesterol esters and triglycerides in most tissues of the body [2]. Wolman's disease is autosomal recessive, occurs in infancy, and is nearly always fatal before 1 year of age. There is failure to thrive, diarrhea, and marked hepatosplenomegaly. The adrenals are markedly and symmetrically enlarged with retention of normal shape. Both adrenals contain multiple punctate calcifications which are radiographically visible (Fig. 3.16). The zona glomerulosa and zona fasciculata are relatively well preserved, but the central zone is expanded and contains haphazardly arranged cells with foamy cytoplasm and cells with cytoplasmic clefts representing cholesterol crystals (Fig. 3.17). There are foci of necrosis, fibrosis, and small lipid cysts. Calcific deposits are prominent. ACTH-stimulation studies have demonstrated decreased adrenal responsiveness. Cholesteryl ester storage disease appears to be a milder form of Wolman's disease and may not be detected until adulthood. Adrenal calcification is only rarely observed.

Congenital Adrenal Hypoplasia

This is a rare cause of adrenal insufficiency in infants and children. There is a primary or cytomegalic form and a secondary or miniature adult form [23]. The cytomegalic form is considered to be sex linked, affecting males. In both forms of congenital adrenal hypoplasia, the clinical signs and symptoms of affected infants include poor feeding, failure to thrive, hyperpigmentation, fever, vomiting, diarrhea, and vascular collapse. A fatal outcome is frequent. The combined adrenal weight is usually less than 1 g (Fig. 3.18). In the cytomegalic form, there is absence or diminution of the

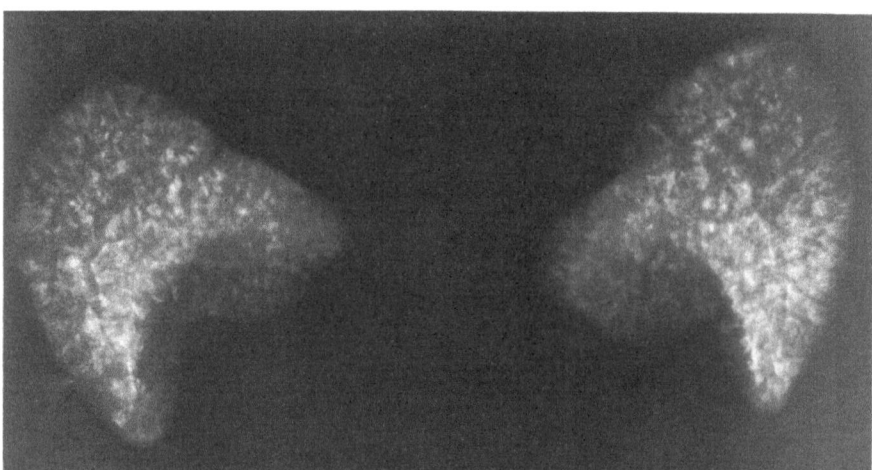

Fig. 3.16. Three-month-old female with Wolman's disease. Radiograph of adrenals obtained at autopsy shows bilateral calcifications.

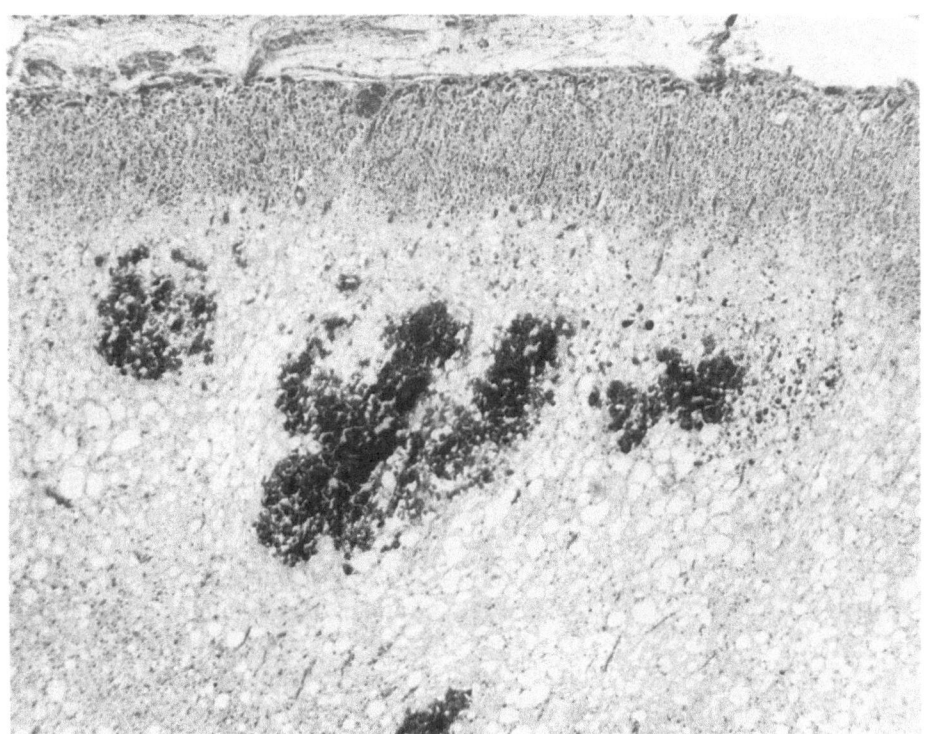

Fig. 3.17. Inner zone of cortex is greatly expanded and contains small "lipid cysts" and foamy cells. Note foci of coarse calcification. H & E, × 52

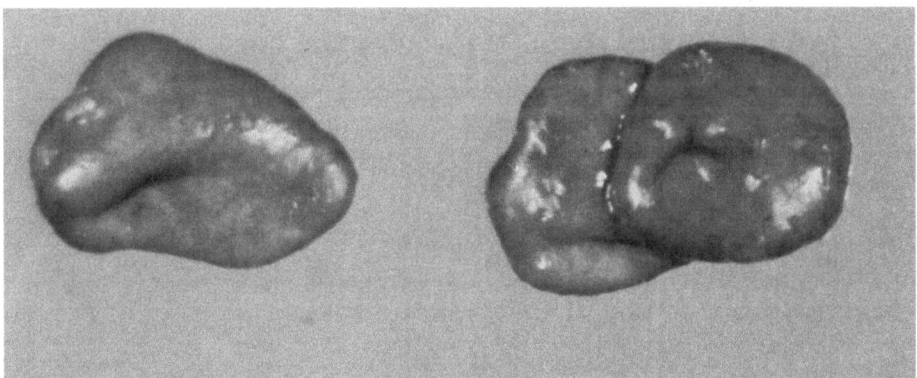

Fig. 3. 18. Eight-day-old male with congenital adrenal hypoplasia. Combined weight of both adrenal glands was 0.5 g. One of the glands is dysmorphic with bilobate appearance.

definitive and provisional cortex, with the cytomegaly affecting provisional cortical cells (Fig. 3.19). The secondary form of congenital hypoplasia may be sporadic or inherited in an autosomal recessive manner. The adrenals are small with a relatively normal definitive zone but absence of the provisional zone.

Adrenal Hemorrhage

Unilateral or bilateral adrenal hemorrhage is a common finding in stillborns and infants dying in the immediate postnatal period, but massive hemorrhage into one or both glands is much less common [5]. The pathogenesis is unclear, but the fol-

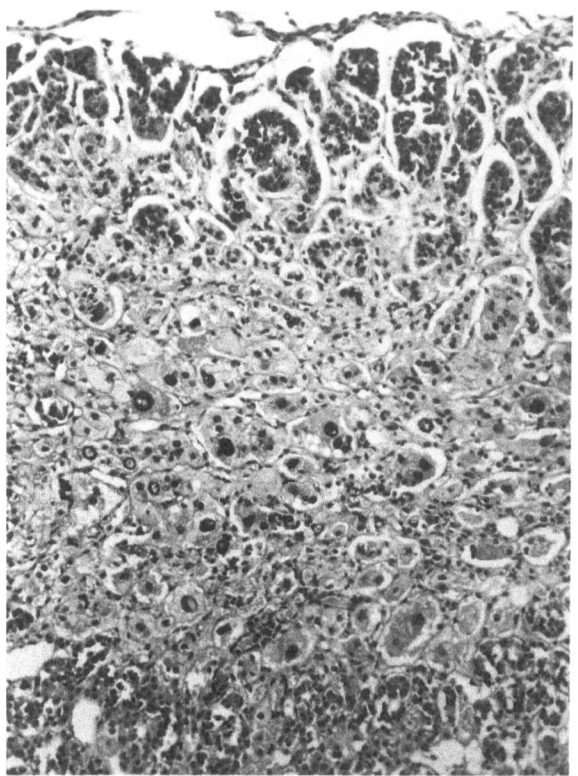

Fig. 3.19. Primary or cytomegalic form of congenital adrenal hypoplasia. There is thinning of cortex and cytomegalic change of provisional cortical cells. H & E, × 95

lowing are predisposing factors: prolonged deliveries or placental bleeding, large birth weight, prematurity with intrapartum anoxia, septicemia, thrombocytopenia, and disseminated thromboembolic disease. In most cases of adrenal hemorrhage in newborns, the diagnosis is made only at autopsy (Fig. 3.20). With massive hemorrhage, there is extension into the retroperitoneal space or rupture into the coelomic cavity followed by shock, abdominal distension, and death. Resolution, if it occurs, may be accompanied by scarring and calcification. Adrenal hemorrhage has also been reported in adults on anticoagulant therapy.

Adrenal Hemorrhage and Necrosis

Waterhouse–Friderichsen Syndrome This is a well-defined clinical and pathologic entity, characterized by the abrupt onset of vascular collapse and shock in association with septicemia. There is usually a petechial rash as a manifestation of disseminated intravascular coagulation. It is classically associated with meningococcal sepsis but has also been seen with bacterial septicemia due to organisms

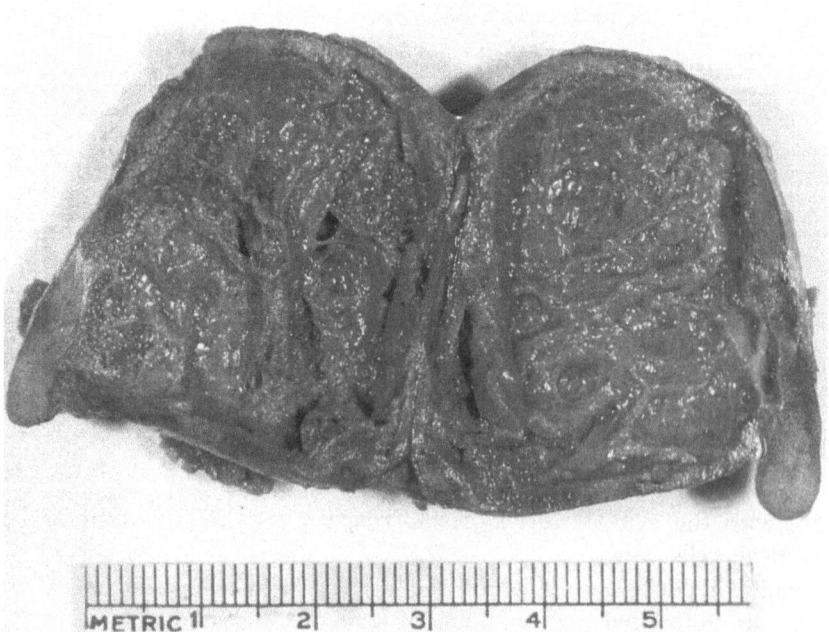

Fig. 3.20. Twenty-three-day-old female with coarctation of aorta and thrombosed aneurysm of the ductus arteriosus. There were numerous thromboemboli in multiple organs, presumably ductal in origin. The right adrenal is enlarged and on cross-section shows extensive hemorrhage and necrosis.

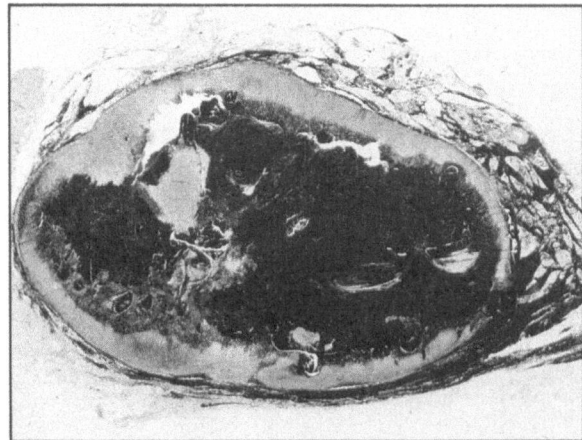

Fig. 3.21. Adrenal gland from an adult with Waterhouse-Friderichsen syndrome shows distension of the gland by acute hemorrhage with some extension into periadrenal fat. H & E, × 4

such as *Hemophilus influenzae* and *Streptococcus pneumoniae*. The fully developed syndrome usually proves rapidly fatal, often within 24 h of onset. At autopsy, the adrenals may or may not be enlarged; but hemorrhage is invariably present in both adrenals and is usually confined to the cortex. The hemorrhage may be so marked that the adrenals are converted to a "bag of blood" (Fig. 3.21). Rarely, blood may extend beyond the capsule into retroperitoneal tissues. Small fibrin thrombi are often seen within vascular sinusoids of the cortex but this is not a universal finding.

The cause of adrenal hemorrhage in the Waterhouse-Friderichsen syndrome is probably related to the action of bacterial endotoxins on vascular endothelium. This, coupled with a marked "stress reaction" within the gland itself, may predispose to acute hemorrhage and necrosis. Although the profound shock has been attributed to acute adrenal failure, it is more likely due to endotoxemia.

Similar adrenal hemorrhage and necrosis can occur during pregnancy. Predisposing factors include eclampsia, abruptio placentae (premature placental separation), and puerperal sepsis. Disseminated intravascular coagulation is reported to be the underlying mechanism. On occasion, adrenal vein thrombosis may lead to hemorrhage and necrosis. Occasionally, it has been described as a sequel to adrenal venography. Adrenal necrosis can also be seen in association with renal vein thrombosis.

Chronic Adrenal Insufficiency (Addison's Disease)

This clinical syndrome was described by Thomas Addison in 1855 and is characterized by weakness, hypotension, pigmentation of skin and buccal mucosa, hypoglycemia, and electrolyte disturbances [31]. Because of the functional reserve of the adrenals, the characteristic features are not observed until about 90% or more of the adrenal cortical tissue is destroyed or ablated. Intercurrent illness or stress, however, may place the individual with borderline function at risk for acute adrenal insufficiency (Addisonian crisis). One of the most common causes of Addison's disease used to be tuberculosis with extensive necrosis of both glands. Currently, the most common etiology is autoimmune which includes many cases previously classified as idiopathic [31]. Some cases are iatrogenic due to exogenous steroid administration with suppression of the hypothalamic–pituitary axis. Marked adrenal cortical atrophy can result from hypophysectomy or destruction of the adenohypophysis by various disease processes. Metastatic tumors in the adrenal glands only rarely cause adrenal insufficiency [40].

In the autoimmune or idiopathic form of Addison's disease, the adrenal glands are "wafer thin" and markedly atrophic (Fig. 3.22a, b). The combined weight of both glands is often less than 3 g. When the atrophy is pronounced, they can be very difficult to identify grossly at autopsy. Histologically, the cortical band is very thin and may be discontinuous with small nodules of cortical cells. The cells may be enlarged and haphazardly arranged with compact acidophilic cytoplasm. Small collections of lymphocytes are usually present, and there may even be lymphoid follicles with reactive germinal centers. Some of the larger nuclei may contain "pseudo inclusions" due to herniation of cell cytoplasm. A nonspecific chronic lymphocytic thyroiditis is occasionally seen with idiopathic Addison's disease, and when associated with primary hypothyroidism the term Schmidt's syndrome is sometimes used.

Congenital Adrenal Hyperplasia (Adrenogenital Syndrome) [29]

The adrenal glands synthesize and secrete three major classes of steroids—glucocorticoids, mineralocorticoids, and sex steroids. A number of

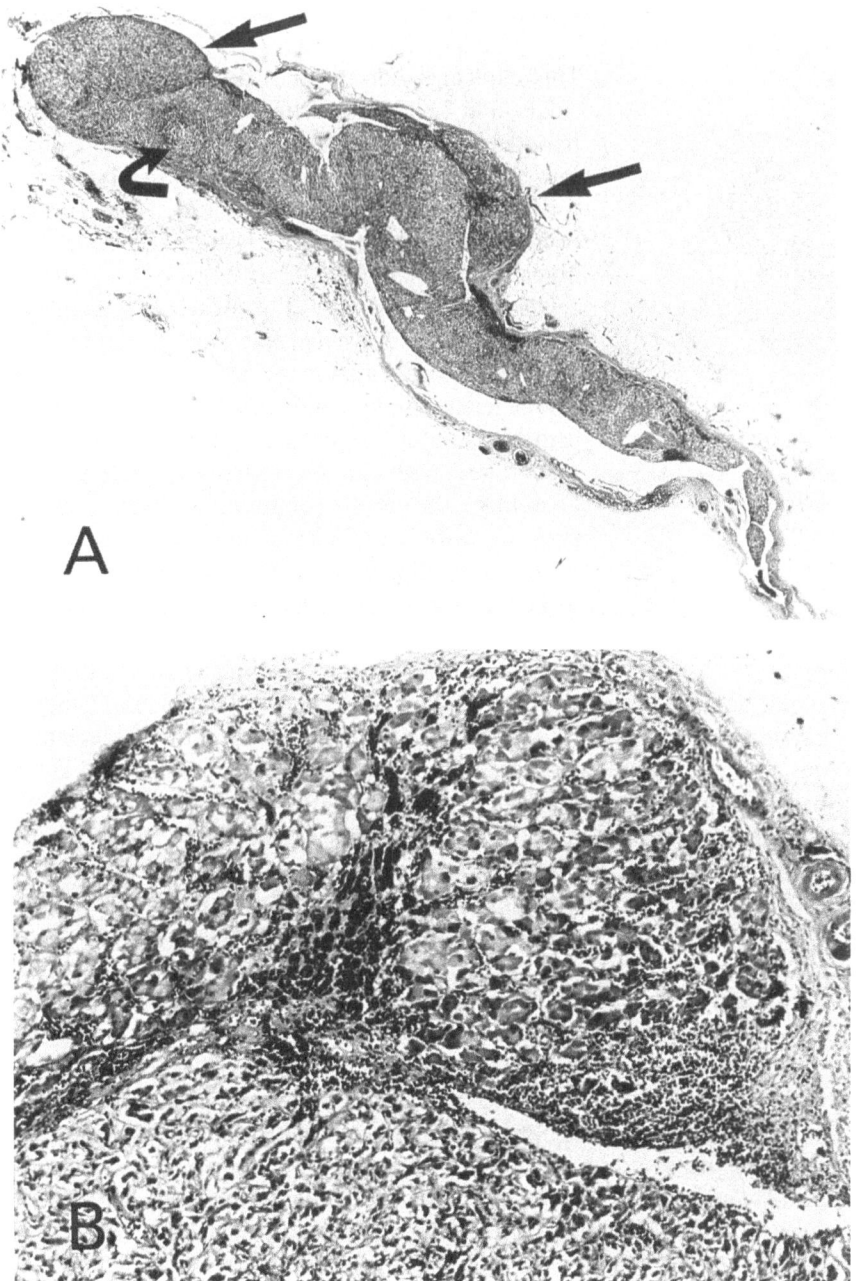

Fig. 3.22. a "Wafer-thin" adrenal gland from an adult with idiopathic Addison's disease shows extreme atrophy of cortex which is discontinuous and represented only by a few nodules of cortical cells (*straight arrows*). Occasional lymphoid follicles are present (*curved arrow*). Adrenal weighed less than 1 g. H & E, × 11.5. **b** Representative micronodule of disorganized cortical cells. Most cells are relatively large with compact lipid-depleted cytoplasm. There is a moderate infiltration by chronic inflammatory cells, mostly lymphocytes. Adrenal medulla at *bottom* is relatively prominent. H & E, × 80

enzymes are involved in their synthesis (Fig. 3.23). Congenital adrenal hyperplasia (CAH) is due to an enzymatic defect in steroid synthesis which is inherited as an autosomal recessive trait. Due to deficient cortisol output, there is loss of the normal feedback inhibition on the hypothalamic–pituitary axis, and increased levels of ACTH cause adrenal cortical hyperplasia with excess secretion of precursor substances proximal to the level of enzymatic block.

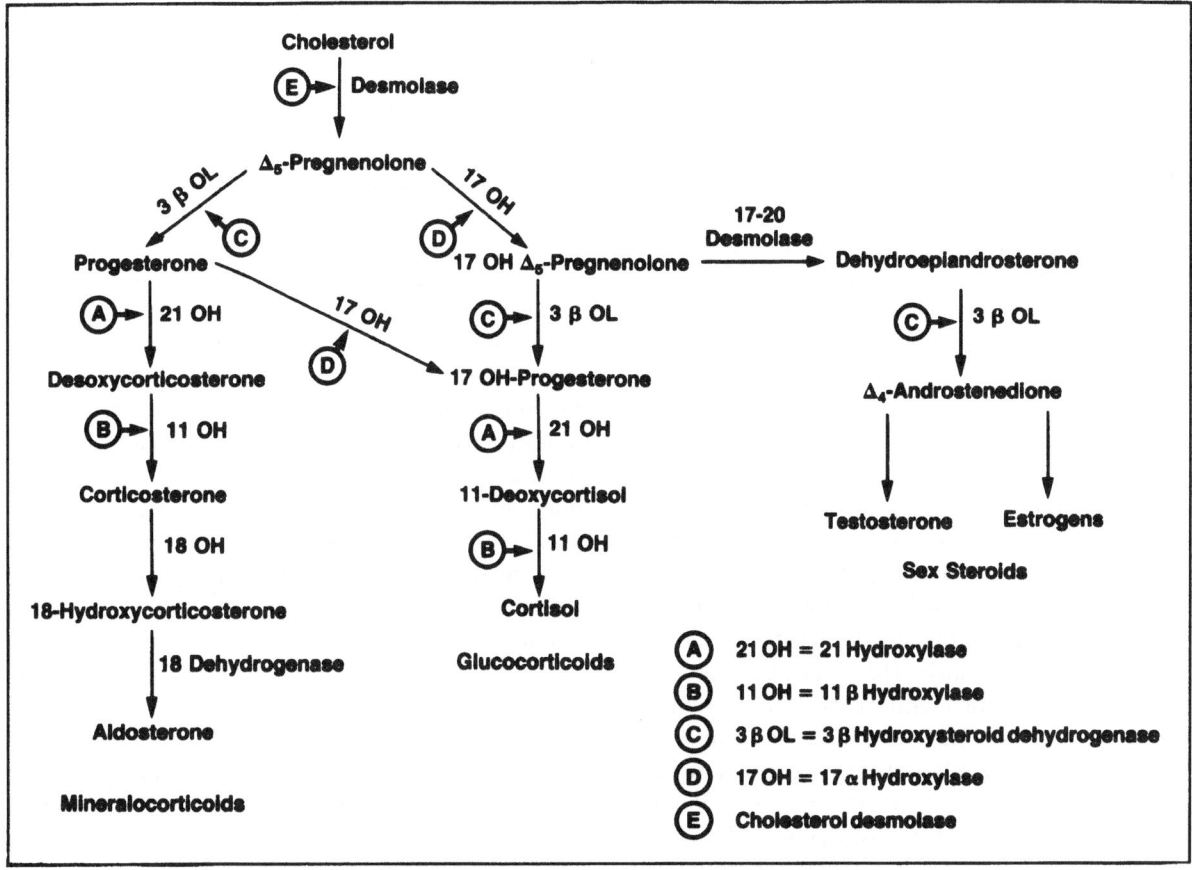

Fig. 3.23. Synthetic pathways for the three major classes of adrenal steroids. Modified after [29].

21-Hydroxylase Deficiency. This is the most common enzymatic defect in CAH and accounts for roughly 90% of cases. Affected females typically show signs of virilization with ambiguous genitalia, clitoromegaly, and fused labioscrotal folds. Affected males may appear normal at birth, and the disorder may be overlooked unless they have a salt-losing variant. If left untreated, children of both sexes will develop progressive virilization, advanced bone age, and premature closure of the epiphyses. Virilization results from an excess of testosterone since the androgen synthetic pathway is not affected by the enzymatic defect. When the enzyme deficiency is mild, decreased synthesis of mineralocorticoids does not clinically manifest itself except perhaps in times of severe stress. There is a severe form of 21-hydroxylase deficiency, however, where virilization is accompanied by marked salt-losing due to deficiency of aldosterone, and there is a more severe deficiency of cortisol.

11β-Hydroxylase Deficiency. Defects in this enzyme

result in decreased cortisol production and consequent ACTH stimulation of the adrenals. There is buildup of desoxycorticosterone in the mineralocorticoid pathway with secondary salt retention and hypertension. Stimulation also causes virilization.

3β-Hydroxysteroid Dehydrogenase Deficiency. This results in an early block in synthesis affecting all three major classes of steroids. There is marked decrease in cortisol, aldosterone, and testosterone. Females are mildly virilized due to overproduction of dehydroepiandrosterone, a steroid with male androgenic properties. There is incomplete virilization in males because of enzyme deficiency in the testes.

17α-Hydroxylase Deficiency. There is decreased synthesis of cortisol and sex steroids. In affected males, the external genitalia are ambiguous with underdevelopment of androgen-dependent parts. There is no interference with Müllerian inhibitory hormone so that males do not develop internal female organs. There is also oversecretion of desoxycorticosterone resulting in salt retention and possible hypertension.

Cholesterol Desmolase Deficiency. This is a very proximal enzymatic defect affecting synthesis of all three classes of steroids. It is probably fatal if adequate hormone replacement is not given. The affected male presents special problems in diagnosis since there is characteristically no ambiguity of external genitalia.

Adrenal Pathology. The pathology of the adrenal glands is similar in all forms of CAH except that due to deficiency of cholesterol desmolase. Both glands are markedly enlarged with a convoluted, almost cerebriform, surface (Fig. 3.24). The adrenals usually weigh 10–12 g each, but some may be over 30 g. The glands are usually darker in color, almost like the zona reticularis. Histologically, the cortex is markedly thickened with hyperplasia of relatively compact cells (Fig. 3.25a, b). In cholesterol desmolase deficiency, the adrenals are reportedly nodular in appearance with abundant lipid. Deficiency of 18-hydroxylase and 18-dehydrogenase also occurs, but there is no adrenal hyperplasia because synthesis of cortisol and sex steroids is unaffected.

Endocrinopathies Due to Adrenal Cortical Hyperfunction

Cushing's Syndrome

This is a well-known clinical entity characterized by centripetal obesity with "moon facies" and "buffalo hump," hypertension, hirsutism, muscle weakness, cutaneous striae with easy bruisability, poor wound healing, osteoporosis, and glucose intolerance. In adults, it occurs in four distinct clinical settings with varied pathogenesis: (1) about 60%–70% of cases are due to adrenal cortical hyperplasia; (2) approximately 20%–25% are "adrenal Cushing's syndrome" due to an adrenal cortical tumor, i.e., adenoma or less commonly carcinoma; (3) 10%–15% are secondary to ectopic production of ACTH or some related hormone with biologic activity; and (4) iatrogenic Cushing's syndrome due to long-term use of exogenous glucocorticoids or ACTH [16]. In very early childhood, Cushing's syndrome is usually attributable to an adrenal cortical tumor [15].

Pituitary Cushing's Syndrome. Most patients with Cushing's syndrome due to adrenal cortical hyperplasia have a pituitary abnormality ("pituitary Cushing's syndrome"), either an adenoma composed of ACTH-secreting cells or a microadenoma

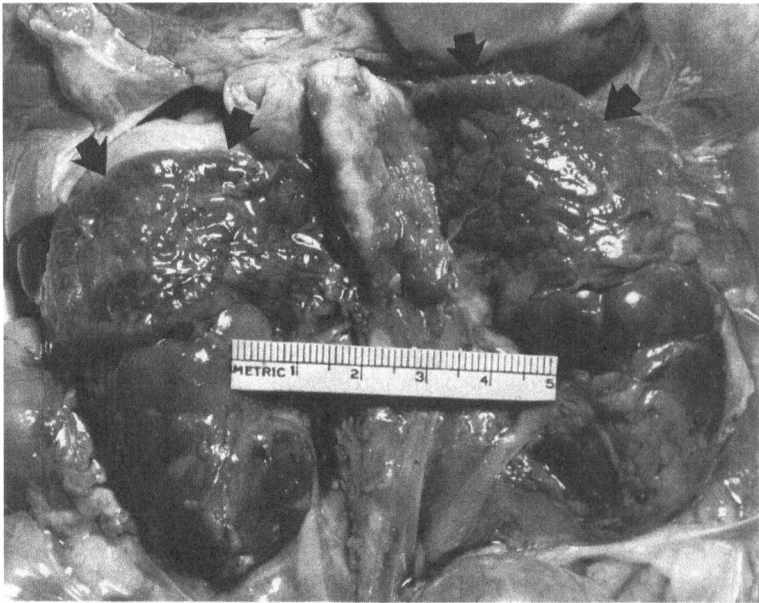

Fig. 3.24. Six-week-old female with congenital adrenal hyperplasia. Superior poles of both kidneys are capped by enlarged adrenals (*arrows*) with exaggerated cortical convolutions. The combined weight of both glands was 16 g. The child had clitoromegaly and ambiguous genitalia and probable salt-losing tendency.

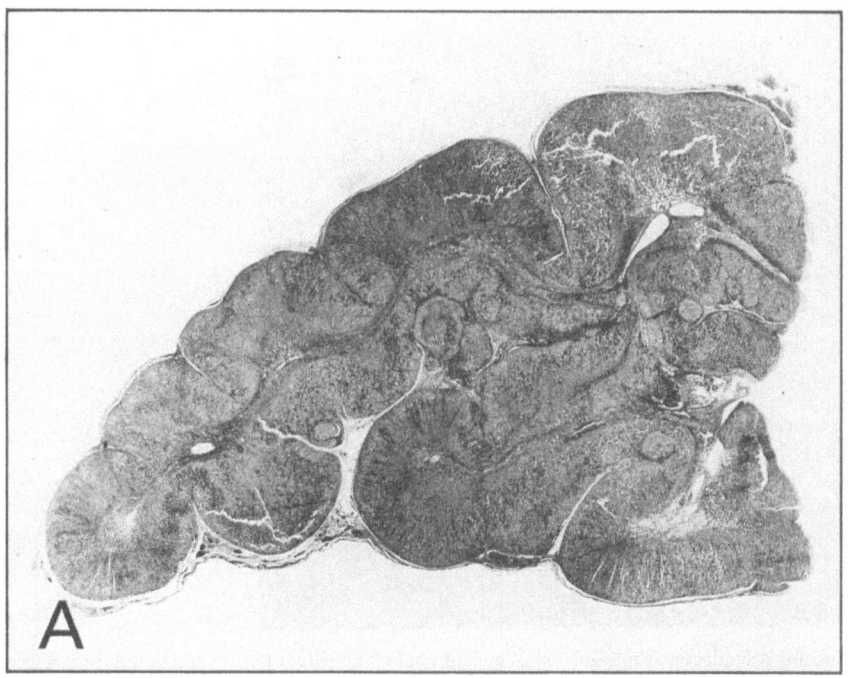

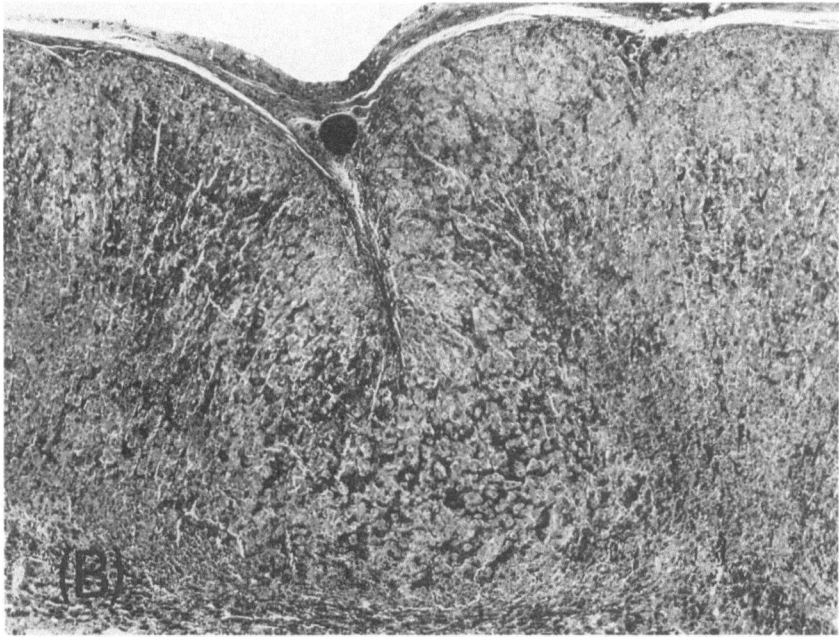

Fig. 3.25. a Cross-section of adrenal gland showing cerebriform convolutions of cortex. There is marked hyperplasia with diffuse widening of cortex. H & E, × 6.5. **b** Cortex is markedly thick and irregular with proliferation of compact cells resembling those of the zona reticularis. Mallory alinine blue, × 40

which is discovered histologically. When there is an underlying pituitary tumor, the condition is often referred to as Cushing's disease. A minority of patients have no detectable pituitary tumor, and some have attributed Cushing's syndrome in this situation to an abnormal "set point" at the level of the hypothalamus. This has led to the concept of "hypothalamic Cushing's syndrome," but pituitary microadenomas or foci of corticotroph hyperplasia have usually not been excluded in a rigorous fashion. In pituitary Cushing's syndrome, there is usually a measurable increase in plasma ACTH and the hypercortisolism can almost always be suppressed by large doses of glucocorticoids such

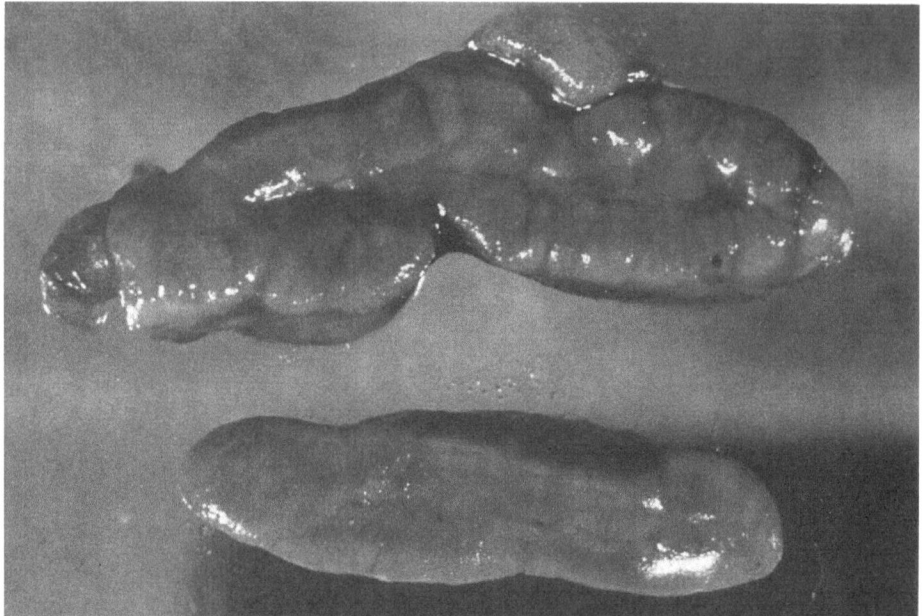

Fig. 3.26. Eight-year-old child with Cushing's syndrome. Cross-section of one adrenal gland shows diffuse and nodular thickening of cortex. Gland weighed 3.5 g.

as dexamethasone. Occasionally, ACTH is not elevated, and this raises the possibility that adrenal cortical cells might have an unusual sensitivity even to normal levels of tropic hormone. Occasionally, patients who undergo bilateral adrenalectomy develop intense skin pigmentation and are found to have a pituitary tumor (Nelson's syndrome) [31].

Adrenal Cortical Hyperplasia. The adrenal glands from patients with "pituitary" or "hypothalamic" Cushing's syndrome show bilateral enlargement due to cortical hyperplasia (Fig. 3.26). Each gland shows only modest enlargement in contrast to that seen in the adrenogenital syndrome. According to Neville and Symington [32], only 12% of patients had individual adrenal weights greater than 12 g. In 78%, the individual weight was less than 10 g and in 53% it was less than 8 g [32]. In the diffusely hyperplastic gland the cortex is thicker than normal (i.e., >2 mm). In nodular hyperplasia there are one or more intracortical nodules of hyperplastic cells measuring up to several centimeters in diameter, and they are almost invariably bilateral. It is sometimes difficult or impossible to distinguish a hyperplastic nodule from an adenoma. Occasionally, the adrenal glands may have a "normal" appearance, but stringent criteria must be used since only very occasionally does the individual gland weigh over 6 g.

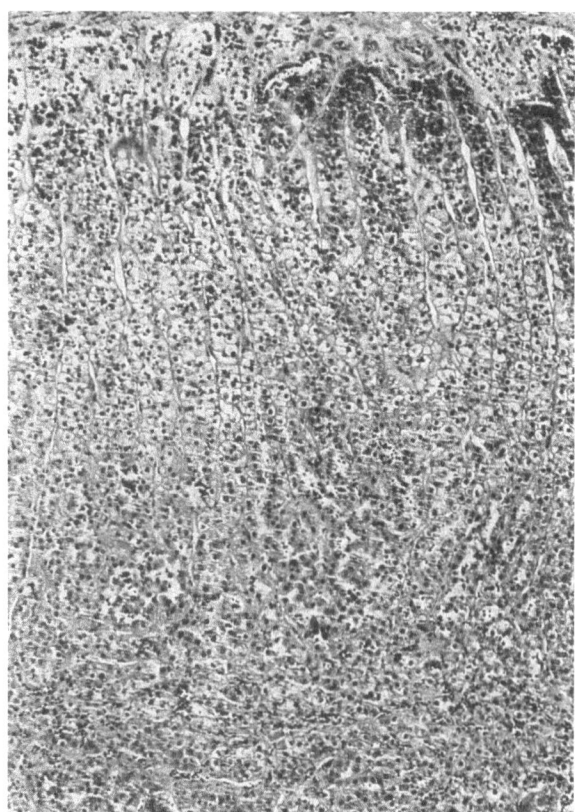

Fig. 3.27. The zona fasciculata is hyperplastic with both clear lipid-rich cells and compact cells. The zona glomerulosa appears as a small indistinct layer at *top of field.* H & E, × 50

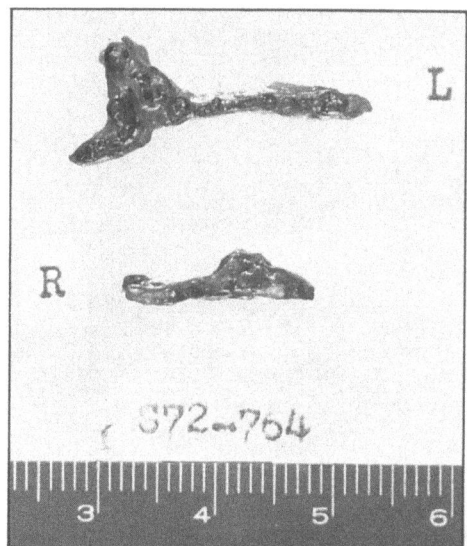

Fig. 3.28. Twenty-three-year-old female with Cushing's syndrome. Both adrenals contained multiple intracortical nodules which were dark-brown to black. The left adrenal weighed 3.1 g and the right 0.9 g.

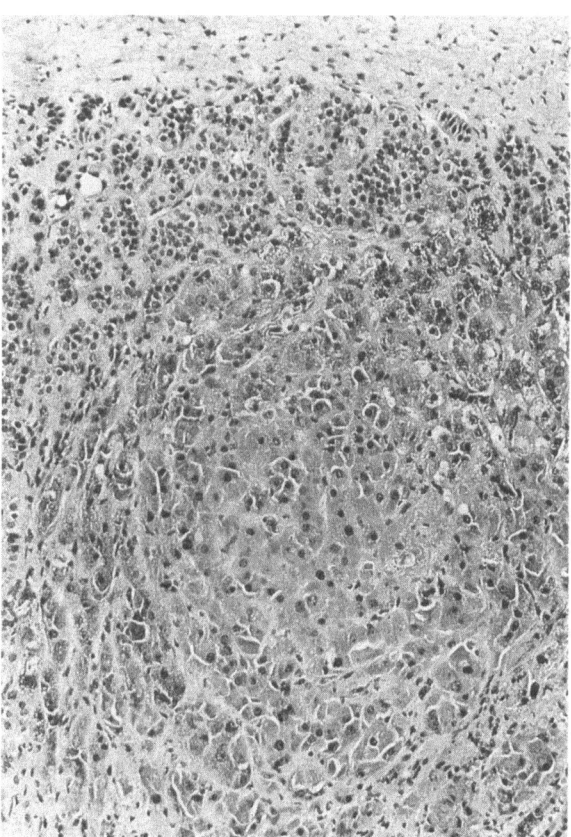

Fig. 3.29. Intracortical nodule is small, expansile, and composed of relatively large compact cells with coarse cytoplasmic pigment resembling lipofuscin. H & E, × 120

Microscopically, the hyperplastic cortex is composed of a compact cell layer occupying the inner third of the cortex and an outer lipid-rich zona fasciculata (Fig. 3.27). Myelolipomatous change can occur within nodular or diffuse areas of hyperplasia. Occasionally, the cortical hyperplasia is ACTH independent and primary in one or both adrenals. A peculiar form is referred to as pigmented nodular adrenocortical disease [41] (Fig. 3.28). The adrenal weights may be less than normal, normal, or slightly increased. Grossly, there are numerous dark-brown to almost jet-black cortical nodules usually measuring 1–3 mm in diameter. The nodules are composed of compact cells with granular brown pigment representing lipofuscin (Fig. 3.29). Some nodules may show myelolipomatous metaplasia. An identical condition has been reported in childhood as primary adrenocortical nodular dysplasia [27].

Ectopic Cushing's Syndrome. This paraneoplastic syndrome is usually secondary to a bronchogenic carcinoma, especially small ("oat") cell carcinoma. The circulating plasma levels of ACTH tend to be very high, probably because of unregulated production by tumor and increased amounts of biologically inert forms of the hormone which are measured in radioimmunoassay procedures. Although plasma ACTH levels tend to be higher in "ectopic" compared with "pituitary" Cushing's syndrome, the distinction between the two usually requires additional investigation [16]. "Adrenal Cushing's syndrome" is associated with low ACTH values. The hyperplasia in patients with ectopic ACTH production is often nodular, and the glands tend to be larger than those of "pituitary Cushing's syndrome."

Primary Aldosteronism (Conn's Syndrome). This syndrome was first described in 1955 in patients with an adrenal cortical adenoma who had hypertension, renal potassium loss with hypokalemic alkalosis, and muscle weakness [31]. A hallmark of the syndrome is an elevation of plasma aldosterone and a decrease in plasma renin levels. The latter serves to distinguish primary from secondary hyperaldosteronism. There is retention of sodium and expansion of the extracellular fluid volume, but, paradoxically, there is no overt edema. Since the initial description, the scope of the syndrome has grown in complexity [49].

The most common pathologic lesion of the adrenals is an adenoma followed by nodular or diffuse hyperplasia of the zona glomerulosa and, rarely, an adrenal cortical carcinoma. In the series reported by Weinberger et al., 77% of cases were caused by adenomas, 22% were attributed to hyperplasia, and there was only one example of carcinoma. The adrenal adenoma or "aldosteronoma" usually affects individuals in the fourth and fifth decades of life and has a predilection for female patients. Some of the cases reported as multiple adenomas may well be examples of nodular hyperplasia. In cases due to cortical hyperplasia, the process may be unilateral or bilateral, and correct preoperative localization is important in patient management. Resection of an adenoma appears to offer the highest rate of cure.

Adrenal Virilization and Feminization

Adrenal virilization in older children and adults is more likely to be caused by an adrenal cortical tumor than by adrenal hyperplasia. As with adrenal feminization, adrenal virilization may be part of a mixed endocrinopathy in conjunction with Cushing's syndrome, and in this setting the underlying adrenal tumor is most likely malignant. The presence of hirsutism alone should not be used as a criterion of virilization since it may be seen with Cushing's syndrome. Adrenal feminization is less common than virilization and, when part of a mixed endocrinopathy, is again suggestive of an underlying malignancy.

Adrenal Cortical Neoplasms

Adrenal Cortical Adenoma

Adenomas resected at surgery are usually small neoplasms which are hormonally active. The affected patient usually has a pure endocrinopathy such as Cushing's syndrome (vide supra). Distinguishing between a cortical adenoma and a hyperplastic cortical nodule can be very difficult. Examination of the remaining gland may provide helpful clues. In cases of Cushing's syndrome caused by an adenoma, the uninvolved cortex may be atrophic due to suppression of ACTH. Hyperplastic cortical nodules are often multiple or bilateral and the intervening cortex may be thicker than normal. In "adrenal Cushing's syndrome" plasma ACTH levels

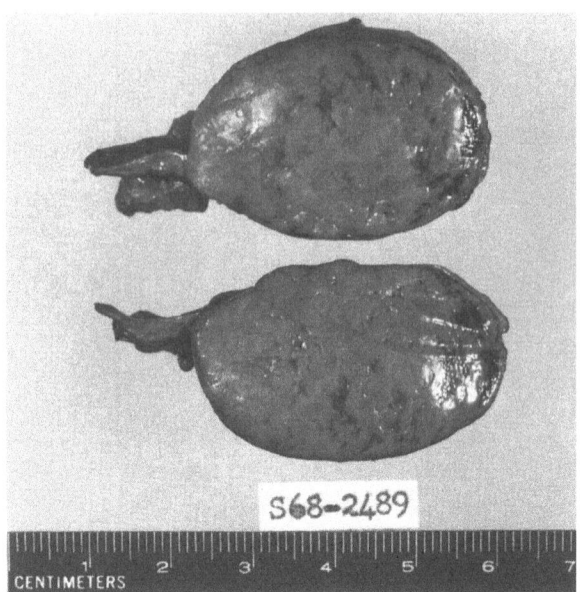

Fig. 3.30. Twenty-two-year-old female with Cushing's syndrome due to an adrenal cortical adenoma which measured 4 cm in diameter. Entire specimen weighed 22 g. Remaining adrenal cortical tissue is atrophic.

are low and the serum cortisol fails to be suppressed by large doses of glucocorticoids such as dexamethasone.

Gross Pathology. Adenomas are typically solitary, well-circumscribed tumors weighing less than 50 g. They are expansile growths with compression of adjacent tissue, but they are seldom if ever truly encapsulated. On cross-section they are yellow with a lobulated bulging surface (Fig. 3.30). The color may vary from tan to brown. Occasionally, there may be hemorrhage or areas of cystic degeneration. In general, when a cortical tumor is small (i.e., < 50 g) and the associated endocrinopathy is pure Cushing's syndrome, the neoplasm is almost always benign. An occasional adenoma, however, may be quite large (e.g., > 100 g) and extremely difficult to differentiate from a cortical carcinoma. Evaluation of other gross features (e.g., local invasion or necrosis) along with careful histologic study is essential in trying to make the distinction.

Adrenal cortical adenomas causing primary aldosteronism (so-called "aldosteronomas") are usually small neoplasms measuring less than 4 cm in diameter and on cross-section tend to have a "canary yellow" to orange color due to high lipid content (Fig. 3.31). The left adrenal gland seems to be affected more often than the right [49]. Rarely, an adrenal adenoma is darkly pigmented and is re-

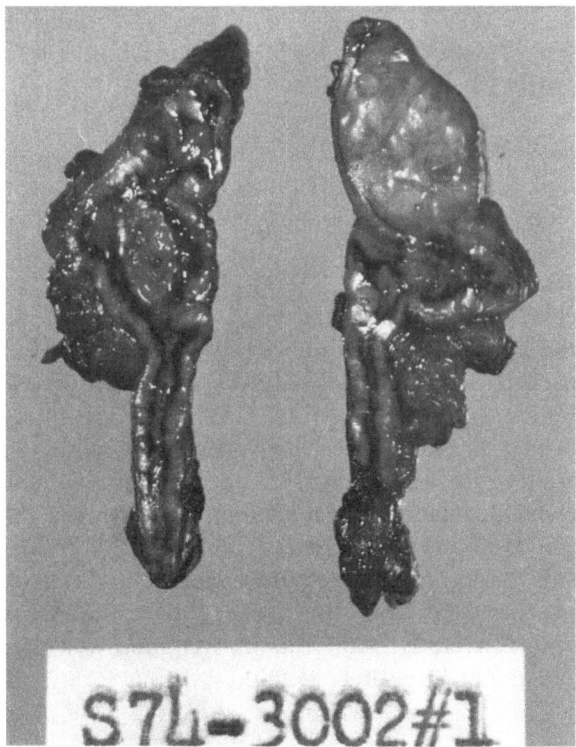

Fig. 3.31. Forty-six-year-old male with primary aldosteronism (Conn's syndrome) due to an adrenal cortical adenoma measuring about 1 cm in diameter. The entire gland weighed 8 g.

ferred to as a pigmented ("black") adenoma. They are usually small (e.g., 2–4 cm) and nonfunctional, but rare examples have been reported in association with Cushing's syndrome or primary aldosteronism.

Microscopic Pathology. Most adrenal cortical adenomas have a compressed rim of cortical tissue but usually lack a well-defined capsule (Fig. 3.32). Adenomas associated with Cushing's syndrome usually contain two cell types—clear, vacuolated lipid-rich cells resembling zona fasciculata and more compact cells like those of the zona reticularis. Enlarged hyperchromatic nuclei may be present but this feature alone is not indicative of malignancy. There may even be a few multinucleated giant cells. Aldosterone-secreting tumors ("aldosteronomas") are also tumors which lack complete encapsulation. Microscopically, they may contain clear cells arranged in small nests or cords with delicate strands of connective tissue (Fig. 3.32). Not uncommonly, there is an admixture of clear and compact cells along with cells intermediate between the two. Ultrastructural study may confirm this mixture of cells, some of which resemble cells of the zona glomerulosa, while others are more characteristic of

zona fasciculata (Fig. 3.33). It should be emphasized, however, that there is a rather poor correlation between the histology of the tumor and the type of steroids elaborated.

Adrenal Cortical Carcinoma

Adrenal cortical carcinoma is a relatively rare malignancy. Based on data compiled in the Third National Cancer Survey, these tumors accounted for only 0.023% of all cancers [24]. The tumor affects patients of all ages and shows a slight predilection for females (3:2) [19, 24]. Symptoms are usually related to the presence of an intraabdominal mass or the effects of excess steroid production. Occasional patients present acutely with abdominal pain and shock because of tumor rupture with retroperitoneal hemorrhage. In a study of "nonhormonal" adrenal cortical tumors (mostly carcinomas), Lewinsky et al. [25] concluded that the

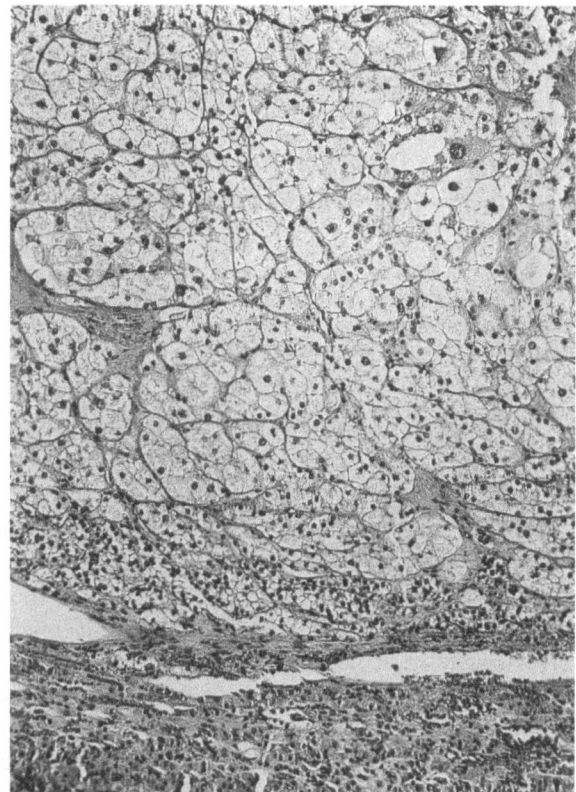

Fig. 3.32. Adrenal cortical adenoma shows expansile growth with compression of adjacent cortex at top. Tumor cells have a vague nesting pattern and have clear lipid-rich cytoplasm. There are occasional enlarged nuclei. Patient had primary aldosteronism (Conn's syndrome). H & E, × 210

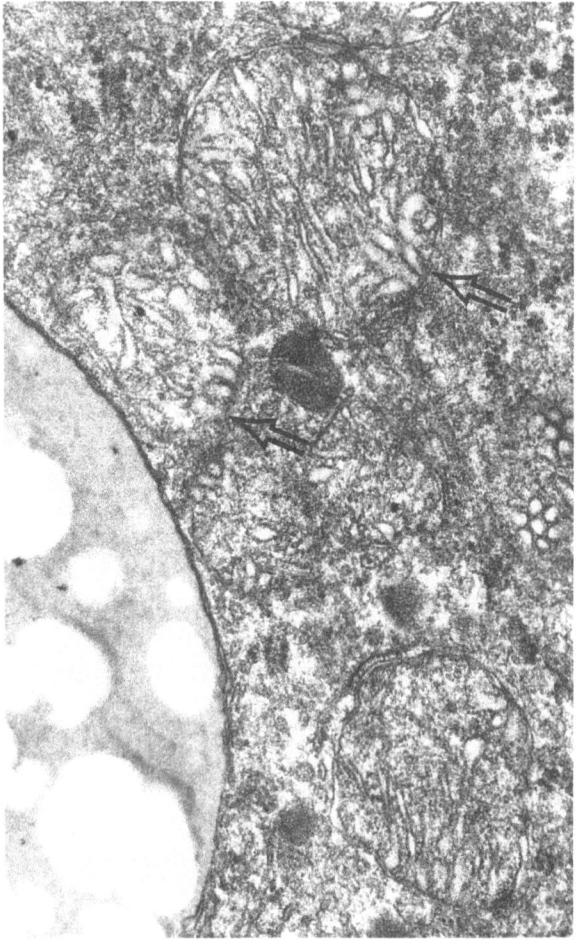

Fig. 3.33. Electron micrograph of an "aldosteronoma" with some cells having mitochondria with tubulovesicular cristae (*arrows*). Other cells contained mitochondria with lamellar cristae, which is more characteristic of the zona glomerulosa. Large membrane-bound lipid droplet is present *in lower left*. There was also abundant smooth endoplasmic reticulum which is typical for steroid-secreting cells. × 30 000

tumor may live considerably longer. Predilected sites of metastasis include lungs, liver, lymph nodes, retroperitoneum, and bone.

Gross Pathology. Cortical carcinomas tend to be bulky tumors, often weighing 1000–4000 g. In a recent review, the average tumor weight was 849 g (range, 33–3100 g) and the average size was 12.4 cm (range, 5–28.5 cm). Tumors which were clinically nonfunctional were slightly larger than the hormonally active ones [24]. On cross-section carcinomas frequently have areas of friable hemorrhage and necrosis (Fig. 3.34). They may display locally aggressive growth with invasion of adjacent organs or extension into the inferior vena cava. In determining malignancy, the size of the tumor alone is very important [47], but it is not the sole discriminating feature. Small cortical neoplasms (e.g., ≤ 50 g) may prove to be malignant and, conversely, some tumors weighing well over 100 g may be entirely benign.

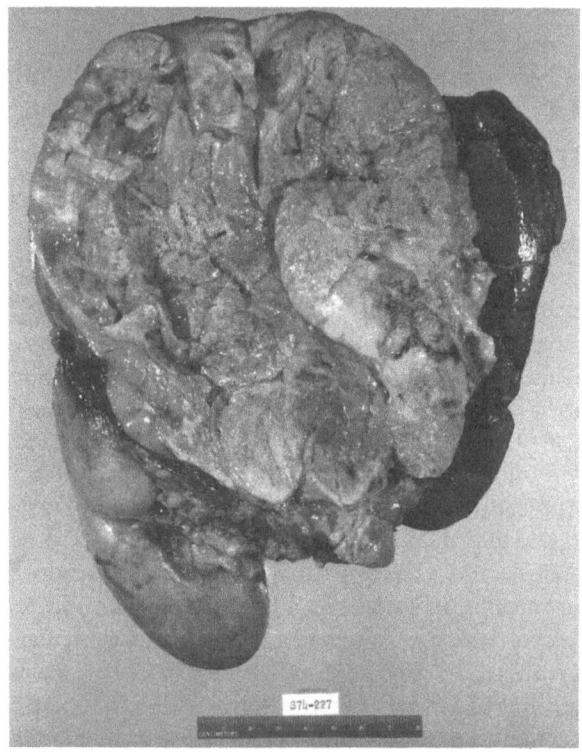

Fig. 3.34. Spleen, kidney, and left adrenal cortical carcinoma resected from a 27-year-old woman with virilization. Tumor was adherent to spleen and kidney and had metastasized to the liver. On cross-section the tumor varied from bright-yellow to dark-red and had extensive areas of necrosis.

tumors were capable of elaborating precursor steroids without hormonal activity and hence were not in fact "nonfunctioning."

In vivo stimulation with ACTH reveals that approximately one-half of all adenomas and only a small minority of carcinomas respond [34]. Detection of significant elevations of 11-deoxysteroids relative to 11β-hydroxysteroids may be useful in distinguishing the majority of functionally active cortical carcinomas in vivo [34]. Most carcinomas prove to be aggressive tumors, with the mortality ranging from 70% to 85% [19,24]. Tumor-related deaths usually occur within 2 years of diagnosis, but some patients with recurrent or metastatic

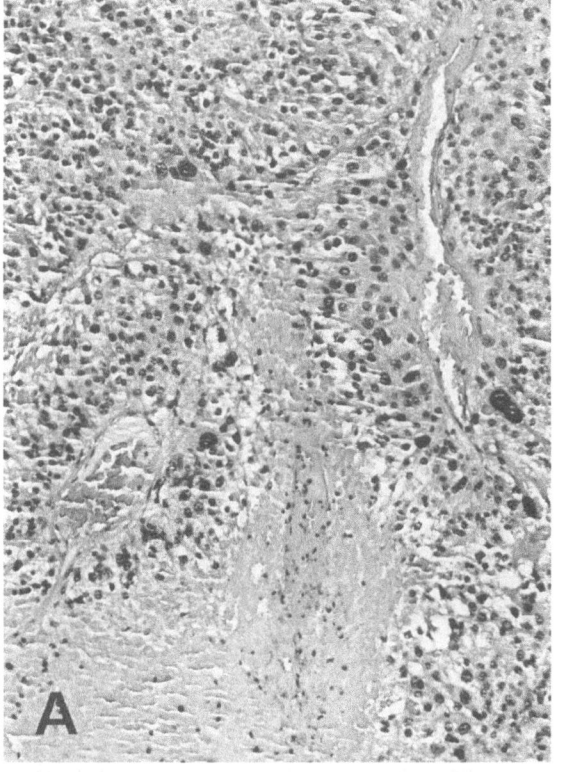

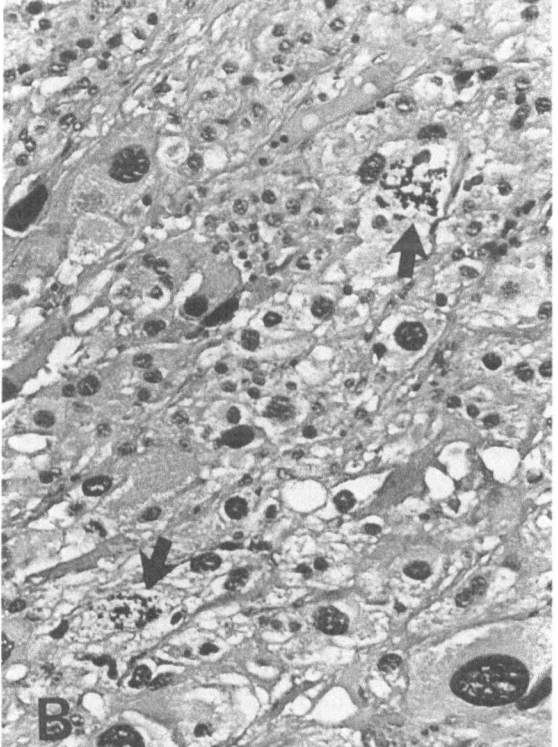

Fig. 3.35. a Adrenal cortical carcinoma with acute tumor necrosis and cells with mildly pleomorphic nuclei. Vascular invasion was seen in other areas. H & E, × 130. **b** More solid growth pattern with pleomorphic nuclei and several atypical mitotic figures (*arrows*). H & E, × 200

Microscopic Pathology. Adrenal cortical carcinomas often display features of frank malignancy such as geographic tumor necrosis, vascular invasion, and conspicuous mitotic figures with some atypical forms (Fig. 3.35a, b). A trabecular growth pattern is frequently seen in cortical carcinoma with broad anastomosing columns of tumor cells separated by delicate sinusoidal spaces (Fig. 3.36). A solid or diffuse pattern may also occur. Paradoxically, some tumors have little in the way of cellular pleomorphism, while in others it is a conspicuous feature. Again, nuclear pleomorphism per se is not a reliable criterion for malignancy. Occasionally, an adrenal cortical carcinoma may be difficult to distinguish from a pheochromocytoma. Characteristic features of cortical tumors include a yellow or orange color on cross-section, the presence of intracytoplasmic lipid, a negative chromaffin reaction, and absence of dense-core neurosecretory granules on ultrastructural study.

Criteria for Malignancy. With regard to criteria for malignancy, Hough et al. [17] evaluated 12 histologic and nonhistologic parameters and found that the most significant features were weight loss, diffuse growth pattern, vascular invasion, tumor necrosis, and tumor mass. Different conclusions were reached in a more recent study by others where tumor weight and mitotic activity were found to be the most useful single discriminators of malignancy. Calculation of a histologic index was found to be more predictive [43]. In summary, there is still a lack of uniform consensus regarding pathologic criteria for malignancy in adults and children [7,48].

Adrenal Medulla

Microscopic Anatomy

Cells of the adrenal medulla are derived embryologically from the neural crest and are part of a more widely dispersed APUD (*A*mine *P*recursor *U*ptake and *D*ecarboxylation) cell system originally proposed by Pearse [35]. Primitive neuroblastic cells appear in the adrenals between the 7th and 12th weeks of intrauterine life. These cells develop into what in essence is a condensed portion of the sympathetic autonomic nervous system analogous to postganglionic neurons. The developmental

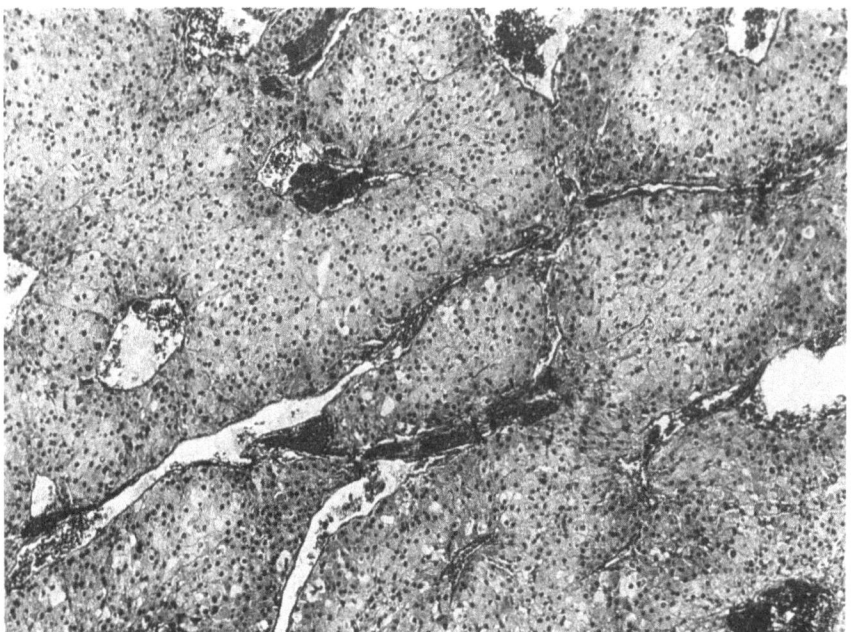

Fig. 3.36. Adrenal carcinoma with broad irregular trabeculae and angular sinusoidal spaces. Note relative uniformity of tumor cells. H & E, × 80

capacity of the primitive neuroblasts is shown in Fig. 3.37 along with the hypothetical tumors which can occur.

The term chromaffin has been applied to cells of the medulla because of the brown color produced by exposing fresh tissue to oxidants such as dichromate or iodate. This chromaffin reaction is due to oxidation of catecholamines. The chromaffin cells are concentrated in the head and body of the gland and are arranged in nests and twisted cell cords with a richly vascular stroma. The medulla constitutes about 10% of the adult adrenal gland [37]. A notable but normal feature in some adult glands is the presence of enlarged hyperchromatic nuclei. Round or oval hyaline globules can be seen in about 80% of patients over the age of 15 years, and in about 5% of cases they can be numerous [10]. In the normal gland from adults, 85% of catecholamine content is epinephrine and the remainder is norepinephrine. In the newborn adrenal gland, med-

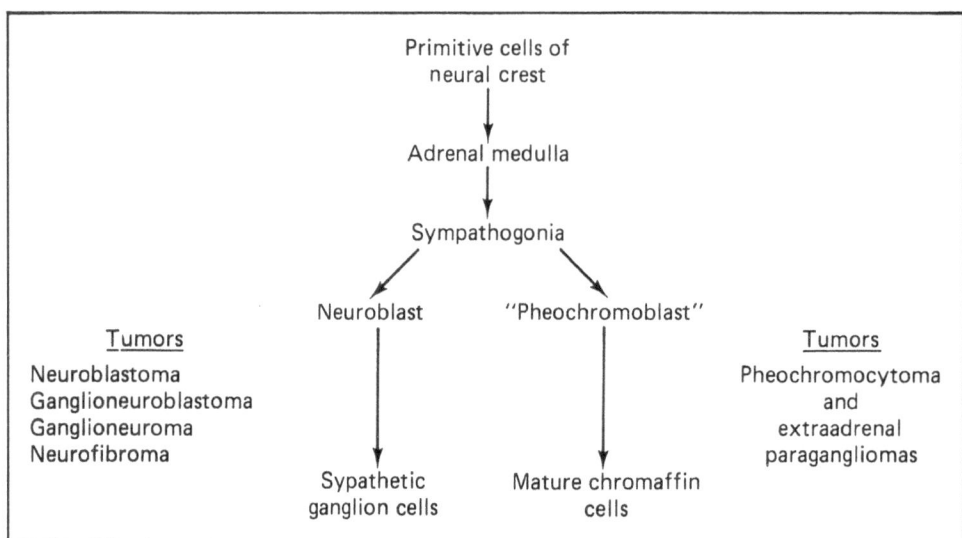

Fig. 3.37. Migration of primitive cells from neural crest and maturation pathways in adrenal medulla.

ullary issue is relatively inconspicuous, and one may occasionally see small nests of immature cells resembling neuroblasts.

Pathology

Adrenal Medullary Hyperplasia

Under normal conditions, medullary tissue is confined to the head and body of the gland with no appreciable extension into the tail or alae. Quantitation of medullary tissue has been difficult because it is entirely enveloped by cortex. Using planimetry on representative tissue sections, the ratio of surface area occupied by cortex relative to medulla is reported to be 10:1 with slightly higher values in the body and lower ones in the head. Some patients with multiple endocrine neoplasia type 2a (Sipple's syndrome) have a combination of nodular or diffuse hyperplasia of the adrenal medulla (Fig. 3.38), which is regarded by some as a precursor of unilateral or bilateral pheochromocytoma. The gland with medullary hyperplasia is heavier than normal and shows a decrease in the ratio of surface areas of cortex to medulla. Other features include some cellular enlargement, increased numbers of hyaline globules, occasional mitotic figures, and increased total catecholamine content [11].

Nodules of proliferating cells greater than 1 cm in diameter have been arbitrarily classified as pheochromocytoma [8]. Bilateral adrenal medullary hyperplasia may also be a clinicopathologic entity unto itself without being a precursor of pheochromocytoma. A number of patients have been reported in which symptoms mimicked those of a pheochromocytoma [39].

Pheochromocytoma (Adrenal Medullary Paraganglioma)

Pheochromocytoma is a distinctive tumor of the adrenal medulla with an estimated incidence rate of 0.8 per 100 000 population [3]. It has a peak frequency in the fourth and fifth decades, but it can affect individuals of all ages, including children. Probably fewer than 0.1% of hypertensive individuals harbor a pheochromocytoma. The term pheochromocytoma has been used in a restrictive sense for tumors arising from the adrenal medulla, but paragangliomas with identical histology may arise in a number of extraadrenal sites in close relation with the sympathetic nervous system. It has been reported that, for every pheochromocytoma diagnosed during life, two will be discovered incidentally at autopsy and that 75% of these tumors are clinically unsuspected [45]. Pheo-

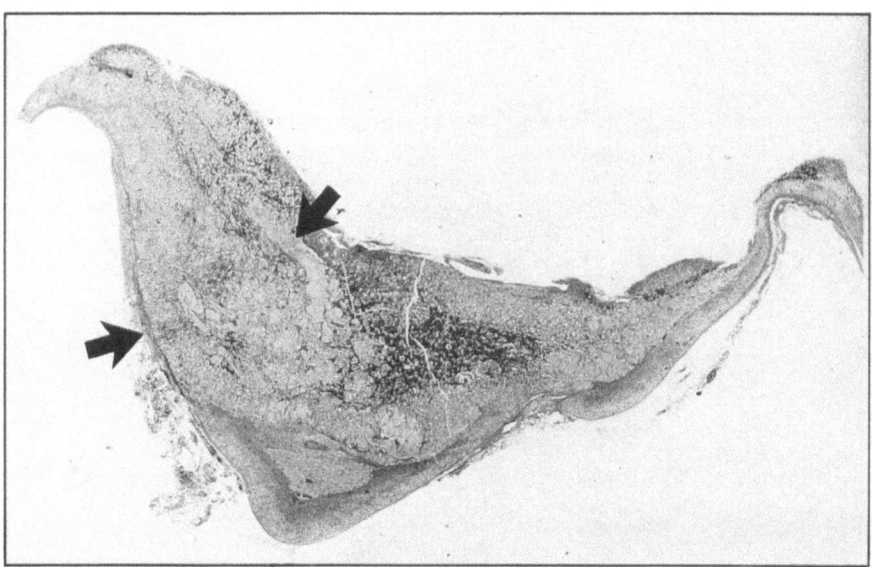

Fig. 3.38. Cross-section of adrenal gland from a patient with multiple endocrine neoplasia type 2a. Medulla is hyperplastic with nodular areas. Dominant nodule *between arrows* probably represents an early pheochromocytoma. H & E, × 6.5

chromocytoma has been referred to as the "10% tumor"—10% being bilateral, 10% occurring in extraadrenal sites, and 10% being malignant. In sporadic cases the incidence of malignant behavior is probably less than 10%. In one series, only 2.4% of intraadrenal pheochromocytomas were malignant, while the incidence of malignancy was much higher with extraadrenal tumors (30%) [28].

It has been estimated that 20% of all pheochromocytomas occur in the pediatric population. In the literature, the great majority of pheochromocytomas (70%–80%) in children have arisen in the adrenal medulla. In approximately one-third of the cases, the tumors are multiple or bilateral. The incidence of malignant behavior appears to be less than that reported in adults [22].

Pheochromocytomas can be remarkably protean in their clinical manifestations. The tumors have the capacity to elaborate and secrete catecholamines in large amounts and produce a variety of symptoms, some of which can be rather alarming. The paroxysm or crisis is a classic symptom complex and includes headache, diaphoresis, palpitations, and tachycardia. The presence of these symptoms in a patient with sustained or paroxysmal hypertension is highly suggestive of a pheochromocytoma; however, a significant number of patients lack these features. A small percentage of tumors cause no symptoms, either because they are nonfunctional or secrete only small amounts of catecholamines. Most pheochromocytomas produce mainly norepinephrine. The rare ones producing only epi-

nephrine are almost all localized in the adrenal. There are a number of diagnostic laboratory tests available. Measurement of plasma catecholamines seems to be as reliable as quantitation of urinary metanephrines in predicting the presence of a pheochromocytoma, particularly when done under rigid standardized conditions [6]. Pheochromocytomas have rarely caused Cushing's syndrome due to ectopic production of ACTH [44]. Other peptides have been identified in pheochromocytomas including leu-enkephalin, met-enkephalin, and substance P [26].

There is an increased incidence of pheochromocytomas in individuals with familial disorders such as von Recklinghausen's disease, von Hippel-Lindau disease, and multiple endocrine neoplasia (MEN) type 2. The latter has an autosomal dominant mode of inheritance and has been separated into two types—MEN type 2a (Sipple's syndrome) and MEN type 2b. MEN type 2a consists of medullary carcinoma of the thyroid, pheochromocytoma, and parathyroid hyperplasia. The pheochromocytomas in this setting are multiple or bilateral in about 50% of cases. In MEN type 2b, there is also medullary carcinoma of the thyroid and pheochromocytoma but usually no parathyroid abnormalities. In addition, there is diffuse ganglioneuromatosis of the gastrointestinal tract and multiple neuromas involving tongue, lips, eyelids, and conjunctivae. A marfanoid habitus may be present as well as other skeletal abnormalities. Pheochromocytomas are responsible for significant mor-

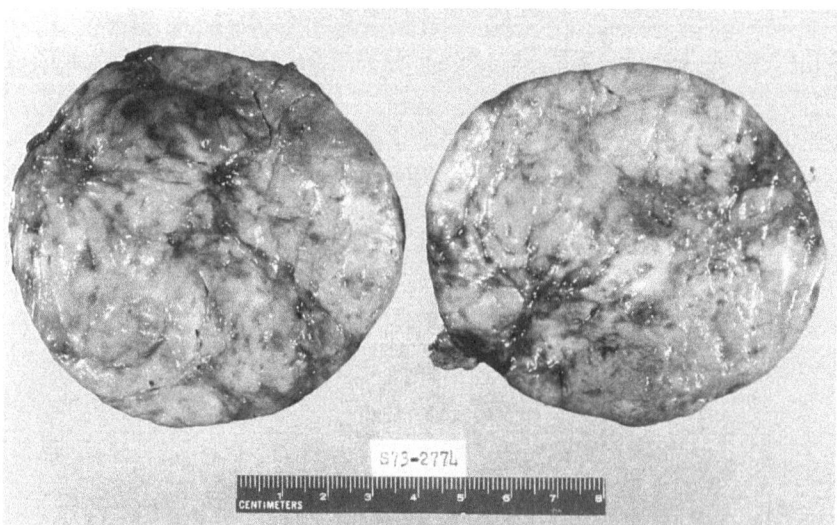

Fig. 3.39. Forty-one-year-old woman with a 9-cm pheochromocytoma weighing 160 g. Bisected tumor is gray to tan with irregular lobulations and speckled areas of hemorrhage.

tality in MEN type 2. In the Mayo Clinic experience, 29% of patients died as a result of the tumor [8]. Another noteworthy finding is that the adrenal pathology may be moderately advanced without producing any clinical or laboratory manifestations or hyperfunction [8]. Malignant pheochromocytomas, both familial and sporadic, metastasize most frequently to regional lymph nodes, liver, lungs, and bone.

Gross Pathology. Pheochromocytomas are variable in size with most weighing between 50 and 100 g; others are considerably larger, weighing well over 1000 g. Tumor size does not seem to correlate with biologic behavior. Tumors are well circumscribed, but when examined microscopically they often lack a complete well-defined capsule. On cross-section they may be pale gray to dark tan with a somewhat lobulated surface (Fig. 3.39). Some have a spongy vascular appearance. In most cases, an adrenal remnant is present either stretched over the surface of the tumor or attached to one pole. There may be areas of hemorrhage and necrosis, and cystic degeneration can be a prominent feature.

Microscopic Pathology. The histopathology of pheochromocytomas has been well described by Sherwin [42]. These tumors are richly vascular with anastomosing cell cords or discrete nests of cells (*Zellballen*) (Fig. 3.40a,b). Sometimes the vasculature is indistinct with tumor cells seemingly growing in a diffuse sheet-like manner. Cytoplasm is characteristically granular and varies from basophilic to acidophilic. There may be considerable nuclear enlargement and hyperchromasia, but this should not be interpreted as evidence of malignancy (Fig. 3.41). There may be intranuclear "pseudo-inclusions" due to herniation of cell cytoplasm. As in the normal adrenal medulla, hyaline globules can be found, and at times they are numerous (Fig. 3.42). In less than 5% of pheochromocytomas, one can identify a component resembling ganglioneuroblastoma or neuroblastoma. Too few of these composite tumors have been described to permit definitive comment with regard to prognostic significance.

Mitotic figures are uncommon but may be seen in both benign and malignant pheochromocytomas. Some tumors contain lakes of eosinophilic colloid material with peripheral scalloping. When fresh tumor is exposed to appropriate fixatives (e.g., Zen-

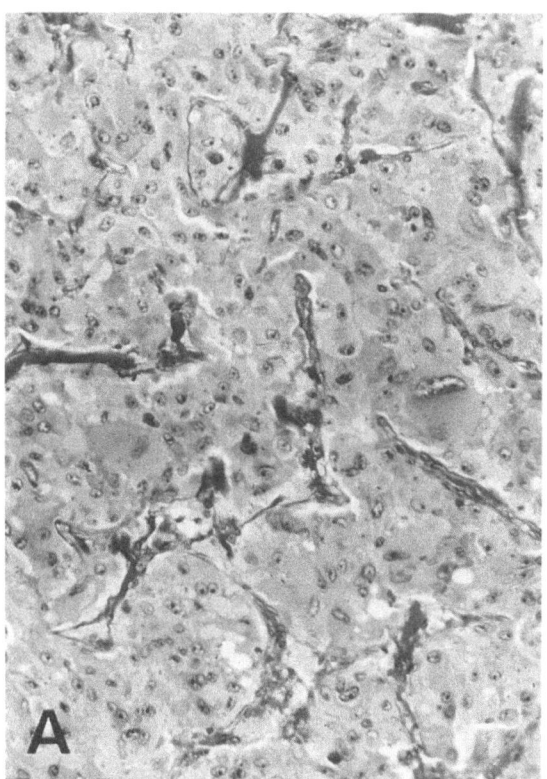

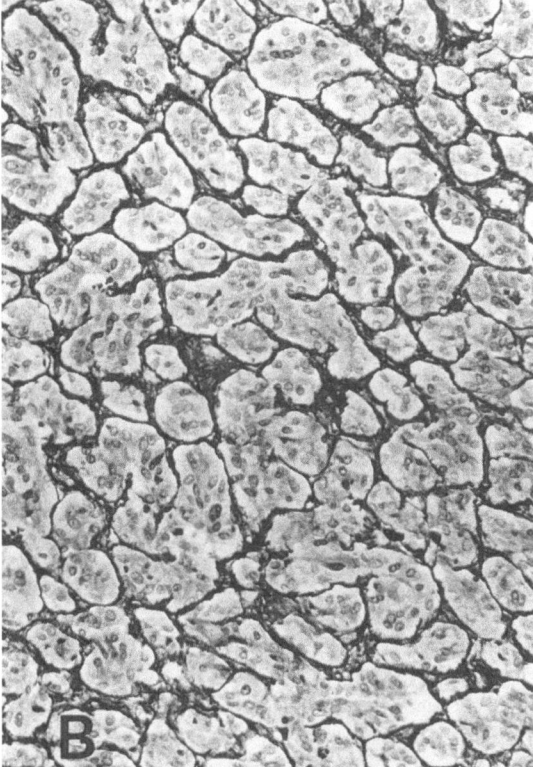

Fig. 3.40 a Anastomosing cords of cells with ample finely granular cytoplasm and moderate nuclear pleomorphism. Note delicate capillary channels. H & E, × 180. **b** Pheochromocytoma with more discrete nests of cells. Snook's reticulin stain, × 180

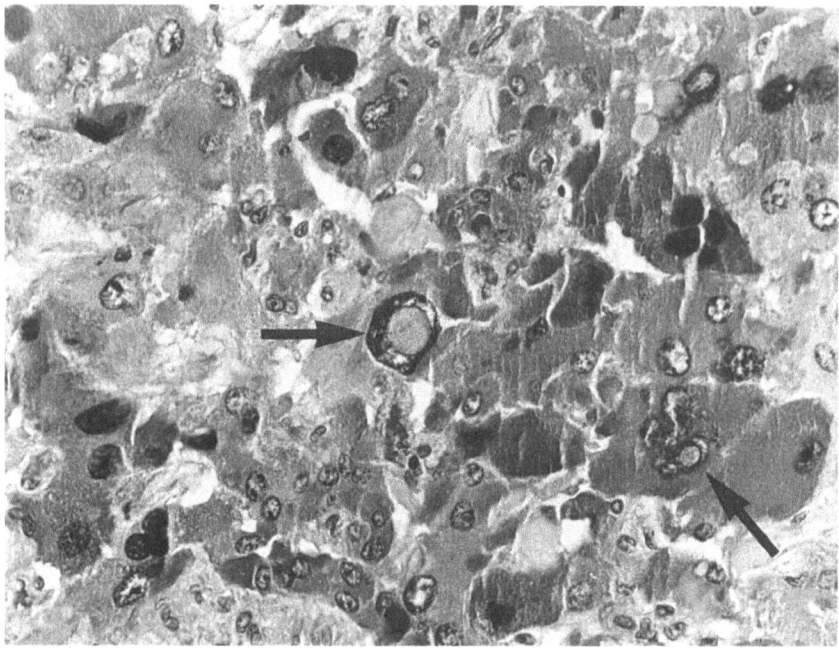

Fig. 3.41. Pheochromocytoma with nuclear pleomorphism and occasional "pseudoinclusions" (*arrows*). Tumor shows a positive chromaffin reaction with brown discoloration of cell cytoplasm. H & E, × 330

ker's or Orth's), a positive chromaffin reaction can be elicited. This is evidenced grossly by a dark-brown color and microscopically by yellow-brown discoloration of cell cytoplasm (Fig. 3.41). Another useful diagnostic technique is demonstration of pinpoint cytoplasmic granules using argyrophilic stains. Cells are characteristically argentaffin nega-tive. Ultrastructurally, the tumor cells contain dense-core granules which usually range from 100 to 300 nm in diameter (Fig. 3.43). The diagnosis of malignancy is extremely difficult in the absence of proven metastases. Features which are suggestive include numerous mitotic figures, multifocal tumor necrosis, and vascular invasion.

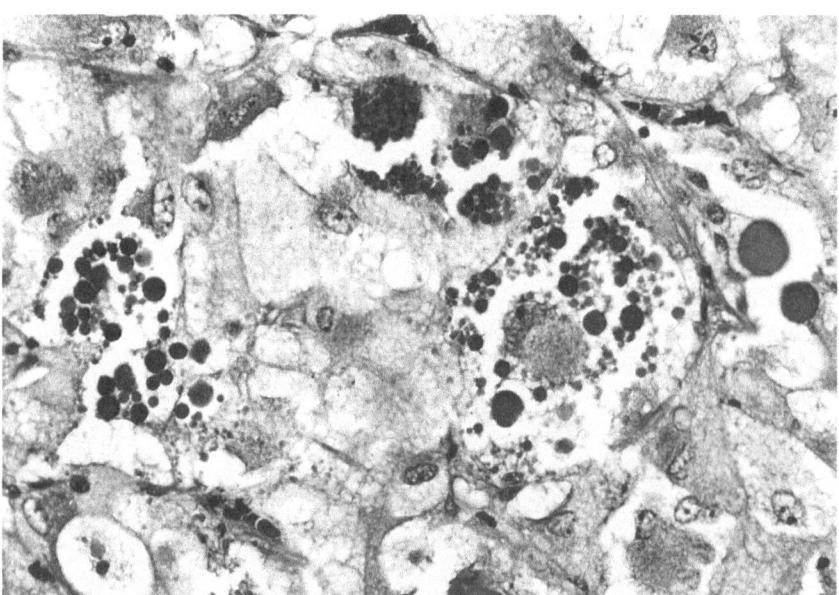

Fig. 3.42. Tumor cells contain numerous hyaline globules which are PAS positive and resistant to diastase digestion. Some globules appear to be extracellular. H & E, × 330

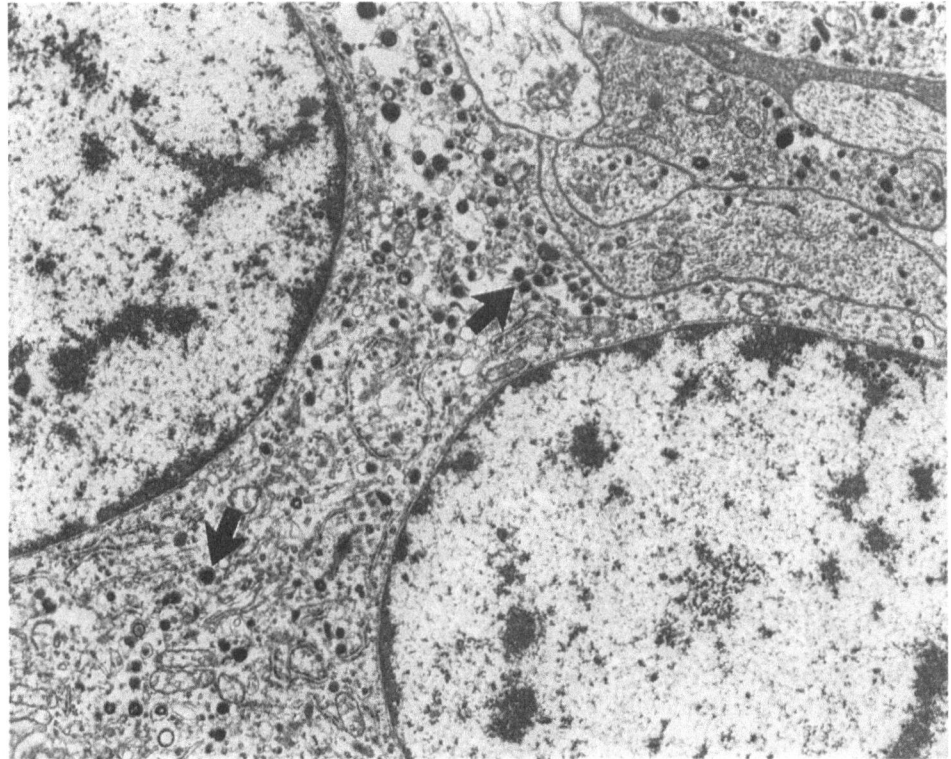

Fig. 3.43. Electron micrograph of a pheochromocytoma showing numerous dense-core neurosecretory granules (*arrows*) with surrounding halo and limiting membrane. There is rough endoplasmic reticulum and scattered mitochondria. × 17 280

Neuroblastoma and Ganglioneuroblastoma

Neuroblastoma is the most common extracranial solid tumor in childhood, ranking third among pediatric malignancies behind leukemia/lymphoma and central nervous system tumors. They usually arise in close relation to the sympathetic chain and adrenal glands. The anatomic distribution of neuroblastomas and ganglioneuroblastomas is shown in Table 3.1. Approximately two-thirds of the tumors arise in the upper abdomen, and of these more than half are adrenal in origin [38]. Fifty to sixty percent of children with neuroblastoma are under the age of 1 year at the time of diagnosis and about 10%–15% are older than 2 years. Those with ganglioneuroblastoma and ganglioneuroma tend to be older. There is no racial predilection and the sexes appear to be equally affected.

Clinically, an abdominal mass is the most common presenting complaint. There may be associated low-grade fever, anemia, and other nonspecific findings. A few children present with intractable diarrhea thought to be related to secretion of vasoactive intestinal polypeptide. There are several other characteristic presenting manifestations described for these tumors, including heterochromia iridis, Horner's syndrome, and opsopolymyoclonus. The latter is a peculiar disorder characterized by darting eye movements, generalized myoclonic jerks, truncal ataxia, and sometimes mental retardation.

The prognosis for children with neuroblastoma depends upon the age at diagnosis and extent of disease or stage. Age at diagnosis is reported to be a more important predictor of long-term disease-free survival than stage, with 93% survival for patients under the age of 1 year and 40% survival for those older than 1 year [38]. The most commonly used

Table 3.1. Distribution of primary sites of neuroblastoma and ganglioneuroblastoma. (Modified from [38])

Cervical	3.4%
Thoracic	20.3%
Adrenal	38.1%
Upper abdomen (nonadrenal)	26.3%
Abdomen (bilateral or multiple)	3.4%
Pelvic	3.4%
Unknown	5.1%
All sites	100%

Table 3.2. Staging of neuroblastoma. [12]

Stage I:	Tumor confined to the organ or structure of origin
Stage II:[a]	Tumors extending in continuity beyond the organ or structure of origin but not crossing the midline. Regional lymph nodes on the homolateral side may be involved
Stage III:	Tumors extending in continuity beyond the midline. Regional lymph nodes may be involved bilaterally
Stage IV:	Remote disease involving skeleton, organs, soft tissues, or distant lymph node groups, etc.
Stage IV-S:	Patients who would otherwise be stage I or II but who have remote disease confined only to one or more of the following sites: liver, skin, or bone marrow (without radiographic evidence of bone metastases on complete skeletal survey)

[a] For tumors arising in midline structures, e.g., the organs of Zuckerkandl, penetration beyond the capsule and involvement of lymph nodes on the same side shall be considered stage II. Bilateral extension of any sort should be considered stage III.

staging classification is that of Evans [12] (Table 3.2). Stage IV-S refers to a subset of children with disseminated disease who have small primaries and distant metastases limited to liver, skin, and/or bone marrow without radiologic evidence of bony metastases. The majority of patients are young infants with adrenal primaries, and over half of the tumors undergo spontaneous regression [13].

In Situ Neuroblastoma. In normal fetal development, nodular collections of neuroblasts are present in the adrenal glands from 7 weeks gestation and increase in size and number thereafter. At about 12 weeks gestation, differentiation into chromaffin cells begins [20]. Beckwith and Perrin [4] reported the incidental occurrence of minute adrenal lesions in autopsies of stillborns and infants up to 3 months of age which were considered identical to neuroblastoma. More than half of the cases of in situ neuroblastoma are less than 3 mm in size and about one-third measure less than 1 mm. The incidence of in situ neuroblastoma was reported to be 1 in 250 autopsies, which is 40 times that of clinically apparent neuroblastoma [4]. This may represent maturation delay in formation of the medulla or spontaneous regression of early neuroblastoma.

Gross Pathology. The tumors vary in size and appearance and may be large and bulky when first detected. While being well demarcated, they usually lack a true capsule. On cross-section neuroblastomas are usually soft and range in color from

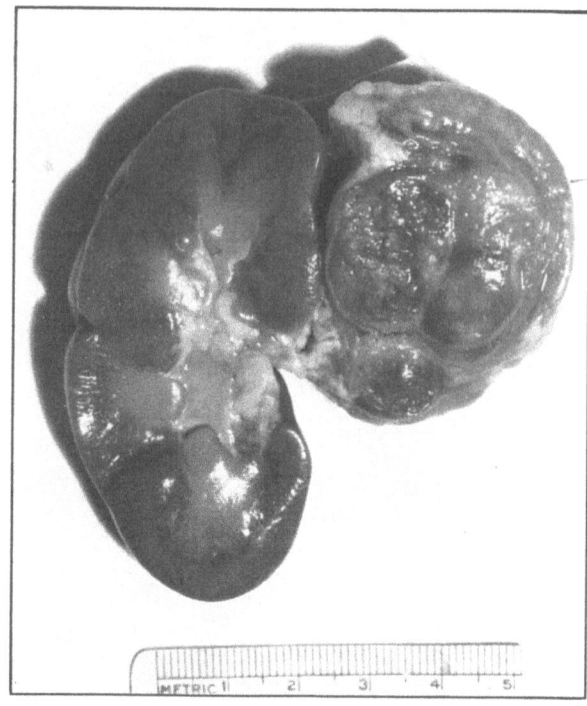

Fig. 3.44. Nine-month-old child with neuroblastoma of left adrenal gland. Tumor is well circumscribed but unencapsulated and has areas of hemorrhage and necrosis on cross-section. Remnant of adrenal gland can be seen on superior aspect of tumor.

light gray to purple; larger tumors may be distinctly lobulated with foci of necrosis which may become cystic (Fig. 3.44). Ganglioneuroblastoma, being a better differentiated tumor, is usually firm, yellow-tan, and more homogeneous on cross-section than neuroblastoma. Soft cellular nodules resembling neuroblastoma may be present (Fig. 3.45).

Microscopic Pathology. Primitive neuroblastoma is composed of nests and sheets of small cells with scant cytoplasm and rounded nuclei (Fig. 3.46). The tumor tends to be subdivided into lobules by delicate connective tissue septa. Maturation is manifest by increasing size of the nucleus, more abundant cytoplasm, and the presence of neurofibrillary processes. Homer-Wright rosettes can often be seen. Secondary changes such as hemorrhage, necrosis, and calcium deposition are common. Evidence of maturation toward ganglion cells is evident in about half of the cases. In rare cases, primary neuroblastoma or its metastases may undergo spontaneous maturation to benign ganglioneuroma. In ganglioneuroblastoma, the ganglioneuromatous portion of the tumor contains ganglion cells with large vesicular nuclei, distinct

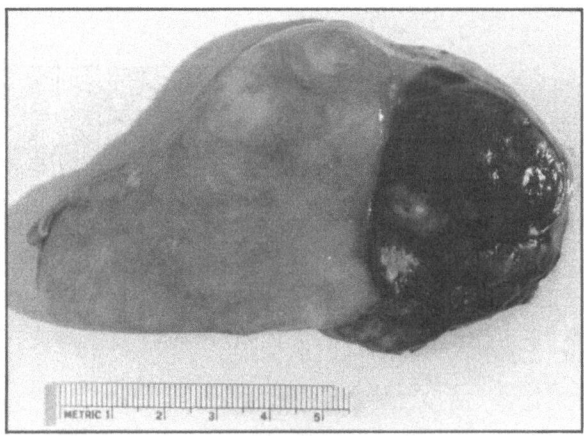

Fig. 3.45. Seven-year-old girl with composite ganglio-neuroblastoma of left adrenal gland. Primitive portion of tumor is sharply demarcated on right side and is dark because of hemorrhage and necrosis. Ganglioneuromatous component is firm and yellowish-white.

nucleoli, and abundant cytoplasm (Fig. 3.47). Ganglioneuroblastomas have been separated into diffuse and composite types (Fig. 3.45).

Ganglioneuroma

This benign tumor is much less common than neuroblastoma and ganglioneuroblastoma. It occurs primarily in older children and young adults and it is rare in early childhood. Only about 10%–15% of tumors arise in the adrenal gland. They are well circumscribed, firm, and rubbery, and on cross-section are gray-white to yellow without hemorrhage or necrosis. There may be small flecks of calcification. Microscopically, they manifest a high degree of differentiation with ganglion cells embedded in a stroma containing Schwann cells, fibroblasts, and neurites (Fig. 3.48). Adequate sampling of the tumor for histologic study is important in order to exclude less-differentiated foci. Neurofibroma has also been reported in the adrenal, but it is extremely rare and almost invariably an incidental finding.

Miscellaneous Tumor-Like Lesions of the Adrenals

Myelolipoma

This is a benign tumor-like lesion which is most often an incidental finding at autopsy. It usually measures less than 5 cm in diameter and is composed of mature adipose tissue and hematopoietic cells. It is probably not a true neoplasm but a type of

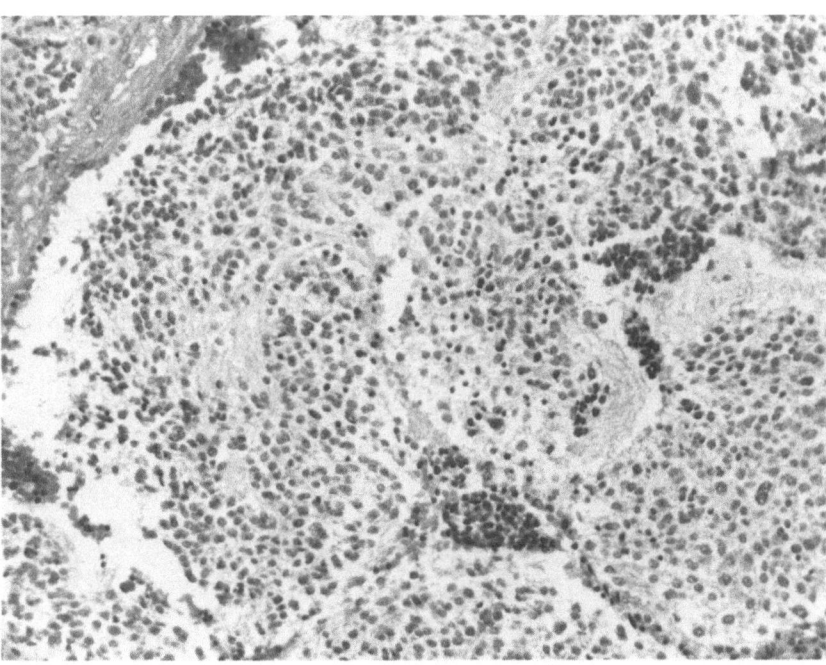

Fig. 3.46. Neuroblastoma with vague nesting pattern and delicate fibrillar material between cells resembling neuropil. In some areas there were Homer-Wright rosettes. H & E, × 180

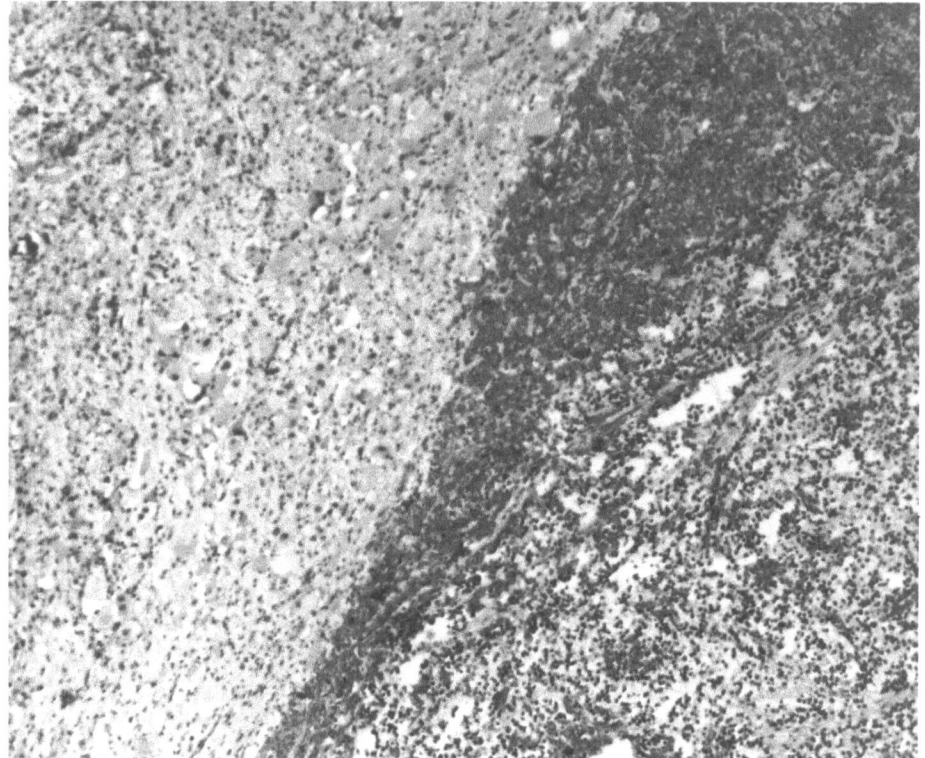

Fig. 3.47. Composite ganglioneuroblastoma with ganglioneuromatous component *on the left* and hemorrhagic neuroblastoma *on the right*. There is an abrupt transition between the two patterns. H & E, × 95

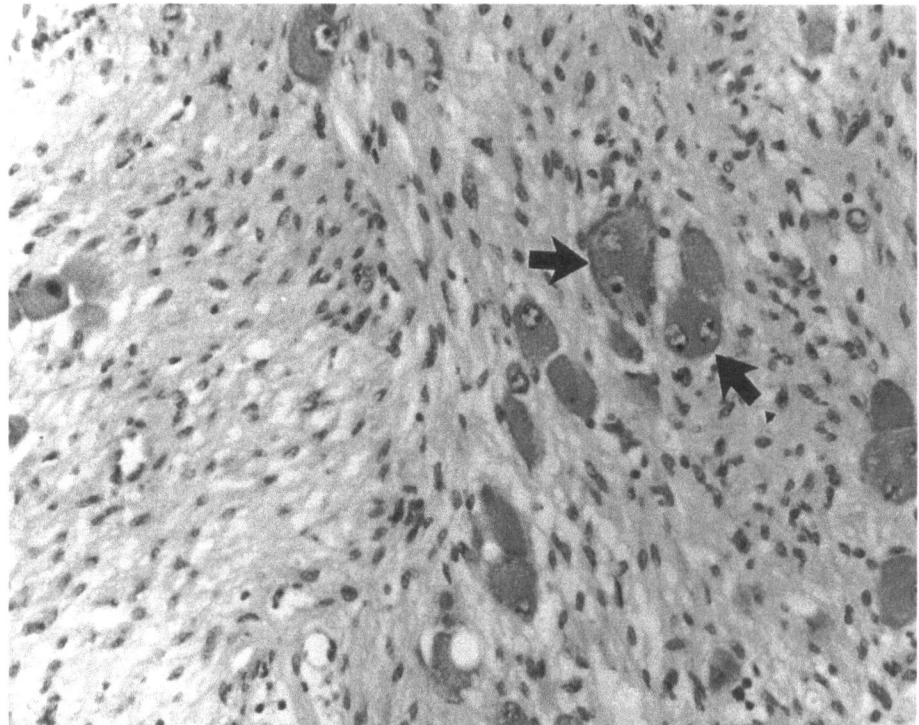

Fig 3.48. Ganglioneuroma with spindle-shaped cells and relatively mature ganglion cells, some of which are multinucleated (*arrows*). H & E, × 200

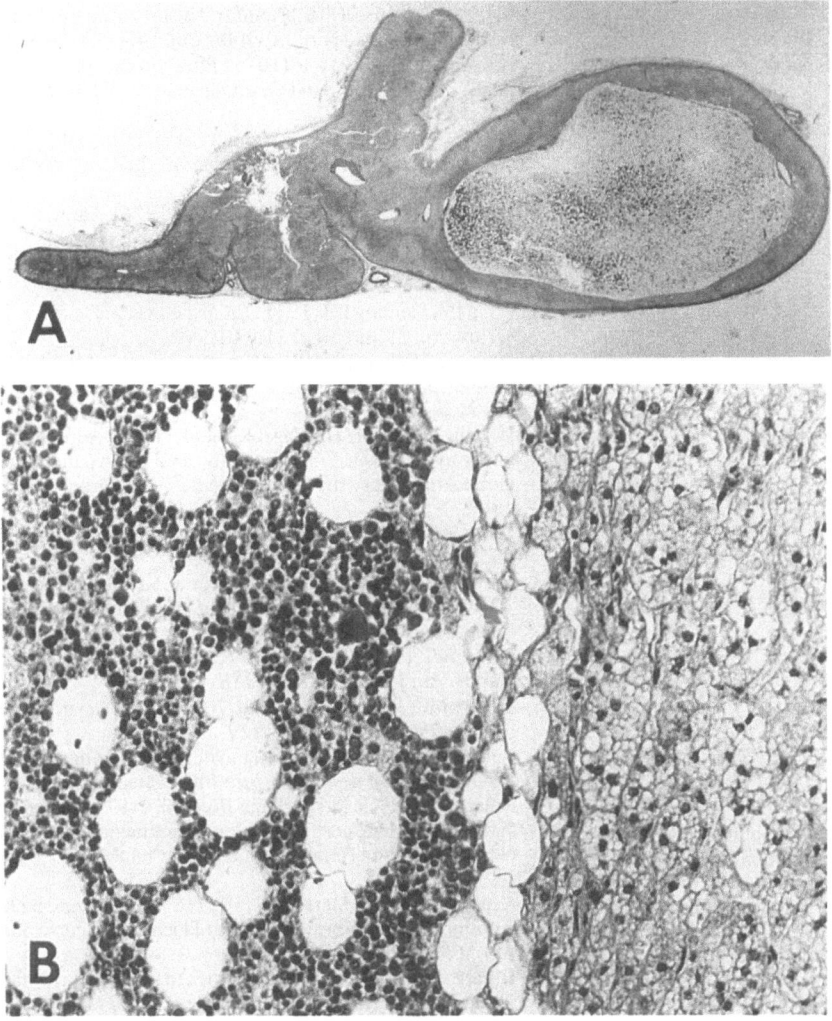

Fig. 3.49. a Myelolipoma of adult adrenal gland discovered incidentally at autopsy. Lesion is sharply delineated but unencapsulated. H & E, × 5. b Higher power view showing admixture of mature fat and hematopoietic elements. Adrenal cortex is *on right*. H & E, × 220

metaplasia. A minority of patients are symptomatic due to the large size of the lesion. It is sufficiently rare as a surgical lesion that it is seldom even considered in the differential diagnosis [33]. The increasing use of high-resolution imaging procedures such as computerized tomography may lead to the discovery of more of these lesions in individuals who are entirely asymptomatic. Rare cases have been reported in association with Cushing's syndrome, but there is lingering suspicion that some of them may be metaplastic foci within adrenal cortical hyperplasia or neoplasia.

Pathologically, the lesions are well demarcated but unencapsulated (Fig. 3.49a, b). Depending upon the relative amounts of fatty and hematopoietic elements, they may range in color from yellow to reddish brown. The hematopoietic component resembles normal marrow with megakaryocytes and myeloid and erythroid cells. Rarely, bony trabeculae may be seen.

Adrenal Cysts

These are usually discovered incidentally at autopsy but may present as a space-occupying suprarenal mass. As with myelolipomas, the use of sophisticated imaging techniques will likely disclose more cases which are clinically unsuspected. Adrenal cysts have been divided into a number of dif-

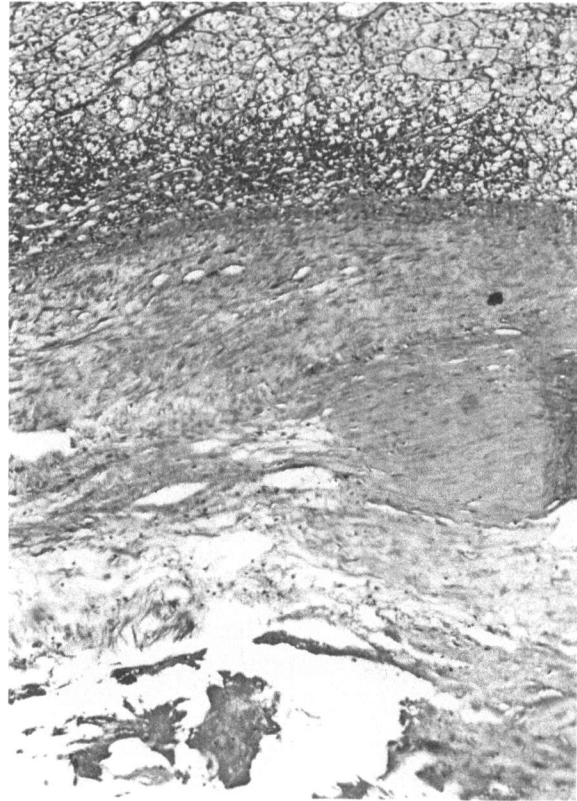

Fig. 3.50. Wall of adrenal cyst is composed of irregular fibrous tissue with edema and minimal inflammation. No lining cells could be identified. Residual cortex is *at top*. H & E, × 75

ferent types with so-called pseudocysts being most common [21]. The wall is composed of collagenized tissue with few inflammatory cells (Fig. 3.50). Occasionally, there may be foci of calcification or metaplastic bone formation within the cyst wall.

References

1. Armin A, Castelli M (1984) Congenital adrenal tissue in the lung with adrenal cytomegaly. Case report and review of the literature. Am J Clin Pathol 82:225–228
2. Assmann G, Frederickson DS (1983) Acid lipase deficiency: Wolman's disease and cholesteryl ester storage disease. In: Stanbury JB, Wyngaarden JB, Frederickson DS, Goldstein JL, Brown MS (eds) Metabolic basis of inherited diseases. McGraw-Hill Book Co, New York, pp 803–819
3. Beard CM, Sheps, SG, Kurland LT et al. (1983) Occurrence of pheochromocytoma in Rochester, Minnesota, 1950 through 1979. Mayo Clin Proc 58:802–804
4. Beckwith JB, Perrin EV (1963) In situ neuroblastomas: a contribution to the natural history of neural crest tumors. Am J Pathol 43:1089–1104
5. Black J, Williams DI (1973) Natural history of adrenal haemorrhage in the newborn. Arch Dis Child 48:183–190
6. Bravo EL, Gifford RW Jr (1984) Pheochromocytoma: diagnosis, localization and management. N Engl J Med 311:1298–1303
7. Cagle PT, Hawkins EP, Kirkland RT et al. (1984) Prognostic criteria of adrenal cortical neoplasms in children. Lab Invest 50:2p
8. Carney JA, Sizemore GW, Sheps SG (1976) Adrenal medullary disease in multiple endocrine neoplasia, type 2. Pheochromocytoma and its precursors. Am J Clin Pathol 66:279–290
9. Craig JM, Landing BH (1951) Anaplastic cells of fetal adrenal cortex. Am J Clin Pathol 21:940–949
10. Dekker A, Oehrle JS (1971) Hyaline globules of the adrenal medulla of man. A product of lipid peroxidation? Arch Pathol Lab Med 91:353–364
11. DeLellis RA, Wolfe HJ. Gagel RF et al. (1976) Adrenal medullary hyperplasia. A morphometric analysis in patients with familial medullary thyroid carcinoma. Am J Pathol 83:177–190
12. Evans AE (1980) Staging and treatment of neuroblastoma. Cancer 45:1799–1802
13. Evans AE, Chatten J, D'Angio GJ et al. (1980) A review of 17 IV-S neuroblastoma patients at the Children's Hospital of Philadelphia. Cancer 45: 833–839
14. Fidler WJ (1977) Ovarian thecal metaplasia in adrenal glands. Am J Clin Pathol 67:318–323
15. Gilbert MG, Cleveland WW (1970) Cushing's syndrome in infancy. Pediatrics 46:217–229
16. Gold EM (1979) The Cushing syndromes: changing views of diagnosis and treatment. Ann Intern Med 90:829–844
17. Hough AJ, Hollifield JW, Page DL et al. (1979) Prognostic factors in adrenal cortical tumors. A mathematical analysis of clinical and morphologic data. Am J Clin Pathol 72:390–399
18. Hsu S-M, Raine L, Martin HF (1981) Spironolactone bodies. An immunoperoxidase study with biochemical correlation. Am J Clin Pathol 75:92–95
19. Hutter AM Jr, Kayhoe DE (1966) Adrenal cortical carcinoma. Clinical features of 138 patients. Am J Med 41:572–580
20. Ikeda Y, Lister J, Bouton JM et al. (1981) Congenital neuroblastoma, neuroblastoma in situ and the normal fetal development of the adrenal. J Pediatr Surg 16:636–644
21. Incze JS, Lui PS, Merriam JC et al. (1979) Morphology and pathogenesis of adrenal cysts. Am J Pathol 95:423–428
22. Kaufman BH, Telander RL, van Heerden JA et al. (1983) Pheochromocytoma in the pediatric age group: current status. J Pediatr Surg 18:879–884
23. Kelch, RP, Verdis R, Rappaport R et al. (1984) Congenital adrenal hypoplasia. In: New MI, Levine LS (eds) Adrenal diseases in childhood. Karger, Basel, pp 156–161
24. King DR, Lack EE (1979) Adrenal cortical carcinoma. A clinical and pathologic study of 49 cases. Cancer 44:239–244
25. Lewinsky BS, Grigor KM, Symington T et al. (1974) The clinical and pathologic features of "non-hormonal" adrenocortical tumors. Report of twenty new cases and review of the literature. Cancer 33:778–790
26. Linnoila RI, Diaugustine RP, Hervonen A et. al (1980) Distribution of [met⁵]- and [leu⁵]-enkephalin-, vasoactive intestinal polypeptide- and substance P-like immunoreactivities in human adrenal glands. Neuroscience 5:2247–2259
27. McArthur RG, Bahn RC, Hayles AB (1982) Primary adrenocortical nodular dysplasia as a cause of Cushing's syndrome in infants and children. Mayo Clin Proc 57:58–63
28. Melicow MM (1977) One hundred cases of pheo-

chromocytoma (107 tumors) at the Columbia-Presbyterian Medical Center, 1926–1976. A clinicopathological analysis. Cancer 40:1987–2004

29. Mininberg DT, Levine LS, New MI (1982) Current concepts in congenital adrenal hyperplasia. In: Sommers SC, Rosen PP (eds) Pathology annual 1982 part 2. Appleton-Century-Crofts, pp 179–195

30. Morgan MWE, O'Hare MJ (1979) Cytotoxic drugs and the human adrenal cortex. A cell culture study. Cancer 43:969–979

31. Nelson DH (1980) The adrenal cortex: physiological function and disease. In: Smith LH (ed) Major problems in internal medicine. WB Saunders Co, Philadelphia, pp 48–64

32. Neville AM, Symington T (1967) The pathology of the adrenal gland in Cushing's syndrome. J Pathol Bacteriol 93:19–35

33. Noble MJ, Montague DK, Levin HS (1982) Myelolipoma: an unusual surgical lesion of the adrenal gland. Cancer 49:952–958

34. O'Hare MJ, Monaghan P, Neville AM (1979) The pathology of adrenocortical neoplasia: a correlated structural and functional approach to the diagnosis of malignant disease. Hum Pathol 10:137–154

35. Pearse AGE (1974) The APUD cell concept and its implication in pathology. In: Sommers SC (ed) Pathology annual. Appleton-Century-Crofts, pp 27–41

36. Powers JM, Moser HW, Moser AB et al. (1982) Fetal adrenoleukodystrophy: the significance of pathologic lesions in adrenal gland and testis. Hum Pathol 13:1013–1019

37. Quinan C, Berger AA (1933) Observations on human adrenals with special reference to the relative weight of the normal medulla. Ann Intern Med 6:1180–1192

38. Rosen EM, Cassady JR, Frantz CN et al. (1984) Neuroblastoma: the joint center for radiation therapy/Dana-Farber Cancer Institute/Children's Hospital experience. J Clin Oncol 2:719–732

39. Rudy FR, Bates RD, Cimorelli AJ et al. (1980) Adrenal medullary hyperplasia: a clinicopathologic study of four cases. Hum Pathol 11:650–657

40. Sheeler LR, Myers JH, Eversman JJ et al. (1983) Adrenal insufficiency secondary to carcinoma metastatic to the adrenal gland. Cancer 52:1312–1316

41. Shenoy BV, Carpenter PC, Carney JA (1984) Bilateral primary pigmented nodular adrenocortical disease. Rare cause of the Cushing syndrome. Am J Surg Pathol 8:335–344

42. Sherwin RP (1959) Histopathology of pheochromocytoma. Cancer 12:861–877

43. Slooten HV, Schaberg A, Smeenk D et al. (1985) Morphologic characteristics of benign and malignant adrenocortical tumors. Cancer 55:766–773

44. Spark RF, Connolly PB, Gluckin DS et al. (1979) ACTH secretion from a functioning pheochromocytoma. N Engl J Med 301:416–418

45. St. John Sutton MG, Sheps SG, Lie JT (1981) Prevalence of clinically unsuspected pheochromocytoma. Review of a 50-year autopsy series. Mayo Clin Proc 56:354–360

46. Stoner HB, Whiteley HJ, Emery JL (1953) The effect of systemic disease on the adrenal cortex of the child. J Pathol Bacteriol 66:171–183

47. Tang CK, Gray GF (1975) Adrenocortical neoplasms. Prognosis and morphology. Urology 5:691–695

48. Weatherby RP, Carney JA (1982) Childhood adrenocortical tumors: pathologic features and prognosis. Lab Invest 46:17p

49. Weinberger MH, Grim CE, Hollifield JW et al. (1979) Primary aldosteronism. Diagnosis, localization and treatment. Ann Intern Med 90:386–395

50. Wilbur OM Jr, Rich AR (1954) A study of the role of adrenocorticotropic hormone (ACTH) in the pathogenesis of tubular degeneration of the adrenals. Bull Hopkins Hosp 93:321–347

Chapter 4

Advances in Diagnosis

T. H. Hsu

The adrenal gland consists of the medulla and the cortex. The medulla, as part of the autonomic system, secretes catecholamines. Its secretory activity is under the direct influence of the central nervous system and responds acutely to internal and external environmental changes.

The human adrenal cortex is further divided into three zones; an outer zona glomerulosa, a middle zona fasciculata, and an inner zona reticularis. The zona glomerulosa produces aldosterone, the most potent mineralocorticoid, under the predominant regulation of the renin-angiotensin system. The zona fasciculata secretes cortisol, the most important glucocorticoid, whereas the zona reticularis is the main source of adrenal androgens and estrogens. The function of the zonae fasciculata and reticularis is normally regulated chiefly by the hypothalamic-pituitary unit through adrenocorticotropic hormone (ACTH) (Fig. 4.1). The rate of cortisol secretion is determined by the net effects of (1) the negative feedback control of cortisol on ACTH secretion, (2) extrinsic stimulations, such as physical or emotional stress, and (3) the intrinsic circadian rhythmicity of ACTH secretion. CNS-controlled corticotropin-releasing factor (CRF) of the hypothalamus regulates the synthesis and release of pituitary ACTH, which is the direct mediator of the secretory activity of the adrenal cortex. In a negative feedback system, high concentrations of plasma cortisol suppress secretion of both ACTH and CRF, whereas low levels enhance their release.

Thus a precise and sensitive control of adrenal corticoid secretion depends upon normal function of the CNS, hypothalamus, pituitary, and adrenal cortex. Extrinsic stimulation by physical or mental stresses such as pain, trauma, hemorrhage, hypoglycemia, febrile reaction, or psychosis may give signals of the hypothalamus to enhance ACTH secretion and hence hypercortisolism. In addition to the negative feedback control mechanism and the extrinsic influences, this regulatory system has an intrinsic rhythmicity. ACTH is secreted episodically; hence the serum levels of cortisol fluctuate accordingly. The main secretory phase occurs during the last 3 h of sleep and the first waking hour. This is followed by intermittent moderate secretory activity throughout the day, reaching a nadir at night. This circadian rhythm is mediated by the hypothalamus according to sleep-wake activity, and is subject to change by altering the sleep-wake cycle.

Unlike glucocorticoids and adrenal sex steroids, the secretion of aldosterone is regulated primarily by the renin-angiotensin system. ACTH and serum potassium also stimulate aldosterone secretion, but normally they are of secondary importance. Aldosterone participates in the maintenance of body sodium balance. When sodium is depleted, contraction of effective blood volume follows. This leads to a decrease in perfusion pressure to the renal juxtaglomerular apparatus, and renin secretion is stimulated. Renin, an enzyme, cleaves the protein angiotensinogen to generate angiotensin I (a deca-

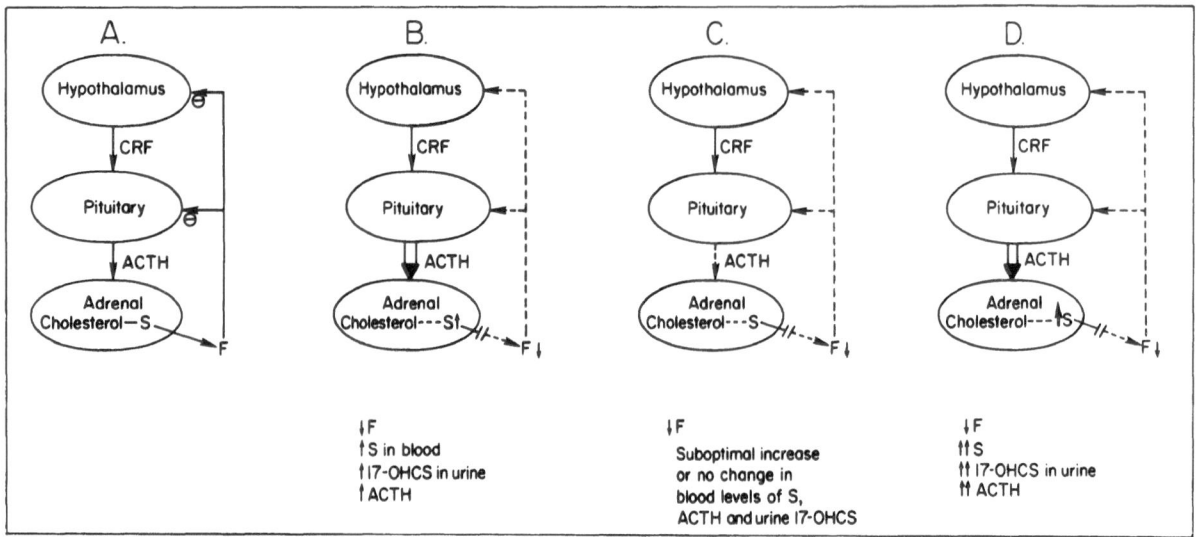

Fig. 4.1. The normal pituitary-adrenal axis control mechanism (A). Pituitary-adrenal response to metyrapone, an 11-hydroxy-lase inhibitor, in the normal subject (B), hypopituitarism (C), and pituitary Cushing's disease (D). Adequate inhibition of 11-hydroxylase by metyrapone results in reduction of cortisol, which triggers further secretion of ACTH in the normal subject. Steroidogenesis is therefore increased, but only to the point of blockade. A rise in ACTH and accumulation of the cortisol (compound F) precursor 11-deoxycortisol (compound S) in plasma and urine is expected. Urinary 17-OHCS levels are also increased because the major metabolite of compound S contributes to its value. No rise or a suboptimal rise in ACTH, compound S, or urinary 17-OHCS after metyrapone indicates impaired ACTH reserve (C). A supranormal response to metyrapone is observed in patients with pituitary Cushing's disease (D).

peptide). This peptide is further hydrolyzed to an octapeptide, known as angiotensin II, by a converting enzyme which is most abundant in the lung. Angiotensin II, in addition to being a vasoconstrictor, is a potent stimulant of aldosterone secretion. Aldosterone in turn increases the reabsorption of sodium from the distal renal tubules to restore body sodium deficit, subsequently normalizing the effective blood volume. Epithelial cells of salivary glands, sweat glands, and the gastrointestinal system also respond to aldosterone by conserving sodium in exchange for potassium. Blood loss or sequestration of blood in the venous system following a resumption of the upright position can also provoke aldosterone secretion by triggering the sympathetic nervous system to stimulate renin secretion and the subsequent renin-angiotensin response [16].

Metabolism and Metabolic Effects of Glucocorticoids

The adrenal steroids once secreted into the bloodstream are carried chiefly by transcortin (corticoid-binding globulin or CBG) to their target cells. Corticoids bound to proteins are metabolically inert and it is the small unbound fraction that is free to exert intracellular biologic effects. Unbound plasma cortisol is readily filtered through the glomeruli and a large portion is reabsorbed by the renal tubules. A small amount excreted into the urine constitutes the free cortisol detected in urine. The measurement of 24-h urinary free cortisol is one of the most practical and accurate parameters for assessing adrenal cortisol function in clinical practice. The major breakdown products of cortisol are measured in the urine as 17-hydroxycorticosteroids (17-OHCS), whereas weak adrenal androgens, such as androsterone and etiocholanolone, are principal constituents of 17-ketosteroids (17-KS) (Fig. 4.2).

Glucocorticoids have many metabolic effects. They promote gluconeogenesis and deposition of liver glycogen. Glucocorticoids at higher doses enhance protein catabolism and inhibit protein synthesis. They also promote fat deposition in faciocervical truncal areas, stimulate appetite, and stimulate hematopoiesis. Glucocorticoids also suppress the synthesis and release of ACTH from the pituitary and/or CRF from the hypothalamus. The metabolic potency of glucocorticoids is variable, but cortisol is the most potent of all naturally occurring products [16].

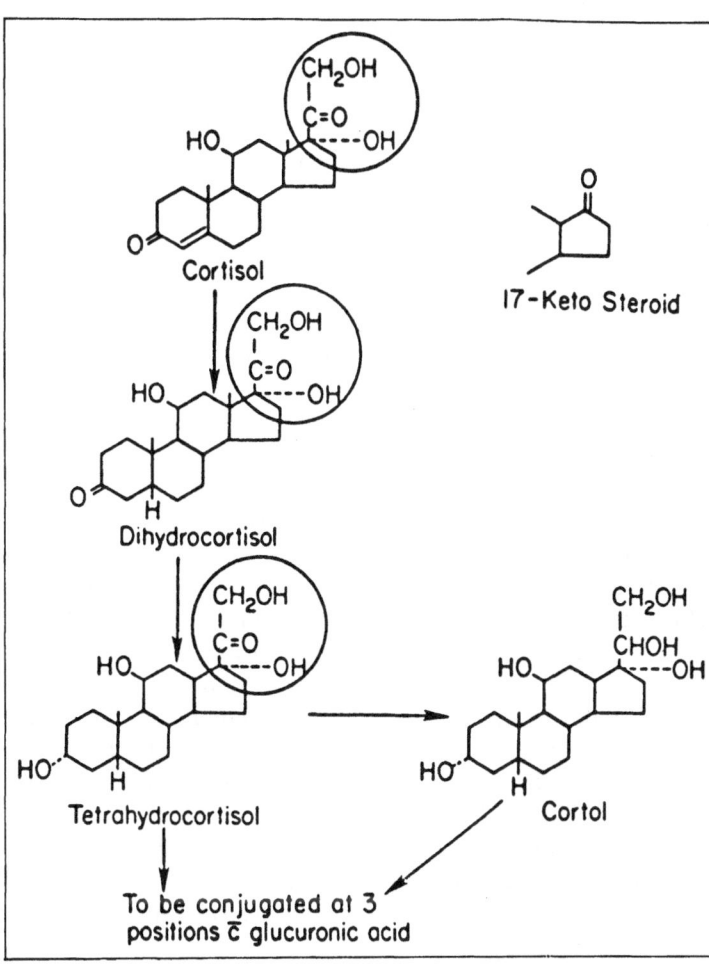

Fig. 4.2. Compounds with a dihydroxyacetone side chain in the 17 position (*encircled*) are measured as 17-OHCS by the Porter–Silber method, compounds that possess a keto group in the 17 position by the Zimmermann reaction. Androsterone, dihydroepiandrosterone, and etiocholanolone are the major constituents of urine 17-KS under normal conditions.

Adrenal Tumors

The adrenal gland, like many other endocrine glands, may develop a neoplastic process. Depending on their cell type (Table 4.1), such lesions may produce sufficient quantities of hormones to cause clinical signs and symptoms referable to hypercortisolism (Cushing's syndrome), hyperaldosteronism (Conn's syndrome), and pheochromocytoma. Some tumors that appear inactive clinically may in fact produce small quantities of hormones when studied carefully in vivo or in vitro. Other adrenal masses such as metastatic malignancies are inactive and clearly nonfunctional.

Nonfunctional Adrenal Tumors

Most benign nonfunctional adrenal tumors are discovered incidentally during radiographic evalu-

ation of the genitourinary system. The widespread use of computed tomography (CT) is leading to an increased detection of small asymptomatic adrenal tumors which would not have been diagnosed pre-

Table 4.1 Classification of common suprarenal masses

Tissue origin	Tumor type	Clinical syndromes
Stroma	Cyst, lipoma, myelolipoma, fibroma, myoma, angioma	Usually nonfunctional
Cortex	Adenoma, carcinoma, nodular hyperplasia	Cushing's syndrome, aldosteronism, virilization, feminization, rarely nonfunctional
Medulla	Ganglioneuroblastoma, neuroblastoma, pheochromocytoma	Catecholamine excess or rarely nonfunctional
Extraadrenal	Metastatic	Space-occupying effects including adrenal insufficiency

viously by conventional imaging techniques. Benign nonfunctioning adrenal tumors, usually less than 5 cm in diameter, are seldom symptomatic. Large ones, however, may present as an abdominal mass or cause ill-defined lumbar pain or nonspecific gastrointestinal symptoms. A strategically located adrenal mass may compress the renal artery and lead to hyperreninemic hypertension [3].

Malignant adrenal mass lesions are usually greater than 7 cm in diameter. They, too, are most frequently discovered accidentally on radiography or present as a palpable mass in an asymptomatic individual. When present, symptoms include nonspecific abdominal pain, backache, anorexia, weight loss, fever, or generalized malaise. If hemorrhage and necrosis occur within the lesion, the clinical presentation may simulate an acute abdominal or pelvic catastrophe.

Metastases to the adrenal glands are more common than primary adrenal tumors; 13%–27% of patients harbor metastatic involvement of the adrenal gland at the time the primary malignant neoplasm is diagnosed [12]. Carcinomas of breast and lung are the commonest primary source of adrenal metastasis. A metastatic adrenal lesion is characteristically multiple and involves both glands [2]. Adrenal insufficiency may occur when the metastatic tumor results in near total destruction of the adrenal cortex.

Functioning Adrenal Tumors

The majority of functioning adrenal cortical adenomas are hypersecretors of hormones which result in Cushing's syndrome. Others produce predominantly aldosterone and cause Conn's syndrome (hyperaldosteronism). Approximately three-fourths of adrenal carcinomas secrete excessive adrenal hormones and cause Cushing's syndrome and/or virilism or feminization. Pheochromocytomas that produce excess catecholamines are neoplasms of the adrenal medulla.

Cushing's Syndrome

The common denominator of spontaneous Cushing's syndrome is an excessive production of cortisol and its resultant metabolic consequences. This syn-

Table 4.2. Clinical manifestations of Cushing's syndrome

	Incidence (%)
Obesity	95
Hypertension	85
Glucosuria and decreased glucose tolerance	80
Menstrual and sexual dysfunction	76
Hirsutism and acne	72
Striae	67
Weakness	65
Osteoporosis	55
Easy bruisability	55
Psychiatric disturbances	50
Edema	46
Polyuria	16
Ocular changes	8

drome may occur at any age in both sexes. A typical patient with Cushing's syndrome, however, is a middle-aged woman with weight gain, hirsutism, plethora, menstrual irregularity, hypertension, acne, weakness, easy bruisability, and emotional disturbances (Table 4.2). The obesity is usually moderate, but it is characterized by abnormal fat distribution, with excessive fat deposits in the face, neck, "dorsal hump" near the base of the neck, supraclavicular area, and trunk. Glucocorticoids produce a variety of catabolic effects resulting in protean clinical manifestations. Relatively specific signs and symptoms that are useful for distinguishing a Cushing's patient from a much more commonly encountered patient with hypertension, obesity, and mild diabetes mellitus include bruisability, proximal muscle weakness, osteoporosis, and truncal obesity.

Causes of Cushing's Syndrome

Hypersecretion of glucocorticoids may be secondary to excess ACTH production or to autonomous secretion of adrenal neoplasms (Table 4.3). Hypersecretion of ACTH may originate from either pituitary or nonpituitary neoplasm.

ACTH-Dependent Cushing's Syndrome

Pituitary Cushing's Disease

The term Cushing's disease (in contrast to Cushing's syndrome) is usually reserved for adrenal hyper-

Table 4.3. Causes of Cushing's syndrome

ACTH dependent	ACTH independent
Pituitary ACTH hyper-secretion with or without pituitary adenoma	Adrenal carcinoma
	Adrenal adenoma
Ectopic ACTH syndrome	Exogenous corticosteroids
Adrenal hyperplasia; some cases of adrenal hyperplasia are independent of ACTH	
Exogenous ACTH	

function due to excess ACTH originating from the pituitary. This is the commonest cause of spontaneous Cushing's syndrome, accounting for 70% or more of all cases. Most patients have pituitary adenoma whereas others do not. As a result of prolonged ACTH hypersecretion, the adrenal cortex appears hyperplastic in most cases.

Biochemical changes of Cushing's disease are characterized by overproduction of cortisol and a relatively high plasma ACTH concentration (Fig. 4.3). In patients with pituitary Cushing's disease, in contrast to all other types of hypercortisolism, the pituitary-adrenal axis is essentially intact except that it operates at a higher set point. Therefore, administration of corticotropin-releasing factor (CRF) to a patient with Cushing's disease leads to an increase in ACTH secretion and cortisol production [9]. Furthermore, ACTH secretion in this circumstance is suppressible by administration of glucocorticoids in an amount that exceeds the pituitary set point. Dexamethasone, an extremely

potent synthetic glucocorticoid, is often employed to test pituitary adrenal suppressibility (see below). Conversely, when cortisol synthesis is inhibited by an adrenal cortex inhibitor such as metyrapone, the hypothalamic-pituitary axis is activated to release more ACTH, which in turn markedly stimulates steroidogenesis up to the point of inhibition (see Fig. 4.1).

Ectopic ACTH Syndrome

A number of neoplasms, principally oat cell carcinoma of lung (50% of cases), thymoma (15%), pancreatic islet cell tumors (10%), and bronchial adenoma (5%), possess the potential to make a hormone that is identical to or similar to the pituitary ACTH. Perhaps because of the short duration of the hypercortisolism and the concurrent catabolic effects of malignancy, classic cushingoid body habitus is often absent in ectopic ACTH syndrome. Rather, these patients often exhibit severe weight loss, hypertension, edema, and hyperpigmentation.

Biochemical derangements of this syndrome are qualitatively similar to those of pituitary Cushing's syndrome but the production rate of cortisol is often higher and extreme elevation of ACTH is the rule. More characteristically, the secretion of ACTH from a nonpituitary source is highly autonomous and usually unresponsive to the suppressive effect of glucocorticoids. Administration of CRF to patients with ectopic ACTH syndrome has no effect on their ACTH and cortisol levels [9].

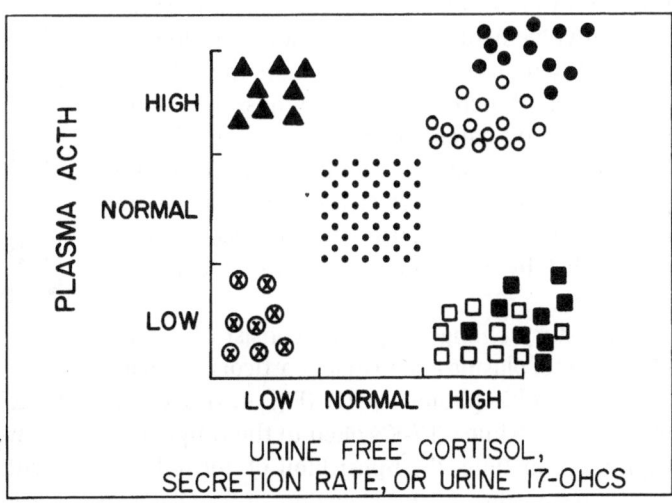

Fig. 4.3. Diagrammatic representation of changes in ACTH and cortisol in different types of Cushing's syndrome and adrenal insufficiency. ▲, adrenal insufficiency; ○, pituitary ACTH deficiency; ○, pituitary Cushing's disease; ●, ectopic ACTH syndrome; □, adrenal adenoma; ■, adrenal carcinoma.

Nodular Adrenal Cortical Hyperplasia

This is an uncommon and heterogeneous form of Cushing's syndrome. Some cases represent multiple adrenal adenomas with autonomous steroid production, others chronic hypersecretion of ACTH leading to diffuse adrenal nodular hyperplasia. Consequently, low plasma ACTH levels are found in some cases, but in others pituitary ACTH dependency is apparent [4].

ACTH-Independent Cushing's Syndrome

Adrenal Carcinoma

Carcinomas of the adrenal occur at all ages and in both sexes, but 80% occur in females, with one peak incidence in the first decade of life and another between 40 and 50 years of age. Pituitary Cushing's disease is uncommon before the age 10 years, but adrenal carcinoma is a common cause of childhood Cushing's syndrome. For unknown reasons, functioning adrenal carcinomas occur slightly more frequently on the left side. Pathologic diagnosis is achieved by demonstrating nuclear and cellular pleomorphism, increased mitotic figures, invasion of the capsule or veins, and presence of metastases. In the absence of these pathologic features one must rely on the clinical course and certain laboratory findings to distinguish carcinoma from adenoma. Even the pathologic features may fail accurately to predict the clinical course of the lesion [6].

The clinical features of adrenal carcinoma are usually inseparable from those of other causes. However, virilization in women or feminization in men can be the dominant clinical presentation. The tumor may present as an abdominal mass and metastatic involvement of kidneys, pancreas, liver, or lungs. When virilization in women is the sole presentation of a functioning adrenal mass, it is almost always due to a carcinoma rather than an adenoma [6]. Very rarely adrenal carcinoma may produce predominantly deoxycorticosterone, a mineralocorticoid, and cause hypertension unaccompanied by other manifestations of Cushing's syndrome.

Laboratory changes typically consist of marked elevations of plasma and urinary corticoids, and low or undetectable plasma ACTH (Fig. 4.3). Extreme elevation of urinary 17-KS often to the range of 50 mg/day (four times the upper limit of normal) and out of proportion to the elevation of 17-OHCS, is found uniquely in Cushing's syndrome due to adrenal carcinomas. Since steroidogenesis is independent of ACTH in patients with adrenal carcinoma, the administration of glucocorticoid (dexamethasone, for testing purposes) does not alter the secretory function of the tumor. Similarly, their low plasma ACTH concentrations are unresponsive to CRF injection [9]. Probably due to severe cellular derangements, adrenal carcinomas are usually incapable of responding to exogenous ACTH. In contrast, at least half of the patients with Cushing's syndrome due to adrenal adenoma are capable of doubling their steroid output following administration of ACTH. Metyrapone administration may alter steroidogenesis qualitatively by a reduction of cortisol and increase of 11-deoxycortisol and its precursors, but total urinary 17-OHCS remains at the same level, proving its independence of ACTH. In patients with the feminization syndrome (gynecomastia, testicular atrophy, and loss of libido), urinary and plasma estrogens are elevated in addition to the above findings.

Adrenal Adenoma

As in the case of adrenal carcinoma, adenoma occurs four times more frequently in females than in males, but the peak incidence occurs at 35 years of age [6]. The tumor is usually unilateral and is well demarcated by a capsule.

The clinical manifestation of functioning adenoma is that of Cushing's syndrome. However, hirsutism and virilization are less frequent and mild when present. Biochemical and radiographic findings of active adrenal adenoma are similar to those of carcinoma. Typically there are elevations of plasma and urinary 17-OHCS, urinary free cortisol, and 17-KS, low plasma ACTH, and a unilateral small (usually less than 5 cm) suprarenal mass. However, the urinary excretions of 17-KS are usually only mildly elevated.

Laboratory Evaluation of Cushing's Syndrome

Once the possibility of Cushing's syndrome is suspected in a patient, two major questions must be answered prior to instituting an appropriate treatment: (1) Does the patient indeed have hypercortisolism? and (2) if so, what type of Cushing's syndrome? For convenience, laboratory approaches to the diagnosis of Cushing's syndrome can accordingly be divided into two major steps: (1) tests to verify the presence of hypercortisolism and (2) tests to evaluate the cause of Cushing's syndrome.

Tests To Verify the Presence of Hypercortisolism

Plasma cortisol levels exhibit frequent fluctuations in both normal subjects and patients with Cushing's syndrome. Furthermore, the level of transcortin, a major steroid carrier in blood, can be significantly altered by nonadrenal factors, such as the use of estrogens, pregnancy, or liver or renal disease. It is therefore difficult to establish or exclude hypercortisolism based on sporadic plasma cortisol value determinations at the basal state. In a study [10], 17% of 182 patients with Cushing's syndrome had normal evening plasma cortisol levels. Conversely, a substantial number of normal individuals have elevated evening plasma cortisol, especially during stress.

The specificity and sensitivity of plasma cortisol assay are, however, substantially enhanced by the concomitant use of the low-dose dexamethasone suppression test. The test is performed by giving 1 mg dexamethasone by mouth between 11 p.m. and midnight and obtaining an 8 a.m. plasma cortisol measurement the following morning. Failure to suppress plasma cortisol below 50% of the basal values, or to less than 5 μg/dl, indirectly indicates the existence of hypercortisolism or an abnormal pituitary-adrenal axis. Nearly 98% of patients with Cushing's syndrome will fail to suppress normally. However, 13%–23% of obese subjects of a hospitalized population may also exhibit a similar abnormal response to 1 mg dexamethasone [10].

Assay of *urinary 17-OHCS* has been the most commonly employed test in the past for adrenal function. In a combined result of 14 separate series of patients, only 89% of 315 patients with Cushing's syndrome had abnormally elevated 17-OHCS values [10]. One of the serious problems encountered in the use of 17-OHCS to diagnose Cushing's syndrome is the fact that 27% of obese subjects had abnormally high urinary 17-OHCS values [17]. Thus the determination of 17-OHCS in urine is not very useful in distinguishing patients with Cushing's syndrome from those with signs and symptoms

mimicking hypercortisolism. It should be recognized that most of the overlapping of 17-OHCS values occurs near the upper limits of the normal range. Extremely high secretion of 17-OHCS strongly suggests the diagnosis of Cushing's syndrome. The value of urinary 17-KS has similar limitations. Extremely high (at least four times the upper limit of normal) urine 17-KS values are a fairly reliable marker of the presence of functioning adrenal carcinoma.

Measurement of *24-h urinary free cortisol* content provides a more reliable parameter in distinguishing patients with Cushing's syndrome from other subjects. In a review of data obtained from 15 independent reports, only 3.3% of 49 lean, obese, or chronically ill subjects had slightly elevated daily free cortisol values in urine, and only 5.6% of 248 patients with genuine Cushing's syndrome had falsely normal urinary free cortisol values [10]. Clearly, because of its specificity, simplicity, and relatively easy accessibility the determination of 24-h urinary free cortisol has become a useful screening test in the diagnosis of Cushing's syndrome [10].

Tests To Evaluate the Cause of Cushing's Syndrome

Once hypercortisolism is assured by reliable laboratory procedures, it is necessary to identify its cause. Etiologic evaluation of Cushing's syndrome is usually achieved by the following procedures:

1. Plasma ACTH determination
2. Study of hypothalamic-pituitary-adrenal dynamics:
   a) High-dose dexamethasone suppression test
   b) CRF stimulation test
   c) Metyrapone test
   d) ACTH stimulation test
3. Imaging procedures

Plasma ACTH Determination

Low levels of plasma ACTH in a patient with hypercortisolism exclude ACTH as the causative factor for the cortisol excess. The cause of Cushing's syndrome in such a case is autonomous adrenal neoplasia. Normal to moderately elevated blood ACTH concentrations are observed in patients with pituitary Cushing's disease. Markedly elevated ACTH levels are usually associated with ectopic ACTH syndrome.

Due to technical difficulties, a reliable ACTH assay method is not widely available. The blood levels of ACTH fluctuate even more acutely than those of cortisol. Therefore, frequent sampling with multiple specimens and a careful analysis of the values are necessary.

Dexamethasone Suppression Test

The high-dose dexamethasone suppression test (2 mg orally every 6 h for eight doses) is the test most commonly relied on in the differentiation of the cause of Cushing's syndrome. When enough dexamethasone is administered to "satisfy" the pituitary set point in patients with pituitary Cushing's syndrome, the secretion of ACTH is suppressed; hence the secretion of cortisol from the adrenal cortex is also reduced. Steroidogenesis is independent of ACTH in patients with autonomous neoplasia, and the secretion of ACTH from ectopic tissues is usually resistant to a negative feedback suppression. Since dexamethasone itself does not add significantly to the values of urinary free cortisol or 17-OHCS, the suppression of ACTH is reflected by the reduction in the values of urinary free cortisol and/or 17-OHCS (see Fig. 4.4).

Corticotropin-Releasing Factor Stimulation Test

Corticotropin-releasing factor (CRF) (1 μg/kg body weight) given intravenously stimulates ACTH and cortisol secretion in normal persons and 95% of patients with pituitary Cushing's disease. Patients with ectopic ACTH syndrone and adrenal neoplasia do not exhibit appreciable response to CRF [9].

ACTH Stimulation Test

ACTH is injected to differentiate the cause of Cushing's syndrome when the results of the dexamethasone suppression test are not clearly discriminatory. The adrenal glands of patients with ACTH-dependent Cushing's syndrome are highly sensitive to administered ACTH and respond to it by producing greater than twice the basal amounts of cortisol. In contrast, the secretion of cortisol from an adrenal carcinoma is almost always unresponsive to ACTH administration, and only about 50% of adenomas will respond to ACTH [6].

Metyrapone Test

Metyrapone is an inhibitor of adrenocortical 11-beta-hydroxylase, an enzyme essential for the synthesis of cortisol. By reducing the plasma levels of cortisol, metyrapone triggers the hypothalamic-pituitary axis to release ACTH, which in turn stimulates the synthesis of steroids by the adrenal to 11-desoxycortisol (compound S), the immediate precursor of cortisol (Fig. 4.1). In the pituitary Cushing's disorder, metyrapone administration will cause an exaggerated rise in ACTH and in compound S. The metabolites of compound S, measured as 17-OHCS, will increase accordingly. In contrast, the pituitary-adrenal axis in adrenal neoplasms and the ectopic ACTH syndrome usually show no such response to metyrapone.

Imaging Procedures in Cushing's Syndrome

Exceptions to the above rules may occur. Therefore, anatomic delineation of masses in the adrenal gland, pituitary areas, and nonendocrine tissues by radiographic techniques contributes indirectly to the identification of the etiology of Cushing's syndrome. Radiographic evaluation of the adrenal gland in patients with pituitary Cushing's disease is usually not necessary when the cause is certain. The adrenal glands may be normal in size or enlarged bilaterally in this disease. One should never equate glandular hypertrophy with hypercortisolism because it may also be observed in patients with congenital adrenal hyperplasia or in patients with long-standing stress.

Identification and localization of an adrenal mass is performed best by computed tomography (see Chap. 5).

By clinical evaluations, skillful use of laboratory techniques, and imaging procedures the diagnosis classification of Cushing's syndrome is usually achievable (see Table 4.4) [13]. The laboratory findings in patients with ectopic ACTH syndrome resulting from occasional benign adenomatous neoplasia

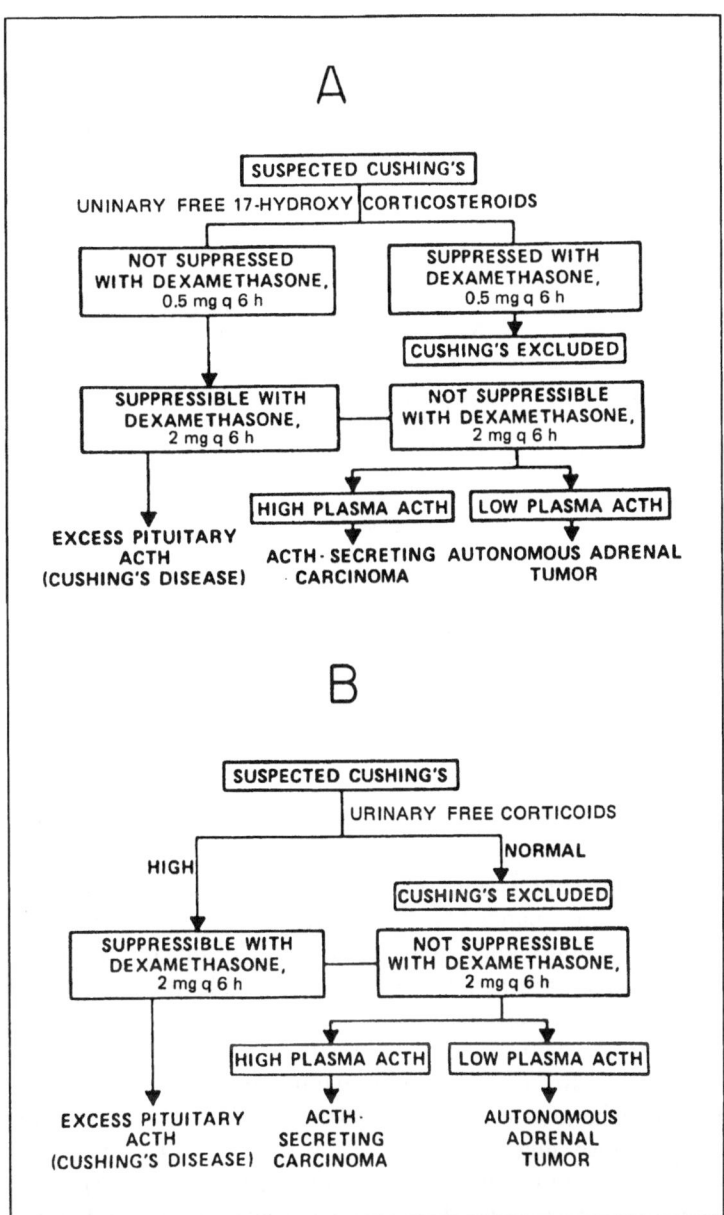

Fig. 4.4. The use of the dexamethasone suppression test and plasma ACTH levels in the differential diagnosis of Cushing's syndrome. Dexamethasone is given for 2 days as outlined above. The low-dose dexamethasone suppression test is usually not necessary when a urinary free cortisol assay is available (B).

are often indistinguishable from those of pituitary Cushing's disease. Bilateral inferior petrosal sinus sampling may be required to establish or to exclude the pituitary as the source of ACTH in extremely difficult circumstances [11].

Primary Hyperaldosteronism (Conn's Syndrome)

The prevalence of this disorder among the hypertensive population has been reported variously as 0.5% to 8%; most data suggest that its incidence is around 0.5%–1% [5]. More women are affected than men by a ratio of 3:1, and the peak incidence is between the third and fourth decades. Pathologically, most of these patients have a solitary adrenal adenoma; between 20% and 30% have bilateral adrenal nodular hyperplasia with apparent hyperactivity of the zona glomerulosa. Among this group of patients a small number have hypersecretion of aldosterone that appears to be ACTH dependent; their hyperaldosteronism is correctable with exogenous glucocorticoid. In a small number of patients hyperaldosteronism is associated with an adrenal cortex of normal appearance.

Table 4.4. Comparison of different types of Cushing's syndrome

Clinical or laboratory changes	Pituitary Cushing's disease	Ectopic ACTH syndrome	Adrenal carcinoma	Adrenal adenoma
Main clinical features	Cushingoid appearance and symptoms	Hyperpigmentation, weight loss, hypertension, hypokalemia	Cushingoid features, hirsutism, weight gain	Cushingoid features
Urine 17-OHCS/free cortisol	Normal to high/high	High/high (may fluctuate from day to day)	High/high	High/high
Urine 17-KS	Normal to high	High	Markedly elevated—four to five times normal value	High
Serum ACTH	Normal to moderate elevation	Markedly elevated	Low	Low
CRF stimulation	ACTH rises	Unresponsive	Unresponsive	Unresponsive
High-dose dexamethasone (8 mg/day)	Steroid production suppressed to 50% of basal value	Not suppressed	Not suppressed	Not suppressed
ACTH stimulation test	Responsive	Responsive	Nonresponsive	50% of cases responsive
Metyrapone administration	Responsive with increased urine 17-OHCS	Variable	Unresponsive	Unresponsive
Typical radiographic appearance	Bilateral hypertrophy; bilateral nodules may appear in nodular hyperplasia	Bilateral hypertrophy	Unilateral suprarenal mass and atrophy of contralateral gland	Unilateral suprarenal mass and atrophy of contralateral gland

The pathophysiologic basis of this disorder is an autonomous excessive secretion of aldosterone despite the suppression of the renin-angiotensin system by an expanded blood volume.

The cardinal clinical manifestations of primary aldosteronism are hypertension and hypokalemia. Large quantities of aldosterone promote the reabsorption of sodium and consequent excretion of potassium. Chronic retention of sodium and hypervolemia lead to arterial hypertension. Hypokalemia and alkalosis give rise to muscle weakness, paresthesia, cramps, tetany, or frank paralysis of limbs. The biochemical diagnosis of primary hyperaldosteronism requires proof of an increased aldosterone production that is not suppressible by intravascular volume expansion or by pharmacologic interruption of angiotension II production and a suppressed renin-angiotensin system that is not activated normally by volume contraction (usually by diuresis).

Since primary hyperaldosteronism is a potentially curable cause of hypertension, every hypertensive patient should have his serum potassium evaluated. Hypokalemia is usually the first clue to clinical suspicion of hyperaldosteronism. Profound spontaneous hypokalemia below 2.7 mEq/liter in the hypertensive patient is highly suggestive of aldosteronism, but a moderate hypokalemia raises many

diagnostic dilemmas. About 4% of a hypertensive population had serum potassium levels below 3.6 mEq/liter, yet primary aldosteronism was found in only 9% [17]. Assay (usually by radioimmunoassay) of blood aldosterone concentration immediately after infusion of saline (2 liters in 4 h) has been found to be a fairly reliable stratagem. Further extensive evaluation as outlined in Chap. 7 becomes necessary when the serum aldosterone concentration is above 8 ng/dl following expansion of the extracellular fluid volume. The diagnosis of primary hyperaldosteronism is virtually certain when increased aldosterone production is proved to occur in the absence of high renin stimulation.

Direct visualization by various radiographic means to localize the tumor has greatly enhanced our ability to diagnose aldosterone-secreting adenoma. Adrenal venography successfully laterized the tumor in about 65% of cases. The limitations of this technique are that its resolution is poor for tumors less than 1 cm in diameter and that it requires highly skilled and experienced radiology personnel. Furthermore, it carries potential serious complications such as perforation of the adrenal veins, hemorrhage, and adrenal infarction. Adrenal imaging with radioiodine-labeled iodocholesterol is a noninvasive technique that can also provide certain functional information of the tumor mass.

Again, it suffers from poor resolution of small tumors less than 1 cm. Computed tomography is currently the most accurate method of imaging aldosterone adenomas. In one review series, a sensitivity of 82% was recorded, with 23 of 28 lesions correctly identified [1].

Pheochromocytoma

Pheochromocytomas are neuroectodermal tumors that secrete catecholamines. Although a rare cause of hypertension, it is usually curable. About 90% of these tumors are located in the adrenal medulla, of which 90% involve one adrenal and 10% are bilateral. Men and women are affected equally. The age of onset varies from early childhood to old age, although its incidence is most common in the third and fourth decades. This tumor may occur sporadically or inherently. The presence of pheochromocytoma should be suspected in all patients with multiple endocrine adenomatosis (MEA) type II (medullary thyroid carcinoma, parathyroid adenoma, and pheochromocytoma) and type III (type II plus marfanoid habitus, mucosal neuromas, and ganglioneuroma).

The clinical presentation of pheochromocytoma may be dramatic. Hypertension is the commonest manifestation and is present in 98% of cases. In contrast to the general impression, true paroxysmal hypertension is seen in only half of the cases. Paroxysms characterized by tachycardia, severe headache, palpitation, pallor or flushing, profuse perspiration, and feeling of "indigestion" occur spontaneously or are occasionally triggered by exercises, bending, urination, defecation, smoking, pressure from abdominal palpation, or induction of anesthesia. Sustained hypertension could mimic essential hypertension and may be accompanied by orthostatic hypotension due to blunted sympathetic reflexes. Other features of catecholamine excess include weight loss, nervousness, carbohydrate intolerance, and even frank diabetes mellitus. In addition to catecholamines, some pheochromocytoma may produce polypeptide hormones such as ACTH, causing Cushing's syndrome.

The laboratory verification of pheochromocytoma is achieved by the determination of catecholamines and their derivatives (metanephrines, normetanephrines, and vanillylmandelic acid (VMA) in timed urine specimens). Over 90% of cases of pheochromocytoma will be diagnosed by a single, properly performed assay of metanephrines and VMA in urine. The measurement of plasma catecholamine is usually reserved for difficult cases where the diagnosis cannot be established by assay of urinary catecholamines. The usefulness of plasma catecholamine assay is enhanced by the application of a suppression test. Both clonidine and pentolinium have no significant effect on blood levels of catecholamine in patients with pheochromocytoma, but decrease them in patients with essential hypertension [7,8]. The principle of the test is based on the fact that clonidine and pentolinium act by diminishing sympathetic activity in the brain stem, and thereby reduce circulating catecholamines in individuals with essential hypertension. Since pheochromocytomas are not innervated, their catecholamine secretory activities are not affected by these drugs. For localization of pheochromocytoma, computed tomography has replaced both angiography and venography as the procedure of choice in recent years (see Chap. 5) [15]. Adrenal medullary imaging can be successfully performed with [^{131}I]iodo-benzylguanidine, but clinical experiences for isotopic scanning of pheochromocytoma are still limited.

References

1. Abrams HL, Siegelmann SS, Adams DF (1982) Computed tomography versus ultrasound of the adrenal gland: a prospective study. Radiology 13:121
2. Abrams HL, Spiro R, Goldstein N (1950) Metastases in carcinoma. Cancer 3: 74
3. Anderson EE (1977) Nonfunctioning tumors of the adrenal gland. Urol Clin North America 4:263
4. Aron DC, Findling JW, Fitzgerald PA et al. (1981) Pituitary ACTH dependency of nodular adrenal hyperplasia in Cushing's syndrome. Am J Med 71: 302
5. Berglund G, Andersson O, Wilhelmsen L (1976) Prevalence of primary and secondary hypertension: studies in a random population sample. Br Med J 2:554
6. Bertagna C, Orth DN (1981) Clinical and laboratory findings and results of therapy in 58 patients with adrenocortical tumors admitted to a single medical center (1951 to 1978). Am J Med 71:855
7. Bravo EL, Tarazi RC, Foud FM et al. (1981) Clonidine-suppression test: useful aid in the diagnosis of pheochromocytoma. N Engl J Med 305: 623
8. Brown MJ, Jenner DA, Allison DJ et al. (1981) Increased sensitivity and accuracy of pheochromocytoma diagnosis achieved by the use of plasma-adrenaline estimates and a pentolinium suppression test. Lancet 1:174
9. Chrousos GP, Schuermeyer TH, Doppman J et al. (1985) Clinical applications of corticotropin-releasing factor. Ann Intern Med 102:344

10. Crapo L (1979) Cushing's syndrome: a review of diagnostic tests. Metabolism 28:955
11. Doppman JL, Oldfield E, Krudy AG et al. (1984) Petrosal sinus sampling for Cushing's syndrome: anatomical and technical considerations. Radiology 150:99
12. Glomset DA (1938) The incidence of metastases of malignant tumors to the adrenals. Am J Cancer 32:57
13. Hsu TH, Nay R (1984) Mass lesions of the adrenal gland: clinical considerations. In Siegelman SS (ed) Computed tomography of the kidneys and adrenals. Churchill Livingstone, New York, p 223
14. King DR, Lack EE (1979) Adrenal cortical carcinoma: a clinical and pathologic study of 49 cases. Cancer 44:239
15. Laursen K, Damgarrd-Pederson K (1980) CT for pheochromocytoma diagnosis. Am J Roentgenol 134:277
16. Nelson DH (1979) Cushing's syndrome: In: DeGroot LJ (ed) Endocrinology. Grune and Stratton, New York, p 1179
17. Streeten DHP, Tomycz N, Anderson GH (1979) Reliability of screening methods for the diagnosis of primary aldosteronism. Am J Med 67:403

Chapter 5

Imaging Techniques

D. R. Bodner, C. L. Schultz, and M. I. Resnick

Imaging of the Adrenal Gland

Accurate imaging of the adrenal glands is of great importance in evaluating abnormalities of these endocrine organs. Diseases affecting the adrenal glands may have profound systemic effects and definitive treatment is based upon careful endocrine evaluation and accurate adrenal imaging. Recent developments in imaging have improved our ability to detect adrenal abnormalities, which has led to more confident surgical management of these lesions. Intravenous urography with nephro-tomography was once the initial screening procedure for adrenal abnormalities, but this has been replaced with computed tomography (CT) and ultrasound. These newer imaging modalities have also diminished the need for invasive vascular studies although angiography is still sometimes needed to study the vascular supply of large tumors prior to surgery, and adrenal venous sampling and venography can be helpful in localizing small functioning tumors. In this chapter we will discuss the imaging techniques which are currently used and widely available for the evaluation of adrenal disorders. We will also examine two emerging techniques: magnetic resonance imaging (MRI) and [131I]metaiodobenzylguanidine (MIBG) scanning for pheochromocytomas.

Anatomy of the Adrenal Gland

The adrenals are composed of two distinct units: the outer cortex and the inner medulla. Each has a separate embryologic origin, the former being derived from mesoderm and the latter from ectoderm. The left gland is semilunar in shape, while the right is triangular (Fig. 5.1). The adrenals lie within Gerota's fascia in the retroperitoneum, superior and anterior medial to each kidney. The left adrenal gland is somewhat more inferior than the right and may extend down to the level of the renal hilum. Each gland is lateral to the adjacent crus of the diaphragm. The right adrenal gland is posterior to the inferior vena cava and the left is posterior to the stomach and pancreas.

The adrenal glands may be thought of as flattened structures folded upon themselves to form two limbs posteriorly and a ridge anteromedially. The appearance of the adrenal glands may vary at different levels on transverse images, such as that obtained with CT, due to prominence of either the medial or the lateral limb at a particular level.

The arterial supply to the adrenal glands originates primarily from three sources. Superiorly, the adrenals are supplied from branches of the inferior phrenic artery. The middle adrenal artery arises directly from the aorta, and the inferior adrenal artery is a branch of the renal artery.

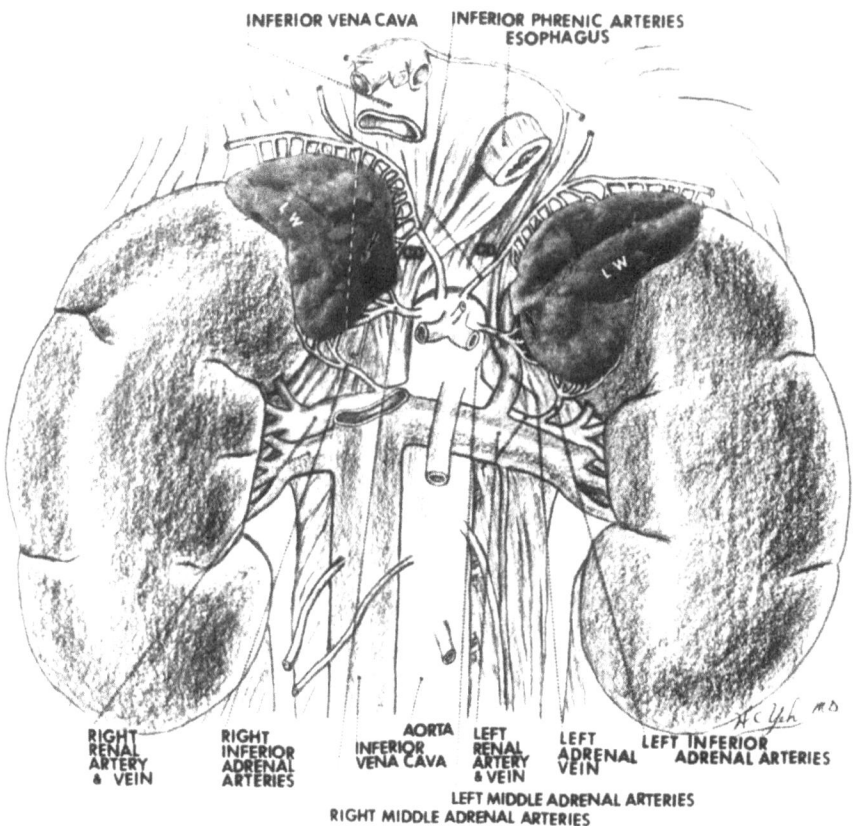

INFERIOR VENA CAVA   INFERIOR PHRENIC ARTERIES
                            ESOPHAGUS

RIGHT   RIGHT   AORTA   LEFT   LEFT   LEFT INFERIOR
RENAL   INFERIOR   INFERIOR   RENAL   ADRENAL ADRENAL ARTERIES
ARTERY   ADRENAL   VENA CAVA   ARTERY   VEIN
& VEIN   ARTERIES   & VEIN
                         LEFT MIDDLE ADRENAL ARTERIES
                    RIGHT MIDDLE ADRENAL ARTERIES

Fig. 5.1. The anatomic relationship of the adrenals to the kidneys, aorta, and inferior vena cava is shown along with its blood supply. *LW*, lateral wings. [36]

Abdominal Radiography, Urography, and Nephrotomography

Abdominal radiography and intravenous urography with nephrotomography were traditionally the initial radiographic screening examinations for adrenal abnormalities. Although these modalities can sometimes provide information about the adrenal glands, they cannot demonstrate normal adrenal glands or small masses and are, therefore, of little value in excluding adrenal abnormalities. An understanding of these modalities in adrenal disease is still important, however, since unsuspected adrenal abnormalities may sometimes first be discovered with these modalities.

Calcification in the region of the adrenal is easily noted on an abdominal radiograph obtained as a separate study or as the initial scout film for excretory urography (Fig. 5.2). It is important to confirm that the calcification is in the adrenal itself and not in adjacent organs; in this regard oblique films are sometimes helpful. It is important to recall that the adrenals are located not only superior but also anteromedial to each kidney. This will help to differentiate adrenal calcifications from calcifications in the kidney, gallbladder, pancreas, spleen, or vasculature.

Calcification is common in neuroblastoma, adrenal carcinoma, and adrenal cysts. The calcification seen in adrenal cysts is usually peripheral and curvilinear, while punctuate or stippled calcifications are more often seen in adrenal carcinoma and neuroblastoma [1,19,24]. Calcification can also be present within adrenal hemorrhage, adrenal adenoma, myelolipoma, pheochromocytoma, and granulomatous disease [13].

For excretory urography, contrast agents are administered in a drip infusion or bolus method after evaluation of the scout film. The bolus technique with adequate amounts of contrast provides optimal images of the kidney. Routine views of the kidney are obtained immediately after injection and at 5, 10, and 20 min after injection. Oblique films and delayed films are obtained as needed. Excretory

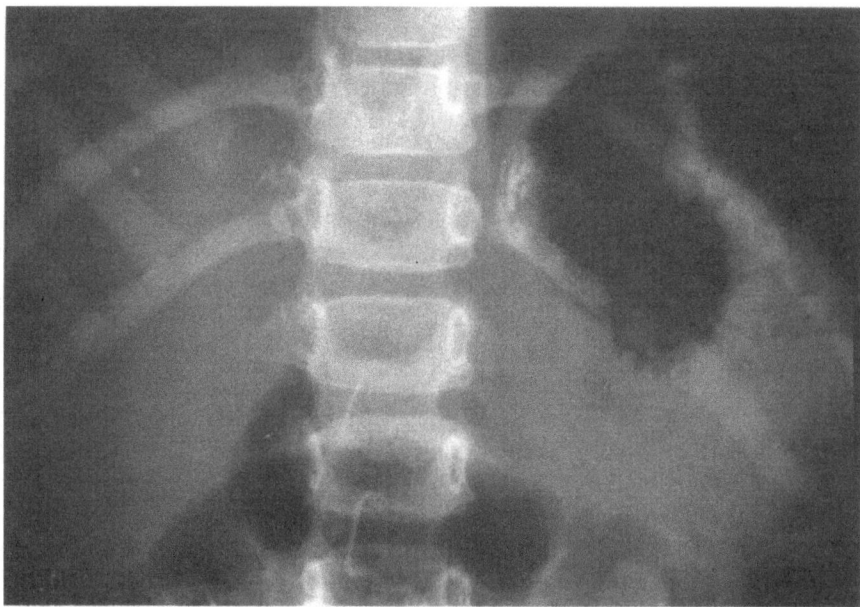

Fig. 5.2. Bilateral adrenal calcification noted on plain film of the abdomen secondary to neonatal adrenal hemorrhage.

urography is of little value in imaging the normal adrenal. However, with nephrotomography and adequate volumes of contrast material injected, the normal adrenal can be visualized in up to 50% of cases [8]. Adrenal masses can be directly visualized in some cases but are more often detected by their mass effect upon the kidney. A left adrenal tumor causes lateral displacement of the upper pole of the left kidney, whereas a right adrenal tumor will tend to displace the kidney downward (Fig. 5.3). The ability of excretory urography to suggest adrenal masses depends upon the size of the mass. If the

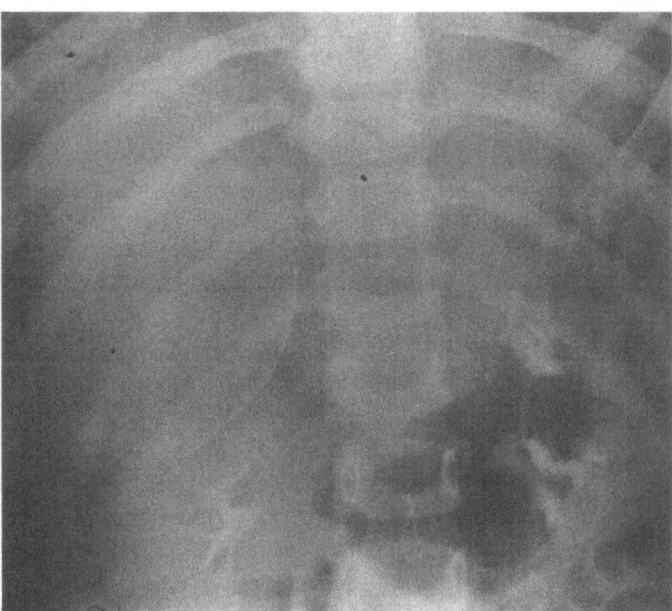

Fig. 5.3. Huge adrenal mass causing inferior displacement of the right kidney.

mass is less than 3 cm in diameter, the pyelogram will often be negative [8]. The detection rate for adrenal tumors such as pheochomocytoma and adrenal carcinoma is about 80% with excretory urography and tomography, but the rate of detection of aldosteronomas is significantly less since these are often small in size [3,19].

Adrenal Arteriography

Adrenal arteriography usually consists of aortography followed by selective cannulization and injection of the three sources of adrenal blood supply: the inferior phrenic artery superiorly, the middle adrenal artery, which originates from the aorta, and the inferior adrenal artery (Fig. 5.4), a branch of the renal artery. The selective catheteriza-

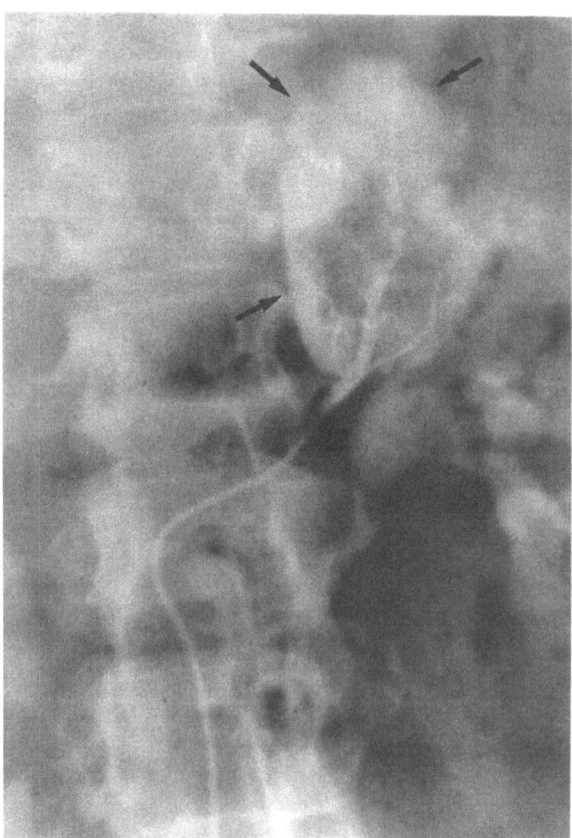

Fig. 5.4. Selective injection of the inferior adrenal artery showing an enlarged adrenal gland secondary to a ganglioneuroma (*arrows*). The collecting system of the left kidney is noted below the mass.

tion of the adrenal arteries is often difficult and requires considerable expertise. Large adrenal malignancies usually demonstrate irregular vessels and neovascularity. The advent of the noninvasive imaging modalities has largely eliminated the need for arteriography in the detection of adrenal disease. Arteriography remains helpful in the preoperative evaluation of the vascular supply of large adrenal tumors.

The diagnosis and localization of small and ectopic pheochromocytomas missed with CT scanning can sometimes be made with selective adrenal arteriography. Although pheochromocytomas can be avascular, they often have a characteristic pattern noted on the arteriogram. The adrenal artery is hypertrophied, undergoes fine reticular branching, and leads to a diffuse homogeneous blush pattern of enhancement [8]. Arterial blood pressure must be monitored carefully during adrenal arteriography, since arteriography can produce a severe hypertensive reaction in patients with pheochromocytoma. Appropriate pharmacologic treatment, such as phenoxybenzamine, must be readily available for these patients.

Adrenal Venous Sampling and Venography

Cannulization of the adrenal vein is performed and venous blood is sampled prior to venography. The venous blood is sent for appropriate analysis and is helpful in confirming the presence and localizing the position of functioning adrenal tumors. This technique is most helpful for aldosterone-producing tumors and is occasionally used in patients with pheochromocytomas [6,9]. In patients with primary hyperaldosteronism, adenomas produce unilateral aldosterone elevation while adrenal hyperplasia results in bilateral elevation of aldosterone. Although only 60%–70% of aldosteronomas can be localized with venography, nearly 100% can be identified when venous sampling [17]. The accuracy of adrenal venous sampling in patients with primary hyperaldosteronism exceeds that obtained with CT, since these tumors are sometimes too small reliably to detect with CT.

Adrenal venography is performed by retrograde injection of the adrenal vein after first obtaining venous blood samples as noted above. Venography

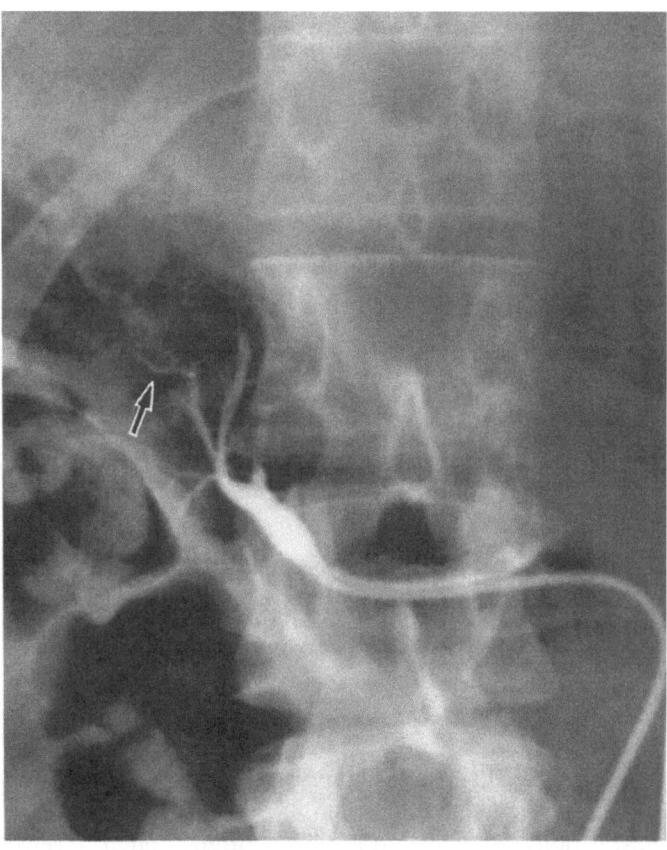

Fig. 5.5. Right adrenal venogram with a small intraadrenal mass displacing a branch of the adrenal vein (*arrow*).

requires only a single injection on each side because of the presence of a single adrenal vein. This is in contradistinction to arteriography, where selective injections of the three adrenal arteries are sometimes necessary. With venography, circumferential curving of the adrenal vein about the mass may be noted (Fig. 5.5). The "spokes of a wheel" may be seen within the mass and the adrenal vein wrapped circumferentially, about the mass. The venographic signs of malignancy include tumor nodules within the vein, which are seldom noted, and the development of accessory draining veins from the tumor [18]. The adrenal tumor may also obstruct or displace the adrenal vein.

The samples obtained for laboratory analysis with adrenal venous sampling are much more important than the images obtained with adrenal venography. The accuracy of adrenal venography is less than that of adrenal venous sampling and serious complications such as adrenal insufficiency or venous thrombosis can result. For these reasons when adrenal venous sampling is performed, a venogram is usually obtained but is now done with only a minimal injection of contrast to reduce the inci-

dence of complications. The radiographs obtained are intended primarily to verify the position of the catheter rather than to aid in tumor detection.

Retroperitoneal Pneumography

Retroperitoneal pneumography is mentioned for its historical importance, as it is no longer performed to image the adrenals. Prior to the development of arteriography and venography, retroperitoneal pneumography was performed after urography and nephrotomography as the next diagnostic test to image the adrenals. A needle was placed either directly into the flank or in the retrorectal space by placing the patient in the knee–chest position with the examiner's fingers in the rectum accurately to localize the retrorectal space. Once the needle was in a good position, 1000–1500 ml gas (air, carbon dioxide, or oxygen) was introduced via the needle into the retroperitoneum. An AP film and nephrotomograms were obtained (Fig. 5.6). The main

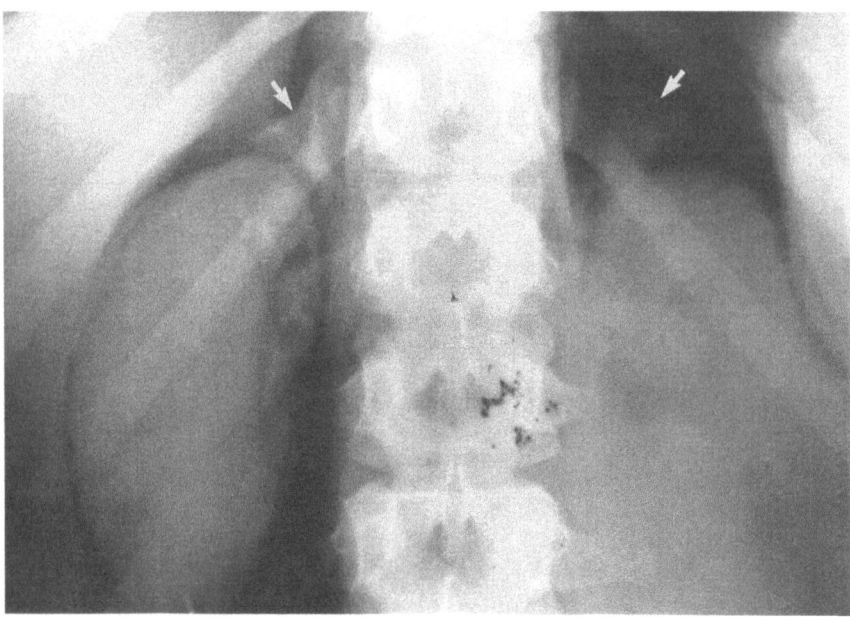

Fig. 5.6. Retroperitoneal pneumography. Both adrenal glands (*arrows*) appear normal on this AP film from a retroperitoneal pneumogram.

problem with the interpretation of this study was in obtaining adequate diffusion of the gas and the most serious complication of retroperitoneal pneumography was air embolism [25].

Ultrasonography

Ultrasound is a noninvasive technique that employs sound waves to image internal structures. The ultrasound transducer acts as both the transmitter and the receiver of the sound waves. The sound waves are initially produced by the transducer and are transmitted, absorbed, and reflected by internal structures. Reflection occurs at the interfaces of tissues with different acoustic impedance and the echoes produced are received by the transducer and recorded on a gray scale. Currently most sonographers employ real-time ultrasound, which provides a continuous display of the ultrasound image.

Ultrasound is the imaging method of choice for evaluating the adrenal glands in neonates, but it is much less useful in evaluating adrenal glands of adults and older children. Visualization of the right and left adrenal glands has been reported as 97% and 83% in neonates, but only 79% and 44% in adults [23,36]. The increased frequency of visu-

alization of adrenal glands in infants is related to their proportionately larger size, the paucity of retroperitoneal fat, and the proximity of the neonatal adrenal glands to the skin's surface. In adults, ultrasound identification of the normal adrenal gland is difficult because of the small size of the gland and because the acoustic texture of the adult adrenal is similar to surrounding structures. The examination is also sometimes limited by obesity or overlying bowel gas. For these reasons even the limited success rate in adults of 79% and 44% for visualization of the right and left adrenal glands requires meticulous scanning technique and considerable expertise and is unlikely to be matched in most institutions.

Ultrasound scans of the adrenals are done in the transverse plane anteriorly with the patient supine, and in the coronal plane through the flank with the patient supine or positioned somewhat obliquely on to the opposite side. The normal neonatal adrenal gland appears as a "V" or "Y" rotated 90° clockwise in coronal scans and shows a curvilinear configuration on transverse scans (Fig. 5.7). The thin echogenic medulla is easily distinguished from the thicker low-echogenicity cortex.

In adults the failure of ultrasound adequately to visualize normal adrenal glands produces a higher false-negative and false-positive rate than with CT [2]. Adrenal masses as small as 1.3 cm have been

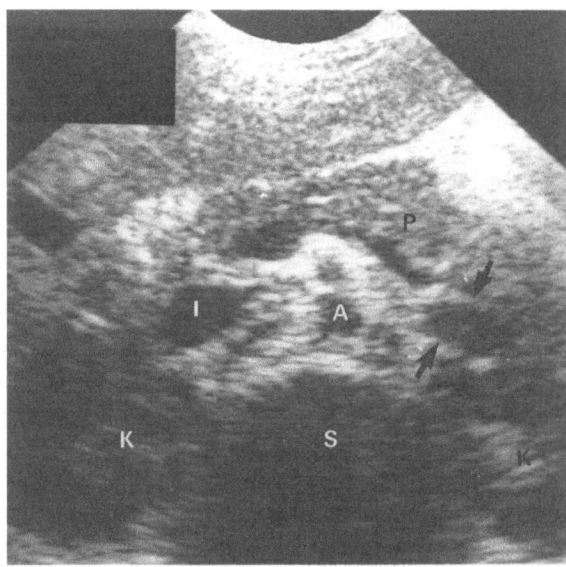

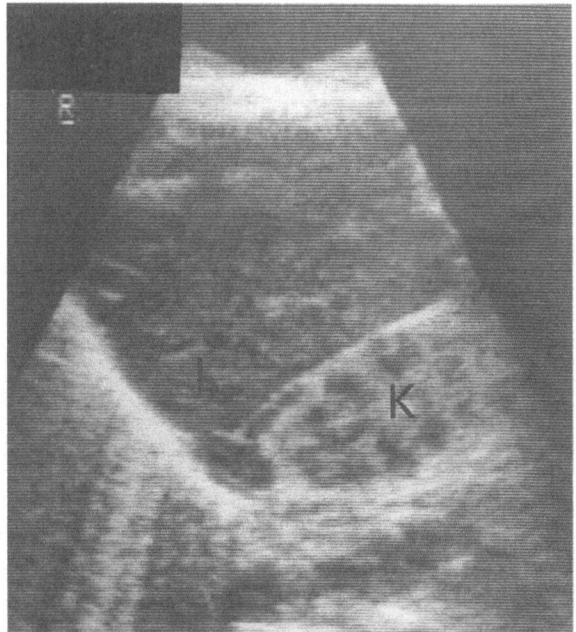

Fig. 5.8. A small left adrenal mass (*arrows*) about 1.4 cm in size is seen anterior to the kidney (*K*) and posterior to the pancreas (*P*). *A*, aorta; *S*, spine; *I*, inferior vena cava.

shadowing. Cystic areas within a mass may be noted and are due to hemorrhage or necrosis. Although most adrenal lesions have a nonspecific appearance, the diagnosis of an adrenal cyst can be reliably made if the lesion has smooth, thin walls, good through transmission of the ultrasound beam, and no internal echogenicity.

Computed Tomography

Computed tomography utilizes ionizing radiation, sensitive radiation detectors, and a computer to generate an image of the internal structures of the body based upon their relative densities. Low-density structures, such as fat and water, appear dark on CT images. High-density structures, such as bone, appear white, and soft tissues appear as varying shades of gray. Although the adrenal glands are similar in density to other nearby organs, in almost all adult patients there is sufficient retroperitoneal fat to allow excellent delineation of the adrenal glands. The characteristic shape and location of the adrenals also aids in their easy identification with CT. Because of CT's ability reliably to delineate normal as well as abnormal adrenal glands, it has become the imaging modality of choice for evaluating the adrenal glands in adults.

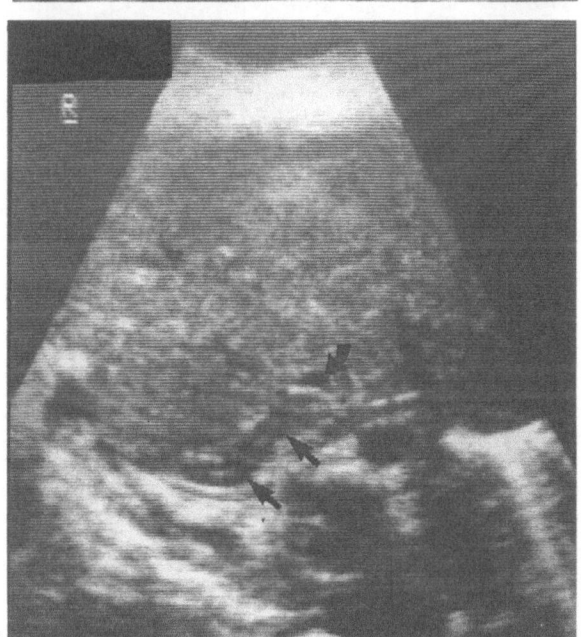

Fig. 5.7 a, b. Normal neonatal adrenal gland. **a** The right adrenal gland is seen posterior to the liver (*L*) and superior to the kidney (*K*) on this coronal scan. **b** A transverse image shows the right adrenal gland (*arrows*) posterior to the inferior vena cava (*curved arrow*). The thin echogenic medulla is easily distinguished from the cortex on this scan.

detected by ultrasound (Fig. 5.8) but reliable detection of adrenal masses usually only occurs with larger masses (greater than or equal to 3 cm) [36]. Most adrenal lesions have a similar appearance on ultrasound with adrenal tumors usually being poorly echogenic. Calcifications within a mass produce areas of intense echogenicity with acoustic

Routine abdominal scans are usually done with 1-cm-thick contiguous sections. Even with this routine abdominal technique, visualization of both normal adrenal glands has been reported to be virtually 100% [28,35]. When evaluating the adrenal glands specifically 4- or 5-mm contiguous or overlapping sections are used to aid in the resolution of small tumors. Intravenous contrast material is not necessary to evaluate the adrenal glands with CT, but is sometimes used to evaluate the relative vascularity of an adrenal lesion. Oral contrast material is also not needed for adrenal evaluation, but is often given since it is harmless and may clarify other regions contained on the CT image. The appearance of the normal adrenal glands can vary from patient to patient and from scan to scan on the same patient. These variations are due to differences in orientation relative to the transverse scanning plane and the relative prominence of the individual adrenal limbs at different levels. The right adrenal gland is most commonly seen as a thin line extending posteriorly from the inferior vena cava between the liver and ipsilateral crus of the diaphragm (Fig. 5.9). The right adrenal gland may also be seen as an inverted "V" or "Y." The shape of the left adrenal gland is usually that of an inverted "Y" or "V" or it may have a triangular configuration (Fig. 5.10). The left adrenal is usually located anterior and superior to the upper pole of the left kidney, posterior to the pancreas, and lateral to the left crus of the diaphragm and aorta (Fig. 5.11).

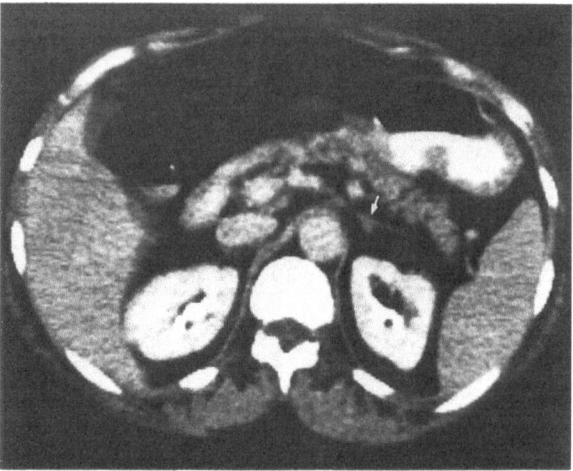

Fig. 5.10. A normal left adrenal gland (*arrow*) is seen as an inverted "V," posterior to the pancreas and anterior to the kidney.

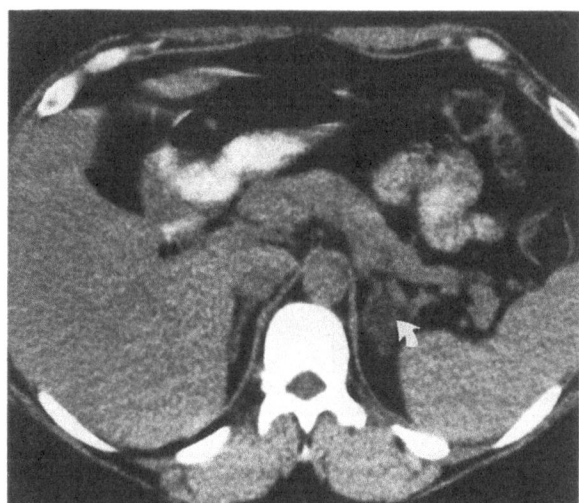

Fig. 5.11. A small left adrenal mass (*arrow*) causes the adrenal gland to appear oval. A normal right adrenal gland is seen.

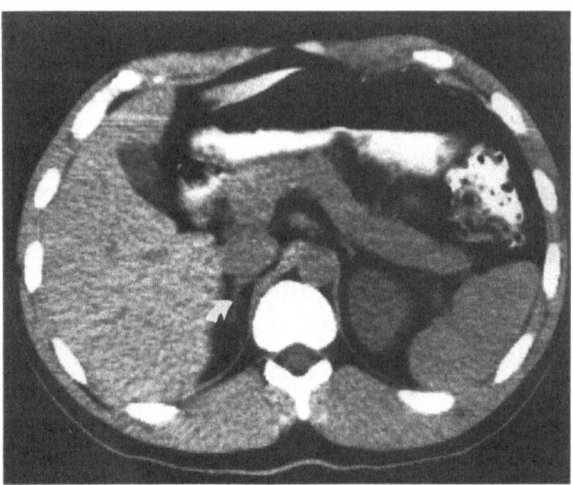

Fig. 5.9. A normal right adrenal gland (*curved arrow*) is seen posterior to the inferior vena cava, medial to the liver, and lateral to the crus of the diaphragm.

Measurements of adrenal size have been made with computed tomography and these measurements are comparable to surgical and autopsy studies [20]. The length (cephalad to caudad dimension) is usually 2–4 cm; the width (anterior to posterior dimension) is usually 1 cm or less, with most adrenal glands being about 5 or 6 mm thick. These measurements are seldom needed in clinical practice to determine if an adrenal gland is normal or abnormal. An assessment of the overall size, shape, and configuration, as well as an evaluation of the margins of the adrenal glands, is more important than actual measurements.

The margins of a normal adrenal gland are straight or slightly concave. Hyperplasia causes a generalized increase in the size of the adrenal glands but does not usually alter the configuration or margins of the glands. Comparison with the ipsilateral crus of the diaphragm is sometimes helpful in identifying hyperplastic glands since the thickness of normal adrenal glands is usually no greater than that of the crus. The distinction between normal and hyperplastic glands can be difficult and is generally not clinically important. Patients with adrenal hyperfunction secondary to a pituitary adenoma may have normal or hyperplastic glands on CT, and are easily distinguished from those patients with an adrenal adenoma as the cause of Cushing's syndrome.

An adrenal mass causes the normally straight or concave margins to become convex, making the gland oval or round. Tumors as small as 5 mm have been reported with CT, although usually a lesion must be 1 cm or greater to be reliably detected [34] (Fig. 5.11). Small masses may be seen on only a single CT section arising from one limb of the gland. Careful scrutiny of multiple sections throughout the entire adrenal gland is, therefore, necessary to exclude a mass. Large adrenal masses are easily detected with CT, but sometimes the origin of a very large mass may not be apparent (Fig. 5.12). Visualization of a normal adrenal gland on the side of the mass excludes adrenal origin, but failure to see a normal adrenal gland does not insure adrenal origin since a large mass may compress and obliterate the normal adrenal gland.

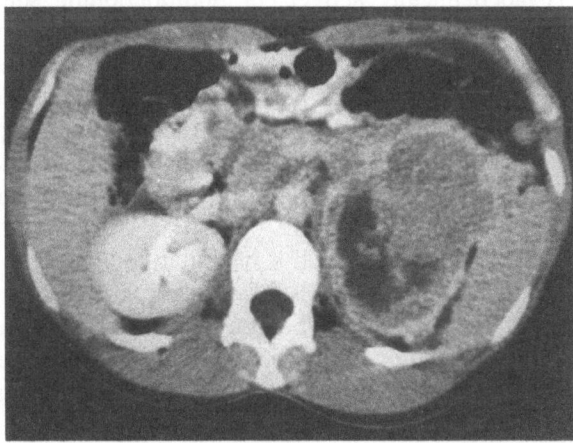

Fig. 5.12. A large left adrenal mass. The site of origin was not readily apparent from the CT scan.

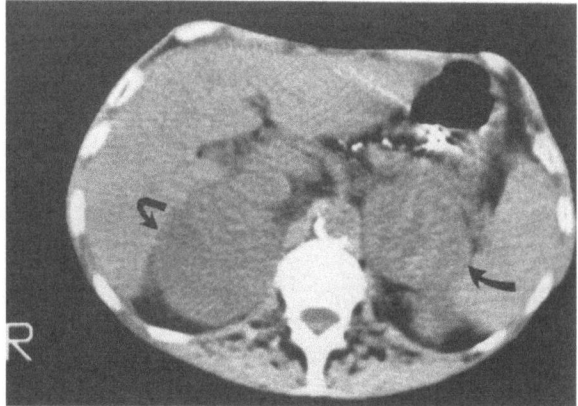

Fig. 5.13. Large bilateral adrenal masses secondary to metastatic disease (*arrows*).

The CT appearance of most adrenal masses is nonspecific, although certain features may suggest the correct diagnosis. The presence of an extremely large mass should raise the possibility of an adrenal carcinoma in an adult or a neuroblastoma in a child. Bilateral masses, in a patient with a primary carcinoma elsewhere in the body, usually represent metastases to the adrenal glands (Fig. 5.13); but bilateral adenomas have also been reported in these patients. An adrenal cyst can be distinguished from other adrenal lesions by its sharp margination, water density, and lack of contrast enhancement. Since adenomas may also appear low in density due to a high lipid content, ultrasound is sometimes needed to confirm the diagnosis of an adrenal cyst. Myelolipoma, which is a rare adrenal tumor composed of fat and bone marrow elements, has a characteristic CT appearance because of its high fat content (Fig. 5.14). The density of these tumors is much less than that seen with other adrenal lesions and is similar to that of subcutaneous or retroperitoneal fat.

With the widespread use of CT scanning and its accuracy in imaging the adrenal glands, the clinical problem arises of how to manage the incidentally discovered adrenal mass [10,16] (Fig. 5.15). Unsuspected adrenal masses are found in 0.6% of upper abdominal CT scans [10]. This is not surprising since nonfunctioning, benign adrenal adenomas have been reported to occur in 1.4%–8.7% of patients in autopsy series [11,14,26,29]. The diagnostic approach to an unsuspected adrenal mass in a patient with no known malignancy elsewhere must determine if the mass is biochemically active and if it is an adrenal carcinoma. If a mass produces symptoms of adrenal hyperfunction, it should

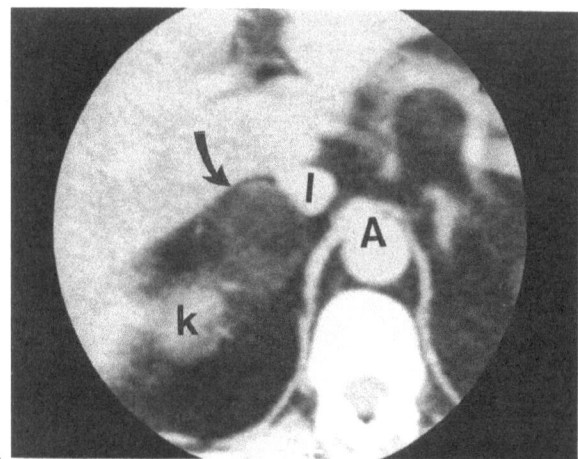

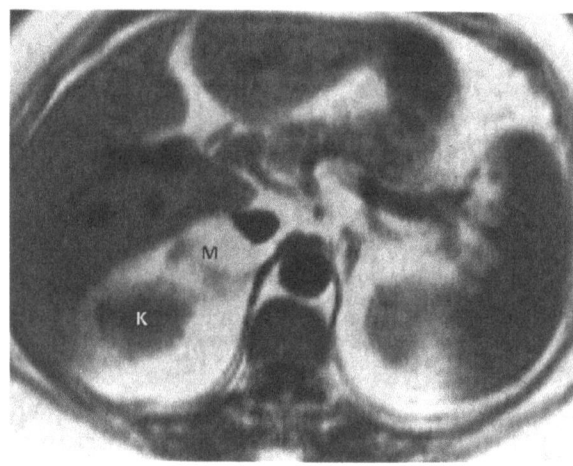

Fig. 5.14 a, b. Myelolipoma of the right adrenal gland. a CT scan shows a right adrenal mass (*curved arrow*) between the inferior vena cava (*I*) and kidney (*K*). The density of the mass is similar to the retroperitoneal fat indicating the fatty content of the tumor. *A*, aorta. b MRI of the same patient again shows the characteristic appearance of a myelolipoma (*M*). *K*, kidney. [33]

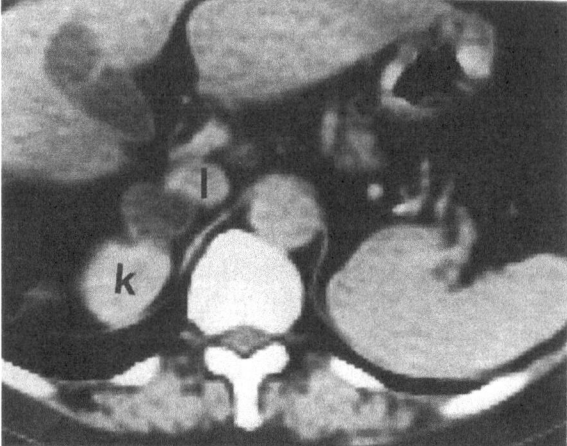

Fig. 5.15. An incidentally discovered adrenal mass between the inferior vena cava (*I*) and kidney (*K*). Subsequent evaluation determined the mass to be a nonfunctioning adenoma.

be removed whether it is an adenoma, carcinoma, or pheochromocytoma. To distinguish between a nonfunctioning adrenal carcinoma and a nonfunctioning adenoma, the most reliable criterion appears to be size. Adrenal carcinomas are extremely rare lesions compared with nonfunctioning adenomas and are usually quite large at the time of discovery. Any lesion 6 cm or greater should be considered a possible adrenal carcinoma.

A rational approach to the evaluation and treatment of unsuspected adrenal masses has been developed by Copeland and is shown in Fig. 5.16 [5]. If clinical signs of Cushing's syndrome, pheochromocytoma, or aldosteronoma are present, surgical removal should be performed once the workup is complete. If the unsuspected adrenal mass is greater than 6 cm by CT and solid in consistency, biochemical assessment and surgical removal should be the approach because of the possibility of carcinoma in this group. If the mass is greater than 6 cm and cystic, cyst puncture under CT guidance should be performed. If the aspirate is bloody, the patient is subjected to biochemical evaluation and surgery, whereas if it is clear, the evaluation is terminated. All masses less than 6 cm should be biochemically evaluated, and surgically removed if found to be active. Following negative biochemical evaluations and for cystic masses, needle aspiration can be performed, but the mass can be assumed to be benign if it shows typical CT and ultrasound characteristics of a cyst. If the cyst is punctured, clear fluid would terminate the evaluation while surgical removal is suggested if a bloody aspirate is obtained. For solid masses less than 6 cm in diameter, biochemical evaluation is performed and surgical removal is preferred when the mass is biochemically active. For nonfunctioning solid masses less than 6 cm in diameter, repeat CT evaluation is performed at 2, 6, and 18 months. If the mass enlarges, repeat biochemical assessment and surgical removal is indicated. If there is no change over this time interval, the mass is assumed to represent a nonfunctioning adenoma and is left alone.

This logical approach is helpful in managing the incidental adrenal mass. Statistically, the majority of adrenal masses are benign and this approach is geared to remove the biochemically active masses and the masses with a higher likelihood of malignancy. This approach does not, however, apply to those patients with a known malignancy. Any size mass in a cancer patient could represent adrenal

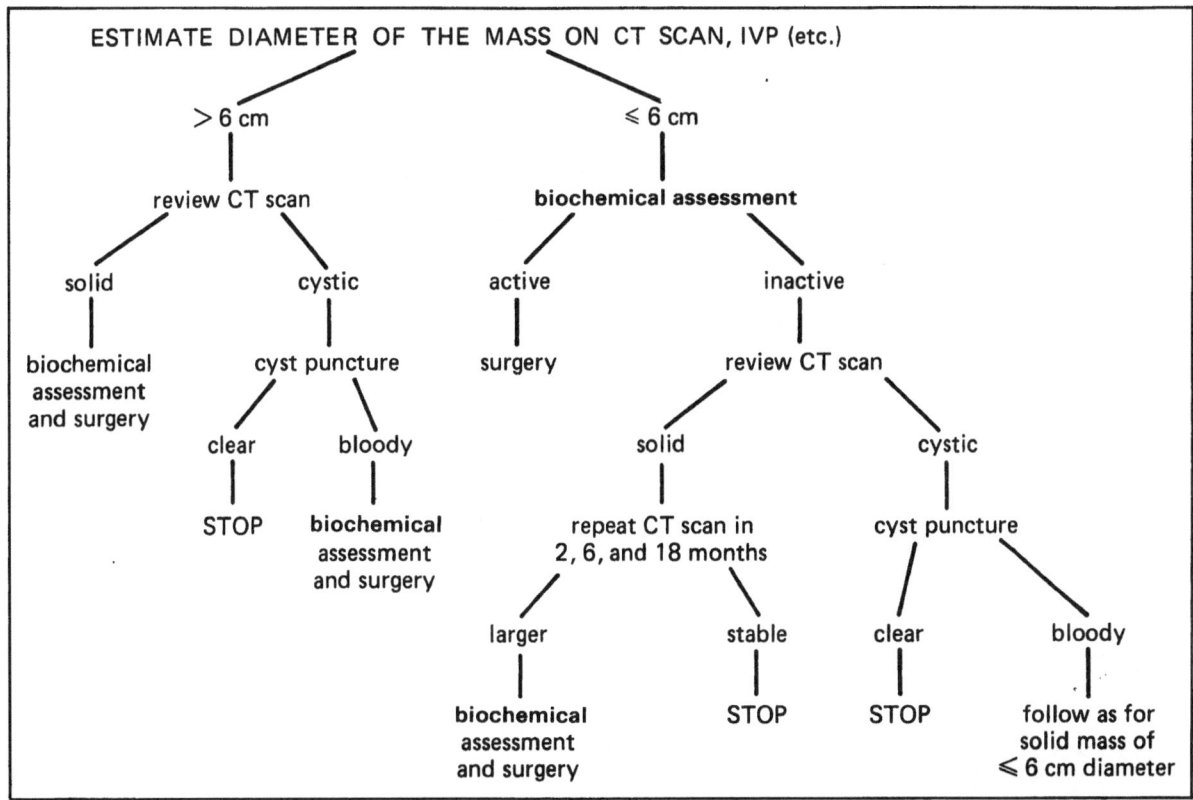

Fig. 5.16. Evaluation of an incidentally discovered adrenal mass. [5]

metastases unless it has the typical appearance of a cyst or myelolipoma. In these patients percutaneous biopsy with CT guidance should be performed if the presence of an adrenal metastasis would affect the patient's therapy [4].

Magnetic Resonance Imaging of the Adrenal

Magnetic resonance imaging (MRI) is the newest of the sectional imaging techniques. This technique uses a magnet and radiofrequency (RF) pulses to create a computer-generated image. The patient is placed within a strong magnet and exposed to strong RF pulses. The patient's magnetic atomic nuclei (primarily hydrogen nuclei) absorb energy from the RF pulses, which changes the direction of their magnetic field. After each RF pulse these nuclei emit energy as RF signals as they return to their equilibrium state. These signals are detected by a

receiving coil and used to produce an image. Advantages of MRI over CT include the lack of ionizing radiation, superior contrast resolution, and the ability to obtain images in the sagittal, coronal, or axial plane.

The configuration of the adrenal glands as visualized with axial magnetic resonance images is identical to that seen with CT. The normal adrenal glands can be consistently visualized with MRI at a rate comparable to CT [21,28]. Normal adrenal glands appear low in intensity and are outlined by the high-intensity retroperitoneal fat (Fig. 5.17). The intensity of the normal adrenal glands is less than that of the liver and renal cortex. In patients with adrenal hyperplasia and in some normal persons, MRI demonstrates corticomedullary differentiation, with the cortex appearing more intense than the medulla due to the higher lipid content of the cortex.

Magnetic resonance imaging can easily demonstrate adrenal lesions that enlarge and distort the gland (Fig. 5.18). As with CT, the MRI appearance of adrenal lesions is not specific except for myelolipomas, which show a characteristic intensity due

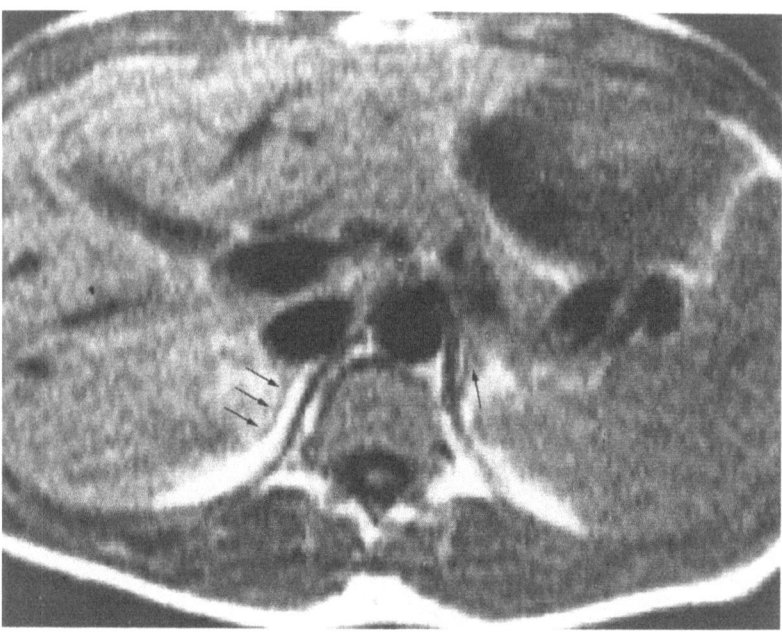

Fig. 5.17. Both adrenal glands are well visualized with MRI (*arrows*).

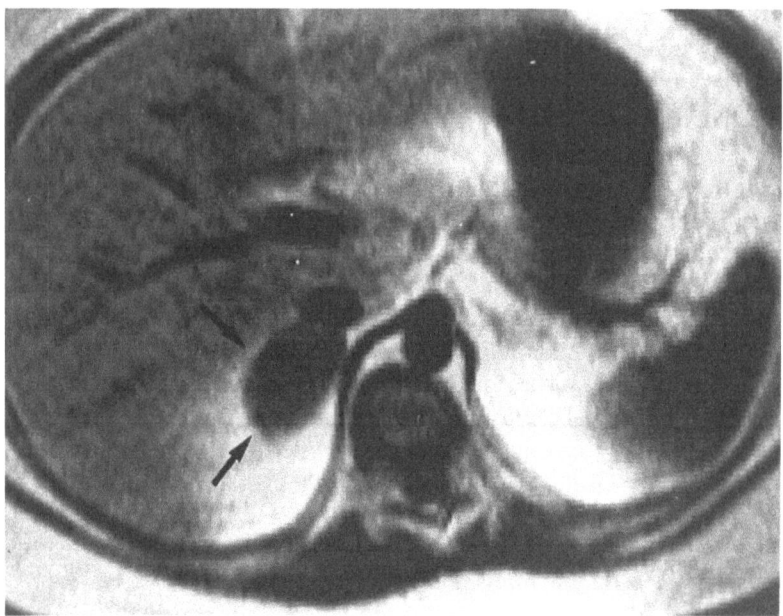

Fig. 5.18. Right adrenal adenoma (*arrows*) as visualized with MRI in a patient with Cushing's syndrome.

to their high fat content (Fig. 5.14b). No prospective comparisons of MRI and CT have been performed for the detection of small masses. The spatial resolution of MRI is currently less than that of CT and abdominal MRI is often degraded by artifact from respiratory motion [27]. For these reasons it is doubtful that MRI will surpass CT in the detection of small adrenal masses without major technical improvements. MRI is also unable to detect calcifications, which is a serious drawback in adrenal imaging, since the presence of calcifications is an important feature in several adrenal lesions (Fig. 5.19). MRI can, however, provide direct coronal or sagittal images which are sometimes useful in surgical planning. Since experience is limited with MRI of the adrenal glands, further studies will be

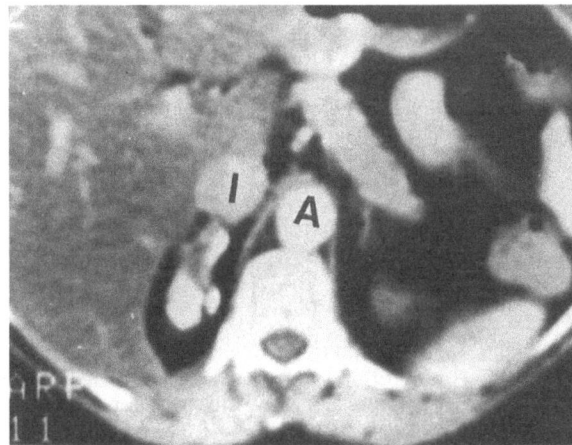

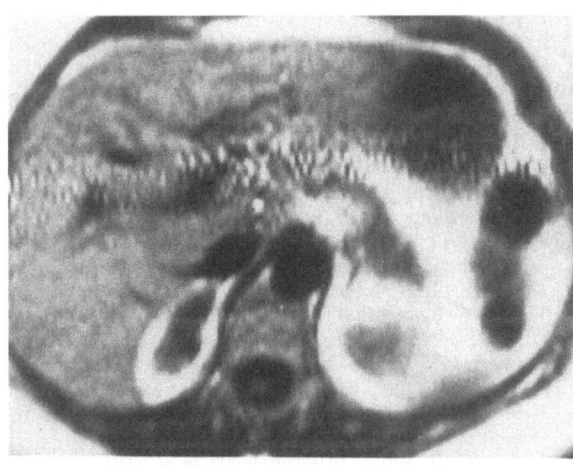

Fig. 5.19. a CT scan shows a right adrenal mass with calcifications secondary to an old adrenal hemorrhage. *I*, inferior vena cava; *A*, aorta. b MRI also shows the right adrenal mass but the calcifications are not apparent.

have been detected as areas of unilateral increased activity with this technique. Adrenal hyperplasia secondary to a pituitary tumor appears as bilaterally symmetric activity. Because of high false-negative rates and the accuracy of CT and adrenal venous sampling in localizing functioning adenomas, there has been little interest in radioisotope scans of the adrenal cortex [12,32].

There have been some recent reports of encouraging results with the localization of pheochromocytomas using [131I]metaiodobenzylguanidine ([131I]MIBG) [30,31]. The molecular structure of this compound resembles norepinephrine and it is concentrated in catecholamine storage areas, such as the adrenal medulla and in pheochromocytomas. Scans of the entire body are obtained at 24, 48, and 72 h after injection. The normal adrenal medulla is usually too small to be seen and so any focal collection of [131I]MIBG will almost always represent a pheochromocytoma. There are advantages to [131I]MIBG in the localization of a pheochromocytoma. Images of the entire body are obtained, which is impractical with CT. Surgical slips and scar tissue, which can make CT recognition of recurrent pheochromocytoma difficult, have no effect on [131I]MIBG. There are, however, several drawbacks to [131I]MIBG scanning. The isotope is not generally available, the examination takes several days to complete, and the radiation dose to the adrenal glands is greater than with CT. False-negatives also occur in about 10%–20% of the cases. For these reasons and because of the high accuracy of CT in detection of adrenal pheochromocytomas, [131I]MIBG is unlikely to replace CT as the initial imaging study [33]. It may prove most beneficial in the evaluation of those patients with well-documented laboratory evidence of pheochromocytoma and negative CT examinations of the abdomen, and in the detection of recurrent and metastatic disease.

required to determine the exact role of this new imaging technique in the evaluation of adrenal pathology.

Radioisotope Scanning

Radioactive cholesterol derivatives, such as [131I]19-iodocholesterol and NP-59, have been used in the evaluation of disorders of the adrenal cortex [22]. Adenomas producing Cushing's syndrome, adrenal remnants following bilateral adrenalectomy, and aldosterone-producing adenomas

Perspective

Great progress has been made in the past 2 decades in adrenal imaging. CT is currently the modality of choice for imaging the adrenal glands in adults, due to its ability reliably to detect normal and abnormal adrenal glands. In infants the best adrenal images are obtained with ultrasound. For children ultrasound should be the initial imaging modality but if a satisfactory evaluation is not obtained or more information is needed, CT is then performed.

Computed tomography and ultrasound have reduced the need for the more invasive diagnostic studies. Arteriography is primarily limited to presurgical planning in large adrenal lesions. Adrenal venous sampling, however, is still required accurately to localize aldosterone-producing tumors when the CT results are negative or equivocal.

Computed tomography and ultrasound have contributed to the safety and success of surgical management of adrenal disorders. The widespread use of these imaging technologies has sometimes led to unexpected clinical problems such as the management of an unsuspected adrenal mass. These patients must be evaluated in a rational manner, and experience clearly indicates that most of these incidental adrenal masses are benign and do not require surgical intervention.

References

1. Abeshouse GA, Goldstein RB, Abeshouse BS (1959) Adrenal cysts. Review of the literature and report of three cases. J Urol 81:711
2. Abrams HI, Siegelman SS, Adams DF et al. (1982) Computed tomography versus ultrasound of the adrenal gland: a prospective study. Radiology 143:121–128
3. Bennet AH, Harrison JH, Thorn GW (1971) Neoplasms of the adrenal gland. J Urol 106:607
4. Bernardino ME, Walther MM, Phillips VM et al. (1985) CT-guided adrenal biopsy: accuracy, safety, and indications. AJR 144:67–69
5. Copeland PM (1983) The incidentally discovered adrenal mass. Ann Intern Med 98(6):940–945
6. Dunnick NR, Doppman JL, Gill JR et al. MF (1982) Localization of functional adrenal tumors by computed tomography and venous sampling. Radiology 142:429–433
7. Dunnick NR, Heaston D, Halvorsen R et al. (1982) CT appearance of adrenal cortical carcinoma. J Comput Assist Tomogr 6: 978–982
8 Ferris EJ, Seibert JJ (ed) (1980) Adrenal gland. In : Urinary tract and adrenal glands: imaging and diagnosis. Grune and Stratton, New York, pp 473–520
9 Geisinger MA, Zelch MG, Bravo EL et al. (1983) Primary hyperaldosteronism: comparison of CT. adrenal venography, and venous sampling. AJR 141:299–302
10. Glazier HS, Weyman PJ, Sagel SS et al. (1982) Non-functioning adrenal masses: incidental discovery on computed tomography. Am J Roentgenol 139:81–85
11. Hedeland H, Ostberg G, Hokfelt B (1968) On the prevalence of adrenocortical adenomas in an autopsy material in relationship to hypertension and diabetes. Acta Med Scand 184:211–214
12. Herwig KR, Sondra LP III (1979) Usefulness of adrenal venography and iodocholesterol scan in adrenal surgery. J Urol 122:7
13. Jarvis JL, Jenkins D, Sosman MC et al. (1954) Roentgenologic observations in Addison's disease: a review of 120 cases. Radiology 62:16
14. Kokko JP, Brown TC, Berman MM (1967) Adrenal adenoma and hypertension. Lancet 1:468–470
15. Kramer DM (1984) Basic principles of magnetic resonance imaging. Radiol Clin N Am 22: 765–778
16. Mitnick JS, Bosniak MA, Megibow AJ et al. (1983) Non-functioning adrenal adenomas discovered incidentally on computed tomography. Radiology 148:495–499
17. Mitty HA, Yeh HC (1982) Aldosteronism. In: Radiology of the adrenals with sonography and CT. Saunders, Philadelphia, pp 116–135
18. Mitty HA, Yeh HC (1982) Cushing's syndrome. In: Radiology of the adrenals with sonography and CT. Saunders, Philadelphia, pp 80–115
19. Mitty HA, Yeh HC (1982) Modalities and techniques. In: Radiology of the adrenals with sonography and CT. Saunders, Philadelphia, pp 17–63
20. Montagne, JP, Kressell HY, Korobkin M, et al. (1978) Computed tomography of the normal adrenal glands. AJR 130:963–966
21. Moon KL, Hricak H, Crooks LE, et al. (1973) Nuclear magnetic resonance imaging of the adrenal gland. A preliminary report. Radiology 147: 155–160
22. Older RA, Moore AV Jr., Glenn JF, et al. (1984) Diagnosis of adrenal disorders. Radiol Clin N Am 22:433–455
23. Oppenheimer DA, Carroll BA, Yousem S (1983) Sonography of the normal neonatal adrenal gland. Radiology 146:157–160
24. Pickering RS, Hartman GW, Weeks RE et al. (1975) Excretory urographic localization of adrenal cortical tumors and pheochromocytomas. Radiology 114:345
25. Ranson CL, Landers RR, McLelland R (1956) Air embolism following retroperitoneal pneumography: a nation-wide survey. J Urol 76:664
26. Russi S, Blumenthal HT, Gray SH (1945) Small adenomas of the adrenal cortex in hypertension and diabetes. Arch Intern Med 76:248–291
27. Schultz CL, Alfidi RJ, Nelson AD et al. (1984) The effect of motion on two-dimensional Fourier transformation magnetic resonance images. Radiology 152:117–121
28. Schultz CL, Haaga JR Fletcher BD, et al. (1984) Magnetic resonance imaging of the adrenal glands: a comparison with computed tomography. AJR 143:1235–1240
29. Shamma AH, Goddard JW, Sommers SC (1958). A study of the adrenal status in hypertension. J Chronic Dis 8:587–595
30. Sisson JC, Shapiro B, Beierwalters WH et al. (1984) Locating pheochromocytomas by scintigraphy using ^{131}I-meta-iodobenzylguanidine. Cancer J Clinic 34:86–92
31. Swensen SJ, Brown MO, Sheps SG, et al. (1985) Use of ^{131}I-MIBG scintigraphy in the evaluation of suspected pheochromocytoma. Mayo Clin Proc 60: 229–304
32. Weinberger MH, Grim CE, Hollifeld JW (1979) Primary aldosteronism. Ann Intern Med 90:386–395
33. Welch TJ, Sheedy PF II, van Heerden JA et al. (1983) Pheochromocytoma: value of computed tomography. Radiology 148:501–503
34. Weyman PJ, Glazer HS (1983) The adrenals. In: Lee JK, Sagel SS, Stanley RJ (eds) Computed body tomography. Raven Press, New York, pp 379–392
35. Wilms G, Baert A, Marchal G et al. (1979) Computed tomography of the normal adrenal glands: correlative study with autopsy specimens. J Comput Assist Tomogr 3:467–469
36. Yeh HC (1980) Sonography of the adrenal glands: normal and small masses. AJR 135: 1167–1177
37. Yeh H (1984) Ultrasound of the adrenal. In: Resnick MI, Sanders RC (eds) Ultrasound in urology. Williams and Wilkins, Baltimore, pp 285–306

Chapter 6

Adrenal Disorders in Childhood

S. A. Chalew

Introduction

Effect of Adrenal Disorders on Normal Growth and Development in Childhood

Growth and development are sensitive indicators of well-being in childhood. Careful monitoring of growth and development in the pediatric patient is an invaluable technique for clinical assessment and follow-up that is unavailable in the evaluation of adult patients. Many abnormalities in childhood may initially come to clinical attention due to a perturbation of normal growth and development. The following discussion focuses on the application of traditional assessments of growth and development with newer endocrine diagnostic and imaging techniques for evaluation of adrenal disorders in children.

Functional Adrenal Units

For the sake of simplicity, the adrenal can be conceptualized as three separate functional units under three independent regulatory mechanisms. Clinical presentation of adrenal disease in childhood often gives symptoms and signs that localize the disorder to one or more of the adrenal functional units.

1. Cortisol, the body's major glucocorticoid, is secreted from the zonae fasciculata and reticularis of the adrenal cortex. Cortisol is essential for life and exerts diverse influence throughout the body, affecting the metabolism of carbohydrate, lipid and protein, immunologic and inflammatory responses, cell growth, integrity of the cardiovascular and central nervous systems, and bone mineral metabolism. Cortisol release from the adrenal is regulated by pituitary adrenocorticotropic hormone (ACTH). ACTH secretion from the pituitary is in turn regulated by higher centers in the CNS. Cortisol exerts a negative feedback on pituitary ACTH secretion. Thus an inability to secrete cortisol leads to a compensatory increase in ACTH secretion. Cortisol secretion has a circadian pattern, and blood levels are generally higher in the morning and decline in the evening hours.

2. Aldosterone, the body's major mineralocorticoid, is secreted from cells in the zona glomerulosa of the adrenal cortex. Aldosterone acts on the distal tubal of the kidney to retain sodium in exchange for potassium. Aldosterone deficiency leads to sodium wasting, hyponatremia, hypovolemia, hyperkalemia, and acidosis. Aldosterone secretion is regulated through the renin-angiotensin system. Hypovolemia, hyponatremia, and hyperkalemia stimulate renin-angiotensin activity for release of aldosterone to restore homeostasis. Impaired secretion of aldosterone leads to a compensatory increase in activity of the renin-angiotensin system. Conversely, mineralocorticoid excess suppresses renin activity.

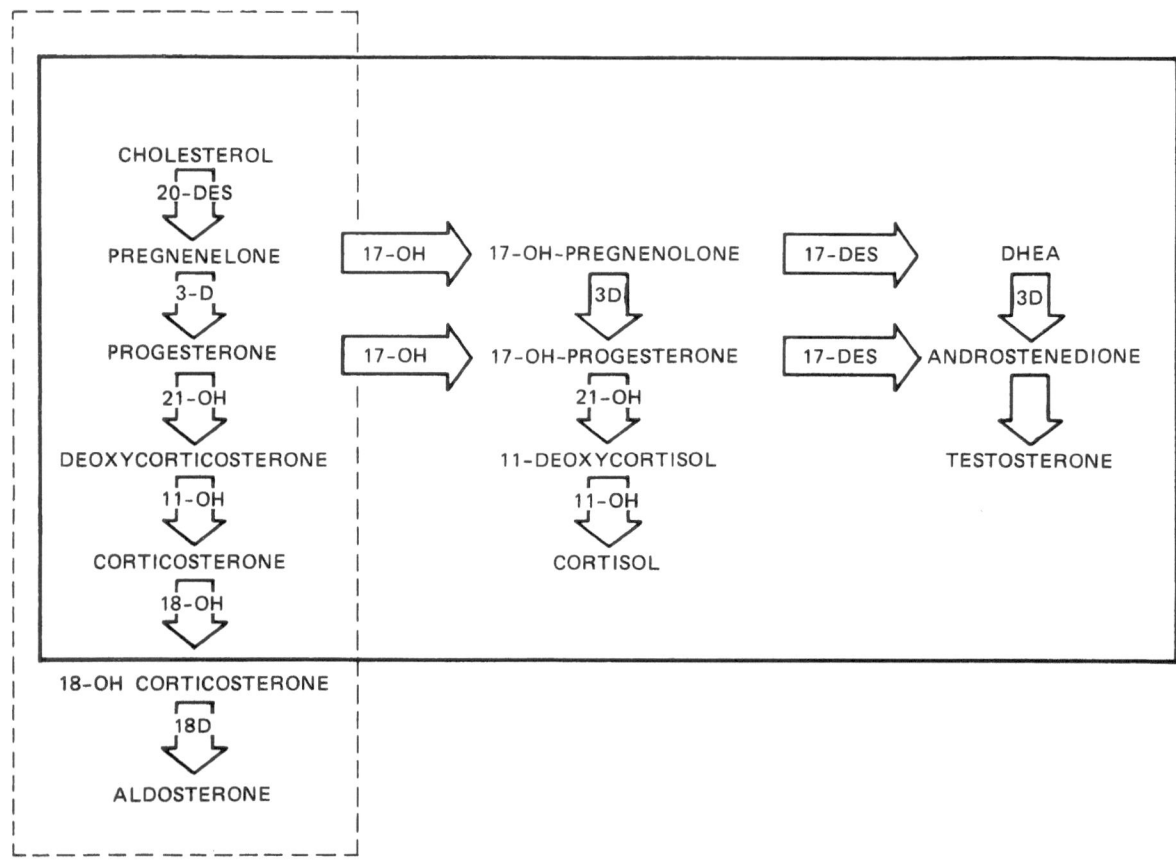

Fig. 6.1. The major steroidogenic pathways in the adrenal. The *solid rectangle* encloses the predominant pathways in the zona fasciculata. *The rectangle with the broken line* encloses the predominant pathway for the zona glomerulosa. Enzyme abbreviations: *17-DES*, 17,20-desmolase; *20-DES*, 20,22-desmolase; *3D*, 3-beta-hydroxy-dehydrogenase; *18D*, 18-hydroxy-dehydrogenase; *11-OH*, 11-hydroxylase; *17-OH*, 17-hydroxylase; *18-OH*, 18-hydroxylase; *21-OH*, 21-hydroxylase.

Although the zona fasciculata contains some of the enzymes necessary to produce mineralocorticoids, the final enzymatic step can only be completed in the zona glomerulosa.

3. Catecholamines, primarily epinephrine, are secreted from the chromaffin cells of the adrenal medulla in response to the sympathetic nervous system regulation. Circulating plasma epinephrine has a role in maintaining cardiovascular tone and carbohydrate metabolism.

Disorders of the Adrenal Cortex

Disorders Due to Impairment of Adrenocorticoid Hormone Secretion

Enzymatic Blocks in Steroidogenesis (Congenital Adrenal Hyperplasia)

21-Hydroxylase Deficiency. The most frequently encountered disorders of the adrenal glands in childhood are caused by defects in the enzymatic production of cortisol and aldosterone. Deficiency of the 21-hydroxylase enzyme is the most commonly encountered enzymatic defect (Fig. 6.1). The 21-hydroxylase enzyme catalyzes the conversion of 17-hydroxyprogesterone to 11-deoxycortisol in the pathway to cortisol, and also catalyzes progesterone to deoxycorticosterone in the steroidogenesis of aldosterone. Thus, deficiency of the 21-hydroxylase

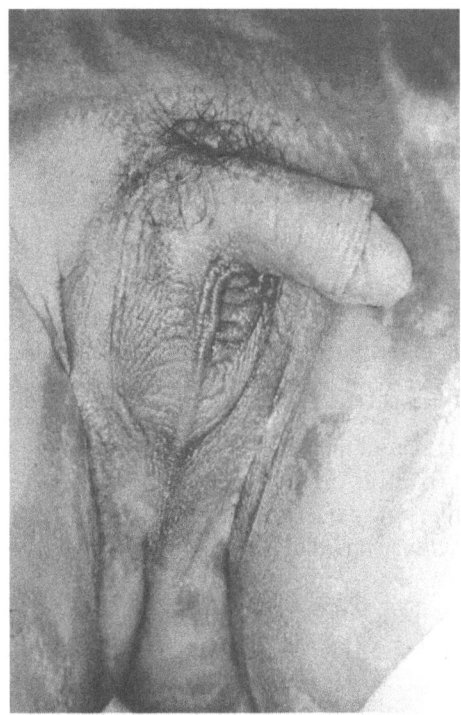

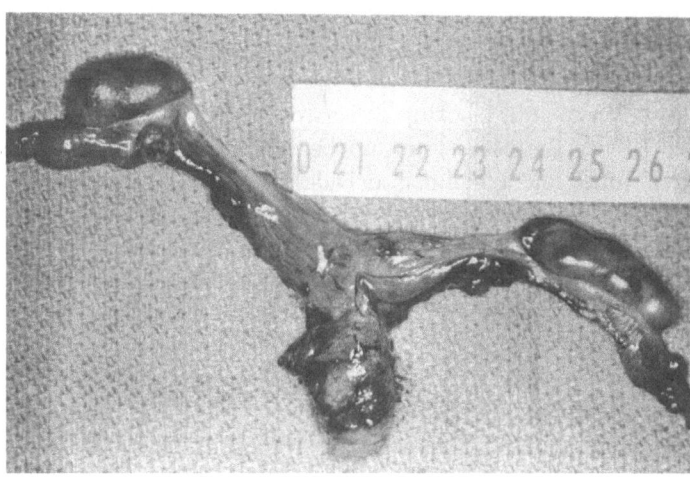

Fig. 6.2. a A genotypic female with 21-hydroxylase deficiency. The external genitalia were completely virilized in utero due to high adrenal androgen secretion. This patient was raised as a male. **b** At laparotomy the patient's uterus and ovaries were removed.

enzyme leads to varying degrees of cortisol and aldosterone deficiency. Inability to secrete aldosterone leads to sodium loss in the urine, hyponatremia, hypovolemia, potassium retention, and acidosis. Hypoaldosteronism brings about a compensatory rise in renin-angiotensin activity. Diminished blood levels of cortisol provoke increased release of ACTH in an attempt to restore adequate glucocorticoid secretion. The excessive secretion of ACTH in turn causes hyperplasia of the adrenal cortex, and accumulation of steroid precursors proximal to the 21-hydroxylase block such as progesterone and 17-hydroxyprogesterone. ACTH promotes increased production of adrenal androgens, whose steroidogenic pathway is unaffected by the 21-hydroxylase block. Plasma levels of these adrenal androgens rise.

The clinical presentation of 21-hydroxylase deficiency can be quite variable. The severity of signs and symptoms depends on the degree of enzymatic block. The most common and dramatic presentations of this disorder are (1) inappropriate virilization due to excessive levels of adrenal androgens and/or (2) salt-losing crisis due to inadequate secretion of aldosterone. Male neonates with 21-hydroxylase deficiency virilization may not be identified at birth, although some male infants may

be large for gestational age and have enlarged genitalia. However, in females intrauterine exposure to androgens usually causes ambiguity of the external genitalia, which allows the disorder to be detected at birth. The virilizing effect of adrenal androgens on the female external genitalia can vary from clitoromegaly, mild posterior labial fusion, to a nearly complete phenotypic male genitalia (Fig. 6.2).

Salt-wasting due to hypoaldosteronism may be unappreciated in the first days of life. In fact, the majority of patients with deficient aldosterone secretion do not have their initial salt-losing crisis until after the 1st week of life.

Male neonates with 21-hydroxylase deficiency who elude detection at birth and have minimal salt-wasting will be chronically exposed to elevated adrenal androgens. The abnormally elevated androgen levels gradually cause penile enlargement and precocious appearance of pubic hair. The testes of these boys are the appropriate size for the chronologic age, indicating a nontesticular source of androgen secretion. In addition to promoting precocious development of secondary sexual characteristics, excessive adrenal androgens accelerate osseous maturation and linear growth. Thus the patient also demonstrates an advanced bone age and may have an accelerated growth curve. This clinical presentation of adrenal hyperplasia must be differentiated from an androgen-secreting adrenal tumor.

With very mild blocking defects of 21-hydroxylase activity, the disorder may not be clinically recognized until late childhood or adolescence. Once again the linear growth may have a gradual but progressive acceleration and osseous maturation may be inappropriately advanced for chronologic age. There may be early appearance of axillary and/or pubic hair and body odor. Adolescent girls may have hirsutism, clitoromegaly, or delayed or irregular menses.

Congenital adrenal hyperplasia should be suspected in neonates with characteristic abnormalities of the external genitalia, where there is a family history of precocious virilization, hirsutism, infertility, irregular menses, or sudden infant death. This diagnosis should also be suspected in neonates with signs and symptoms of salt-wasting: poor feeding, vomiting, failure to gain weight, hyperkalemia, hyponatremia, and acidosis. A complete karyotype should be performed in any child with ambiguous genitalia or an infant with a male phenotype but without palpable testes. Hyperkalemia may be the earliest manifestation of insufficient mineralocorticoid activity and may precede hyponatremia and shock. Hyperkalemia may be overlooked in the newborn period if care is not taken to prevent hemolysis of the blood sample. Diagnosis of 21-hydroxylase deficiency is established by documenting excessive levels of steroid precursors that precede the 21-hydroxylation step. 17-Hydroxyprogesterone, the substrate just proximal to the 21-hydroxylation step, is typically elevated in the plasma of affected patients. Care should be taken to interpret levels of 17-hydroxyprogesterone with respect to the patient's age (Table 6.1). Other steroids, such as progesterone, dihydroepiandrosterone (DHEA), androstenedione, and testosterone, are also usually elevated. Urinary 17-ketosteroids and pregnantriol levels are inappropriately elevated. These abnormalities are corrected by physiologic replacement doses of glucocorticoids.

Plasma renin levels are extremely valuable in identification of patients with salt-wasting. Renin levels are elevated in patients with significant mineralocorticoid deficiency even before the salt-wasting crisis. Elevations in renin may also include a partial defect whereby increased stimulation is able to produce sufficient aldosterone to maintain salt balance. Plasma renin levels must also be inter-

Table 6.1. Reference levels in childhood for renin, aldosterone, 17-hydroxyprogesterone (mean ± 1 SD). (Adapted from [8,9,13])

	Renin (ng/ml/h)	Aldosterone (ng/dl)	17-Hydroxy-progesterone (ng/dl)
Cord blood	. . . . .	22 ± 18	2600 ± 900
Neonates	11 ± 10	25 ± 10	210 ± 80
Infants	4.6 ± 5.9	80 ± 50	50 ± 30
Prepubertal	1.8 ± 0.9	24 ± 20	30 ± 16

preted with respect to age, with neonates having generally higher values than in later childhood and adolescence [15,16] (Table 6.1). Measurement of plasma cortisol and aldosterone levels is not usually of diagnostic value in 21-hydroxylase deficiency because values may overlap the normal range.

In cases with severe deficiency of 21-hydroxylase, 17-hydroxyprogesterone levels and other precursors are unequivocally elevated. However, patients with partial 21-hydroxylase deficiency may not have salient elevations of 17-hydroxyprogesterone on randomly drawn single blood samples. The diagnosis of a partial enzyme deficiency can be made by the ACTH stimulation test [7,11] or 24-h integrated plasma hormone levels [5,14].

Treatment of 21-hydroxylase deficiency is directed at replacing vital hormone activity. Glucocorticoid replacement will restore feedback inhibition on the pituitary and suppress ACTH secretion. In salt-losers, mineralocorticoid replacement will restore vascular homeostasis. The dose of glucocorticoid is approximately 12 mg/m² per day of hydrocortisone parenterally or 25 mg/m² per day orally [3]. Hydrocortisone is usually divided into three doses per day. In cases with salt loss, mineralocorticoid replacement can be started initially with deoxycorticosterone acetate (Percorten acetate) 1–2 mg/day. When the patient is stable, long-term replacement therapy can be accomplished with deoxycorticosterone pivilate (Percorten pivilate) 25 mg intramuscularly every 3–4 weeks. Parenteral administration of mineralocorticoid is preferred in infancy to ensure that the medication is not inadvertently regurgitated. After infancy, mineralocorticoid replacement can be switched to one 9-fluorocortisol (Florinef) at a dose of 0.05–0.1 mg/day.

Therapy should be carefully tailored to the patient [13,14]. Overtreatment with glucocorticoid can lead to retardation of growth and clinical stigmata of Cushing's syndrome. Undertreatment leads to accelerated epiphyseal fusion and progressive virilization. Salt loss and poor growth may continue with inadequate mineralocorticoid therapy; on the other hand, overtreatment with mineralocorticoid can cause hypertension. Therefore, patients should be frequently monitored throughout childhood and doses of medication adjusted to permit reasonably normal growth and development.

11-Hydroxylase Deficiency. 11-Hydroxylase deficiency is a less frequently encountered adrenal enzyme deficit. Deficiency of the 11-hydroxylase step in the zona fasciculata impairs the synthesis of 11-deoxycortisol to cortisol and deoxycorticosterone to corticosterone (Fig. 6.1). Deficient levels of cortisol lead to a compensatory rise in ACTH, excessive stimulation of the adrenal cortex, and a subsequent abnormal elevation of steroids proximal to the 11-hydroxylation step. The clinically important elevated precursors are deoxycorticosterone (DOC), 11-deoxycortisol, and androgens. Due to elevated androgens, female newborns may have ambiguous genitalia; in females with partial enzyme defects, virilization may gradually become apparent. Males may present with signs of precocious puberty, i.e., penile enlargement, sex hair; however, the testes are prepubertal in size. In addition, excessive androgen secretion would cause rapid linear growth and advancement of bone age. Because deoxycorticosterone is a potent mineralocorticoid, affected children may often have low renin hypertension and hypokalemia. Occasionally, gynecomastia is a presenting feature of 11-hydroxylase deficit.

Treatment is directed at replacement of glucocorticoids. Doses of glucocorticoids are similar to those used in treatment of 21-hydroxylase deficiency. Because the 11-hydroxylase block may not affect the glomerulosa, these patients may have adequate aldosterone secretion once appropriate glucocorticoid replacement is undertaken.

3-Beta-hydroxy-dehydrogenase Deficiency and Other Defects. Several other less frequently encountered enzyme deficiencies in adrenal steroidogenic pathways can occur. 3-Beta-hydroxysteroid dehydrogenase deficiency (3HSD) can affect the gonads, as well as the adrenals (Fig. 6.1). 3HSD deficiency causes impaired synthesis of glucocorticoids, mineralocorticoids, and gonadal sex steroids. Affected neonates usually present with ambiguous genitalia regardless of genotype. Lack of aldosterone can lead to salt-wasting associated with hyperkalemia and high levels of renin. Figure 6.3 illustrates the early clinical course of an infant affected with 3-beta-hydroxysteroid dehydrogenase deficiency. Treatment usually requires replacement of glucocorticoids and mineralocorticoids. Due to high gonadotropin levels in infancy, gonadal steroids in 3HSD may be secreted that antagonize mineralocorticoid activity and precipitate salt loss. In those infants who cannot be adequately stabilized with hydrocortisone and DOCA, suppression of gonadal steroid secretion might be considered with luteinizing hormone releasing factor (LHRH) analogues. An alternative in the cases which require gender reassignment would be early surgical gonadectomy.

There are several, even less frequently encountered, adrenal enzyme deficits that have been recognized. In 20,22-desmolase deficiency, adrenal (Fig. 6.1), as well as gonadal, steroidogenesis is impaired. This deficiency is also associated with salt-wasting. Affected males have ambiguous genitalia. 17-Hydroxylase deficiency involves the adrenal, as well as the gonads; males may have ambiguous genitalia. This defect is associated with hypertension. 17,20-Desmolase deficiency (Fig. 6.1) leads to ambiguous genitalia in males but no metabolic deficits.

Adrenal Hemorrhage

Hemorrhage may occur into one or both adrenal glands (Fig. 6.4). Large amounts of extravasated blood produce a palpable enlargement of the affected adrenal and may be accompanied by signs of an acute abdomen and shock. It is believed that newborns are particularly prone to adrenal hemorrhage because of the relatively large adrenal mass and lack of musculature in adrenal veins. Adrenal hemorrhage in infancy may occur as a consequence of birth trauma or fetal hypoxia or may be associated with severe infection or coagulopathy [1]. In older patients, adrenal hemorrhage may also be associated with anticoagulant therapy, extensive burns, or severe renal or cardiac failure [17]. Adrenal hemorrhage needs to be distinguished from renal vein thrombosis that may have a similar presentation. Ultrasonography helps identify an enlarged adrenal hemorrhage above a normal-sized kidney (Fig. 6.5). Treatment includes vigorous therapy of underlying associated abnormalities,

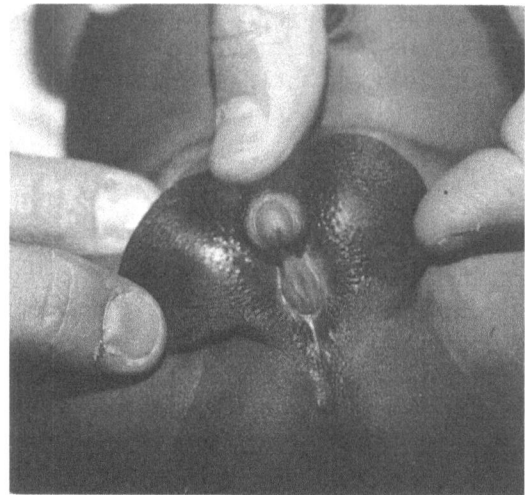

Fig. 6.3. a The external genitalia of a genotypic male with 3-beta-hydroxysteroid dehydrogenase deficiency. The testes were palpable bilaterally in the bifid scrotum. The patient had a severe chordee and urethral meatus was on the perineum. b The infant's early clinical course in the nursery. The infant fed poorly and lost weight during the first 2 weeks of life. Hyperkalemia was the first indication of aldosterone deficiency and preceded significant hyponatremia. The infant's renin level was over 200 ng/ml per hour prior to therapy. After introduction of therapy, hyperkalemia remained difficult to control presumably due to antagonism from steroids secreted from the testes.

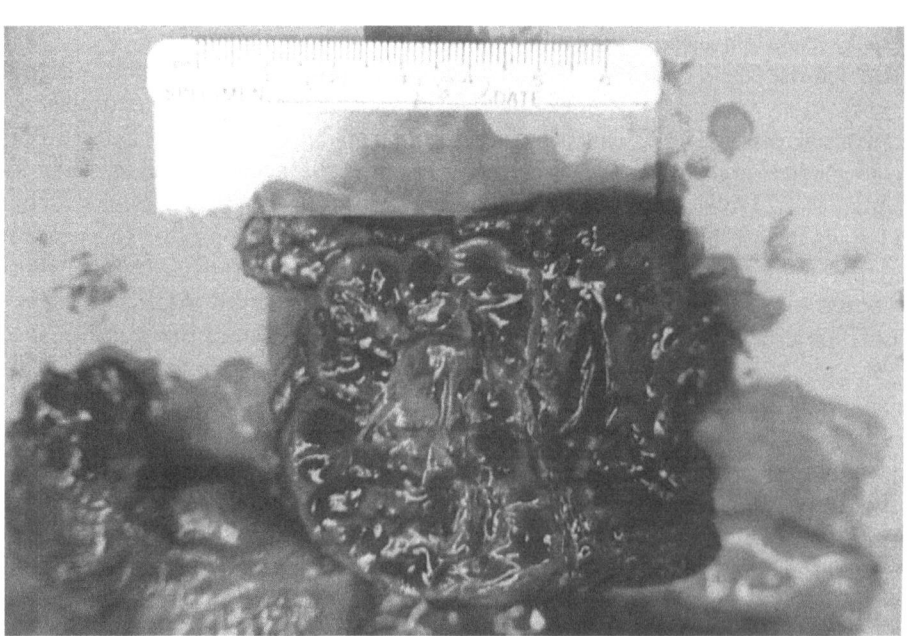

Fig. 6.4. Adrenal hemorrhage in a 2-week-old infant due to fulminant ECHO virus sepsis. The kidney has been sectioned in half for comparison with the hemorrhaged adrenal above it.

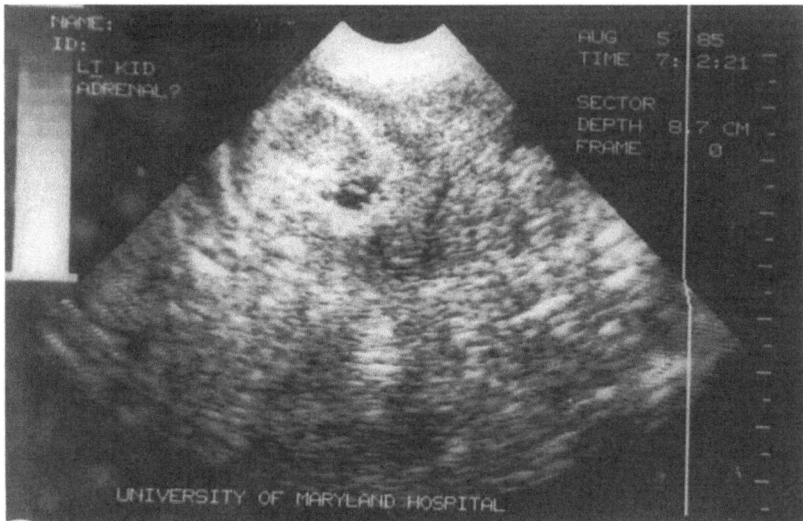

Fig. 6.5. Premortem abdominal ultrasound of the infant from Fig. 6.4 showing an echo-dense enlarged adrenal adjacent to the upper pole of a normal-sized kidney.

volume resuscitation, and stress doses of glucocorticoids. In cases of bilateral adrenal hemorrhage, adrenocortical secretion often recovers if the patient survives. Permanent adrenal calcifications may appear after resolution of the process.

Other Causes of Impaired Adrenal Secretion

Adrenal insufficiency in childhood may occur from a number of other etiologies. In infancy, adrenal agenesis or unresponsiveness to ACTH can cause hypoadrenalcortisolism.

Acquired autoimmune destruction of the adrenal can lead to impaired secretion of both glucocorticoids and mineralocorticoids. This form of Addison's disease may be associated with other autoimmune endocrinopathies, such as hypoparathyroidism, thyroiditis, and diabetes mellitus. These patients may have hyperpigmentation. Impaired secretion of aldosterone leads to elevation of plasma renin levels. It may be possible to demonstrate circulating antibodies against adrenal tissue. Plasma ACTH concentration may be distinctly elevated, and the cortisol response to exogenous ACTH will be blunted.

Adrenal insufficiency has been associated with degenerative disorders, such as familial xanthanatosis and diffuse cerebral sclerosis (adrenoleukodystrophy syndrome).

Disorders Due to Excess Adrenocorticoid Hormone Secretion

Overview

Autonomously secreting tumors causing Cushing's syndrome, virilization, or feminization are exceedingly uncommon. Adrenocortical tumors seem to occur more frequently in females than males, with a 2.3/1 ratio in childhood. These tumors have sometimes been associated with hemihypertrophy syndromes, neurologic tumors, and multiple endocrine neoplasia syndrome type 1 (MEN1). In some cases, adrenocortical tumors may secrete excessive amounts of several adrenocortical hormones, leading to mixed symptomatology. However, the initial presentation may suggest predominant hypersecretion of one type of adrenocortical hormone. The following discussion has been organized according to the predominant syndrome at clinical appearance.

Cushing's Syndrome

Cushing's syndrome is characterized by excessive levels of circulating cortisol.

Endogenous causes of hypercortisolism include autonomously secreting adrenal tumor, excessive pituitary ACTH secretion, or ectopic ACTH production. With the widespread availability of glucocorticoid preparations, exogenously administered steroids should also be suspected in the workup of Cushing's syndrome.

Hypercortisolism is a potent inhibitor of linear growth, and growth failure may be one of the earliest signs of Cushing's syndrome. Growth failure may be a helpful clinical clue to separate Cushing's syndrome from simple exogenous obesity, where linear growth is usually excellent. Other classical features of hypercortisolism may also be present: central obesity, moon facies, striae, easy bruisability, and muscle weakness. Many adrenal tumors may secrete clinically significant quantities of androgens, causing clinical signs of virilization in addition to features of Cushing's syndrome. The growth-promoting effect of androgens may ameliorate the growth-inhibiting effects of cortisol hypersecretion. Hypercortisolism may cause a retardation in the bone age and osteoporosis. Because cortisol has mineralocorticoid activity, hypercortisolism may be associated with low renin hypokalemic hypertension.

Documentation of excessive cortisol production and lack of diurnal variation in cortisol secretion is the key to diagnosis of the disorder. The most sensitive method for diagnosis of Cushing's syndrome is a 6-h (4:00 p.m. to 10:00 p.m.) evening integrated plasma concentration of cortisol (Fig. 6.6) [18]. This procedure can be performed in all but the youngest children. A 6-h integrated concentration of cortisol over 10 μg/dl is diagnostic of hypercortisolism. A 24-h collection of urine should also be obtained for measurement of urinary free cortisol and 17-hydroxysteroids. Measurement of 17-ketosteroids is also useful, particularly if clinical signs of virilization are present (see next section on virilizing tumors). Measurement of urinary steroids should be corrected for body surface area. Urinary steroid levels may give false-negative results so plasma documentation of hypercortisolemia is essential [18]. Blood samples should optimally be collected through an indwelling cannula to prevent artifactually high, stress-related rises in cortisol due to acute venepuncture. Multiple individual blood samples drawn in the evening may permit approximation of an integrated cortisol concentration.

Once the diagnosis of hypercortisolism has been established, the etiology should be localized to the adrenal, pituitary, or ectopic source of ACTH. Documentation of elevated levels of ACTH in the face of hypercortisolism may suggest either excessive

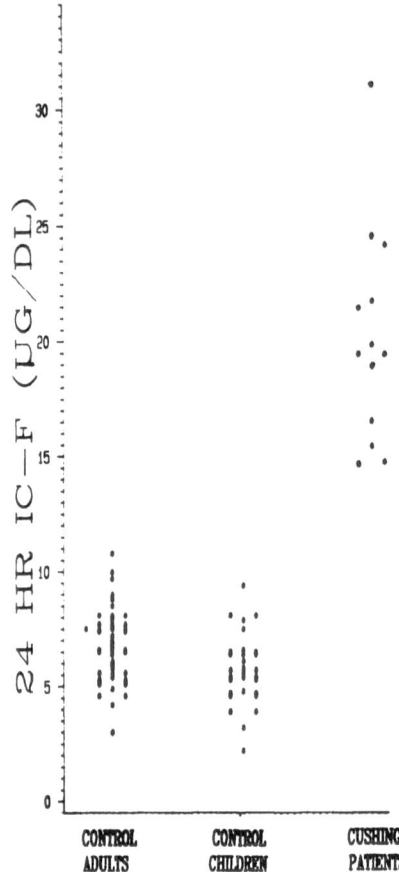

Fig. 6.6. Twenty-four-hour integrated concentration of cortisol from normal subjects compared with adolescents and adults with Cushing's disease. A shorter 6-h version of this test performed in the evening has excellent diagnostic capabilities.

pituitary ACTH secretion or ectopic ACTH secretion. However, low normal levels of ACTH do not necessarily rule out pituitary Cushing's disease. Use of dexamethasone suppression testing may be helpful in differentiating borderline high elevations in plasma cortisol levels or localizing the source of hypercortisolism. In the "low-dose" portion of the test, dexamethasone is administered orally at 1.2 mg/m^2 body surface per day (divided into four doses/day) for 2 days. After 2 days at this dose of dexamethasone, plasma and urinary corticoids will be suppressed by more than 50% in normal children. If there is no suppression on this low dose, a high-dose dexamethasone test at 5 mg/m^2 per day (divided into four doses/day) should be performed over the following 2 days. Suppression after high-dose dexamethasone suggests pituitary hypersecretion of ACTH; failure to suppress is indicative of an adrenal tumor or, more rarely, an ectopic source of ACTH.

Treatment of hypercortisolism in childhood is by surgical removal of the source of autonomous hormone secretion, whether in the pituitary or adrenal, or ectopic. Care must be taken to institute appropriate glucocorticoid replacement therapy prior to surgery and postoperatively because effective surgical removal of the tumor may lead to acute hypocortisolism. In cases of metastatic or unresectable adrenal tumors, therapy with agents that block adrenal synthesis of cortisol, radiation, or other chemotherapeutic agents should be tailored to the specifics of the case.

Virilizing Adrenal Tumors

Virilizing adrenal tumors usually come to medical attention because of the inappropriate appearance of physical signs related to excessive androgen secretion [11]. In males and females, clinical findings may include development of pubic and axillary hair, increase in muscle mass, body odor, acne, accelerated linear growth, and advanced bone age. In males, penile enlargement may be evident; however, the testes are prepubertal in size, indicating that the source of androgen is the adrenal (Fig. 6.7). Girls with a virilizing tumor may present with clitoromegaly. Frequently an abdominal mass is palpable.

Adrenocortical tumors may secrete excessive amounts of other adrenocortical steroids in addition to androgens. Thus some patients may also have clinical features of Cushing's syndrome, as well as virilization if their tumors secrete large amounts of cortisol. In cases with excessive androgens and hypercortisolism, the growth impairment typical of high circulating levels of cortisol may be offset by growth stimulation due to androgens. Very rarely, these tumors have been associated with hypoglycemia.

Endocrine diagnosis rests on documenting abnormally elevated secretion of adrenocortical androgens. Plasma should be assayed for 17-hydroxyprogesterone, cortisol, DHEA, DHEAS, testosterone, androstenedione, aldosterone, and renin. Elevated plasma levels of cortisol may also be documented. Luteinizing hormone (LH) and follicle-stimulating hormone (FSH) are at prepubertal levels. Urine should be collected for measurement of 17-hydroxysteroids, 17-ketosteroids, and urinary free cortisol. There is no significant suppression of excessive adrenal androgens with low-dose dexamethasone suppression as occurs in 21-hydroxylase deficiency. Preoperative visualization of the tumor should be undertaken. Abdominal CT and/or abdominal ultrasound have been helpful in documenting the location and extent of the tumor. Surgical removal of the tumor is the definitive treatment for these neoplasms. The malignant nature of the tumor may be evident if the lesion is locally invasive or metastatic spread to liver, lung, or lymph nodes is apparent. Diagnosis of malignancy based on the histology of the tumor mass is often difficult. If there is no evidence of dissemination and the tumor can be completely resected with amelioration of hormonal abnormalities postoperatively, then other modes of therapy are not advocated. In malignant disease, experience with chemotherapy and/or irradiation is limited in childhood [4].

Adequate glucocorticoid replacement therapy is essential before, during, and after surgery.

Feminizing Tumors

These tumors are characterized by breast development in males and females. These tumors may exhibit manifestations of excessive secretion of other steroid hormones, such as virilization or Cushing's syndrome. There may be accelerated linear growth and advanced bone age. Urinary 17-ketosteroids are elevated, as are plasma levels of estrogens.

Aldosterone-Secreting Tumors

These adenomas secrete high levels of aldosterone that lead to hypertension due to sodium retention and volume expansion [6]. There is often a hypokalemic alkalosis. Renin is suppressed. The ratio of the 6-h integrated concentration of renin to aldosterone is a useful endocrine parameter in support of the diagnosis [20].

Nonfunctioning Tumors

So-called nonfunctioning adrenal tumors are usually capable of some degree of steroidogenesis. However, they do not produce levels of hormones sufficient to produce signs or symptoms of Cushing's syndrome or precocious puberty which would bring

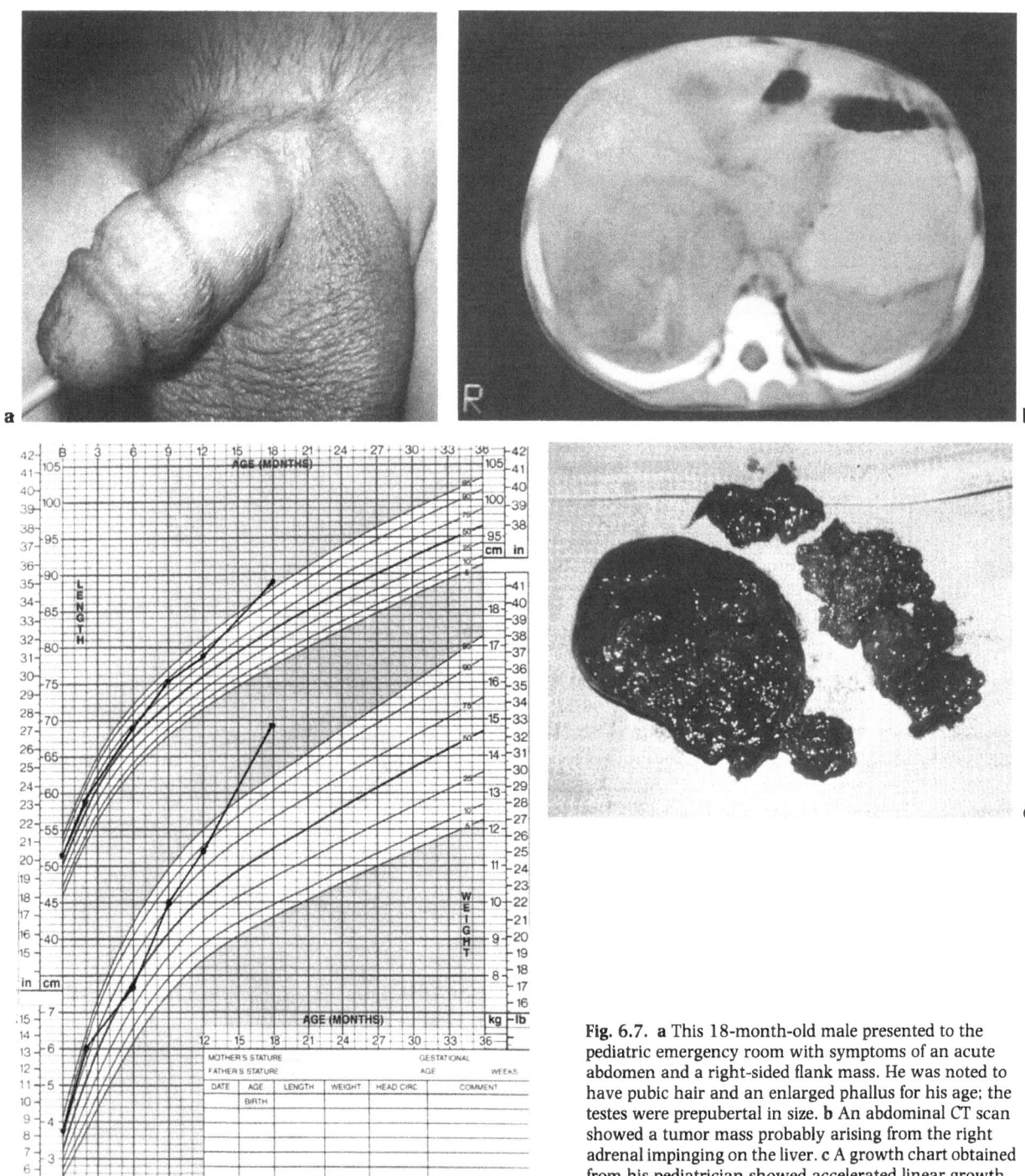

Fig. 6.7. **a** This 18-month-old male presented to the pediatric emergency room with symptoms of an acute abdomen and a right-sided flank mass. He was noted to have pubic hair and an enlarged phallus for his age; the testes were prepubertal in size. **b** An abdominal CT scan showed a tumor mass probably arising from the right adrenal impinging on the liver. **c** A growth chart obtained from his pediatrician showed accelerated linear growth stimulated by tumor androgen secretion. **d** At surgery, an adrenal carcinoma was removed.

the patient to medical attention. Because of the lack of external signs, these tumors are often discovered late, and tend to be quite large. The long-term survival for patients with these tumors has been poor.

Adrenal Cell Rests

In the course of embryonic development, adrenocortical tissue may remain in areas outside the adrenal gland. The most common sites for this ectopic tissue are the ovaries, ovarian pedicule, kidney, adjacent to the adrenal, and testes. This tissue may become hypertrophied and clinically important in situations with elevated levels of ACTH, such as enzyme blocks in biosynthesis of cortisol or tumor secretion of ACTH. A testicular adrenal rest may hypertrophy in a patient with a cortisol biosynthetic defect and may be mistaken for a testicular neoplasm. In these cases, regression of hypertrophied tissue should occur with glucocorticoid replacement therapy.

Disorders of the Adrenal Medulla

Pheochromocytoma

Pheochromocytoma is a tumor derived from chromaffin tissue and can occur wherever this tissue is located. However, the most common site of origin is the adrenal medulla. Approximately 10% of diagnosed pheochromocytomas occur in children. Pheochromocytoma may occur as part of a familial syndrome of multiple endocrine neoplasia.

Pheochromocytomas can secrete catecholamines, and the presence of the tumor is usually recognized by excessive circulating catecholamine levels. Intermittent or sustained hypertension is the most frequent sign of tumor activity. Other symptoms may include headache, palpitations, diaphoresis, pallor, anxiety, nausea, weight loss, acrocyanosis, weakness, visual disturbances, and behavior changes. The patient may complain of episodes of abdominal pain.

Diagnosis of pheochromocytoma is based on documentation of excessive catecholamine secretion. Single blood specimens for plasma norepinephrine and epinephrine levels may be elevated in pheochromocytoma, particularly if drawn at the time of a symptom episode. However, excessive catecholamine secretion can occur episodically; thus, integrated plasma hormone samples are often more useful for diagnostic purposes [19].

Twenty-four-hour urine collection should be obtained for catecholamines, normetanephrine, metanephrine, vanillylmandelic acid, and homovanillic acid. In patients with episodic symptoms, it might be particularly helpful to check a urine collection in the 4 h immediately after an attack. Suppression tests with clonidine [2] or glucagon stimulation tests [12] may be helpful in certain cases. Other causes of elevated catecholamines can include porphyria, Guillain-Barré syndrome, neuroblastoma, astrocytoma, and psychosis. It should be kept in mind that in addition to catecholamines, some pheochromocytomas have been reported to secrete ACTH, dopa, dopamine, serotonin, and somatostatin. CT scanning may pinpoint the anatomic location of the tumor prior to surgery. Recently, successful location of pheochromocytomas using [^{131}I]metaiodobenzylguanidine scanning has been reported.

Neuroblastoma

Neuroblastoma is a malignant tumor of childhood that arises from sympathetic nervous tissue. Seventy-five percent of the tumors presenting are diagnosed in the first 5 years of life. Neuroblastomas of the adrenal often present as an abdominal flank mass. These tumors usually secrete excessive amounts of dopamine and norepinephrine. Neuroblastomas cannot produce epinephrine. If this tumor is suspected, urine should be collected for estimation of norepinephrine, homovanillic acid, and vanillylmandelic acid. Treatment of these tumors may include surgery, radiation, and chemotherapy. Neuroblastomas are discussed in more detail in Chap. 11.

Acknowledgments. The author would like to thank Mrs. Barbara S. Mace for her help in preparation of the manuscript.

References

1. Black J, Williams DI (1973) Natural history of adrenal haemorrhage in the newborn. Arch Dis Child 48:183–190
2. Bravo EL, Tarazi RC, Fouad FM et al. (1982) Clonidine-suppression test: a useful aid in the diagnosis of pheochromocytoma. N Engl J Med 305:623–626
3. Brook CGD, Zachmann M, Prader A et al. (1974) Experience with long-term therapy in congenital adrenal hyperplasia. J Pediatr 85:12–19
4. Chan HSL (1983) Carcinoma of the adrenal gland in children—a study. In: Humphrey GM, Grindey GB, Dehner LP, Acton RT, Pysher TJ (eds) Adrenal and endocrine tumors in children, Kluwer/Nijhoff Publishing, Hingham, Massachusetts
5. Edwin C, Lanes R, Migeon CJ et al. (1979) Persistence of the enzymatic block in adolescent patients with salt-losing congenital adrenal hyperplasia. J Pediatr 95:534–537
6. Ganguly A, Bergstein J, Grim CE et al. (1980) Childhood primary aldosteronism due to an adrenal adenoma: preoperative localization by adrenal vein catheterization. Pediatrics 65:605–609

7. Gutai JP, Kowarski AA, Migeon CJ (1977) The detection of the heterozygous carrier for congenital virilizing adrenal hyperplasia. J Pediatr 90:924–929
8. Hughes IA, Winter JSD (1977) 17-Hydroxyprogesterone and plasma renin activity in congenital adrenal hyperplasia. In: Migeon, CJ, Kowarski AA, Plotnick LP, Lee PA (eds) Congenital adrenal hyperplasia, University Park Press Publishers, Baltimore, pp 203–215 (International symposium on the treatment of congenital adrenal hyperplasia)
9. Kowarski A, Katz H, Migeon CJ (1974) Plasma aldosterone concentration in normal subjects from infancy to adulthood. J Clin Endocrinol Metab 38:489–491
10. Lee PA, Rosenwaks Z, Urban MD et al. (1982) Attenuated forms of congenital adrenal hyperplasia due to 21-hydroxylase deficiency. J Clin Endocrinol Metab 55:866–871
11. Lee PDK, Winter RJ, Green OC (1985) Virilizing adrenocortical tumors in childhood: eight cases and a review of the literature. Pediatrics 76:437–444
12. Levinson PD, Hamilton BP, Mersey JH et al. (1983) Plasma norepinephrine and epinephrine responses to glucagon in patients with suggested pheochromocytomas. Metabolism 32:998–1001
13. Lippe BM, LaFranchi SH, Lavin N et al. (1974) Serum 17-alpha hydroxyprogesterone, progesterone, estradiol and testosterone in the diagnosis and management of congenital adrenal hyperplasia. J Pediatr 85:782–787
14. Meyer WJ, Gutai JP, Keenan BS et al. (1977) A chronobiological approach to the treatment of congenital adrenal hyperplasia. In: Migeon CJ, Kowarski AA, Plotnick LP, Lee PA (eds) Congenital adrenal hyperplasia, University Park Press Publishers, Baltimore, pp 203–215 (International symposium on the treatment of congenital adrenal hyperplasia)
15. Sassard J, Sann L, Vincent M et al. (1975) Plasma renin activity in normal subjects from infancy to puberty. J Clin Endocrinol Metab 40:524
16. Stalker HP, Holland NH, Kotchen JM et al. (1976) Plasma renin activity in healthy children. J Pediatr 89:256–258
17. Xarli VP, Steels AA, Davis PJ et al. (1978) Adrenal hemorrhage in the adult. Medicine 57:211–221
18. Zadik Z, deLacerda L, Kowarski AA (1982) Evaluation of the 6-hour integrated concentration of cortisol as a diagnostic procedure for Cushing syndrome. J Clin Endocrinol Metab 54:1072–1074
19. Zadik Z, Hamilton BP, Kowarski AA (1980) Integrated concentration of epinephrine and norepinephrine in normal subjects and in patients with mild essential hypertension. J Clin Endocrinol Metab 50:842–843
20. Zadik Z, Levin P, Kowarski A (1985) The diagnostic value of the 24-hour integrated concentration of plasma aldosterone. Clin Exper Hyper: Theory and Practice A7:1233–1242

Chapter 7

Primary Aldosteronism

J. H. Mersey

Introduction

Primary aldosteronism was first described in 1954, shortly after the description of a substance isolated from the adrenal that retained sodium and caused potassium wasting. Conn [15] described a patient with hypertension, hypokalemia, and neuromuscular symptoms whose clinical syndrome was reversed by removal of an adrenal adenoma. Urine aldosterone was found to be elevated preoperatively. Other cases were then described, but because of lack of knowledge of the physiology of renin, it was not possible to separate primary from other causes of hyperaldosteronism. With the discovery and acquired ability to measure renin, the biochemical characteristics were further defined as elevated aldosterone, low renin, and hypokalemia in a patient with hypertension [21].

Separation of primary from secondary aldosteronism was only the beginning of establishing the pathogenesis of this syndrome. Subsequently, patients with high aldosterone and low plasma renin but without adrenal tumors were found [17,46]. This condition was subsequently called idiopathic hyperaldosteronism [21]. At about the same time a familial version of hyperaldosteronism in which abnormalities could be suppressed with dexamethasone was described [67,80]. Also patients with adrenocortical carcinomas which secrete aldosterone have been described. And in rare cases ovarian carcinoma has been described to produce excess aldosterone. Finally, many patients have been described with apparent mineralocorticoid excess which was due to medication or foods containing exogenous mineralocorticoids [21]. A classification of primary aldosteronism is shown in Table 7.1.

Based on this classification, one cannot discuss primary aldosteronism as if it were a single entity. While the clinical features are similar if not identical, the pathophysiology of the various causes of hyperaldosteronism differs. Also then, the approach to therapy differs. Only those causes due to unilateral adrenal tumors respond predictably to surgical removal. In this chapter, I will discuss the clinical features, pathophysiology, diagnostic approach, and therapy, in each case based on the type of hyperaldosteronism. The emphasis will be on differentiation among the causes, in order to separate out those that respond to medication versus surgery.

Table 7.1. Classification of primary aldosteronism

1. Aldosterone-producing adrenal adenoma
2. Idiopathic hyperaldosteronism (bilateral hyperplasia)
3. Glucocorticoid-suppressible hyperaldosteronism
4. Adrenal carcinoma
5. Exogenous administration

Clinical Features

Primary aldosteronism, in spite of its notoriety, and contrary to predictions of its occurrence in as many as 20% of hypertensives, remains an uncommon clinical syndrome. Most investigators agree that primary aldosterone excess in all its forms accounts for 1%–2% of all patients with hypertension [27,57,80]. Epidemiologic characteristics do not help separate this condition from essential hypertension. In one series the mean age of patients was 46.5 years, with a range of 18–70 years [20]. Patients with adrenal adenomas show a slight preponderance of females, but idiopathic hyperplasia is without sex preference [21]. Thus, the patients are not recognizable by age or sex from those with essential hypertension. Eighty-five percent of patients with hyperaldosteronism have an adrenal adenoma [85].

Symptoms attributable to primary aldosteronism are in most patients simply those due to the hypertension itself. In other words, most patients are asymptomatic. In addition, rare patients have been described who are normotensive and present only with hypokalemia [68,78,89]. As in other causes of hypertension, the patients may experience headache, dizziness, malaise, and fatigue. The only symptoms which suggest aldosterone excess are those due to hypokalemia. With severe hypokalemia, these may include paralysis, muscle weakness and cramps, or tetany. These neuromuscular symptoms are now rarely observed, presumably due to earlier detection of low potassium. Hypokalemia may also produce polyuria and nocturia and rarely orthostatic hypotension, due to the effect of low levels of potassium on renal tubular sodium resorption [27,30,64].

Physical examination is only remarkable for hypertension. While initially it was thought that these patients had mild hypertension, it has more recently been observed that patients with primary aldosteronism may have any degree of blood pressure elevation, including malignant hypertension [10,30]. Other than the possible addition of orthostasis and muscle weakness or tetany, there are no other specific physical findings [10,64]. In particular edema is not found in these patients. The lack of edema is due to the mineralocorticoid escape phenomenon in which, in spite of continued exogenous or endogenous mineralocorticoid,

sodium retention stops after 3–5 days, and partial natriuresis occurs [27].

Routine laboratory evaluation reveals only the following: hypokalemia, mild hypernatremia, and alkalosis. Patients with adenomas and carcinoma have lower mean levels of potassium, and less patients will be normokalemic. As many as 22% of patients with adenomas may have a normal level of potassium; this is rarely, however, greater than 4 mEq/liter. Sodium is usually in the high normal range, or slightly above, and rarely less than 140 mEq/liter [85]. Bicarbonate levels are also mildly elevated. As expected, urine potassium levels are inappropriately elevated given the serum potassium, and a urine potassium level at a time of hypokalemia in an untreated patient will identify the kidney as the source of potassium loss [29].

As mentioned a significant fraction of patients will have normal levels of potassium on presentation. Almost all, however, will demonstrate hypokalemia when salt loaded or on diuretics [19,27]. Therefore, in the treatment of any hypertensive it is important to obtain a potassium level before and after treatment with diuretics [19,27], both for the safety of the patients and for identification of possible mineralocorticoid excess.

Glucocorticoid-suppressible hyperaldosteronism differs clinically from the other forms only in that there is a dominant inheritance and therefore a strong family history of similar problems [25].

Adrenal carcinoma producing aldosterone is extremely rare, but should be identifiable by extreme levels of hormone excess, excretion of other adrenal hormones in excess, or tumor size, which is usually quite large, and much larger than aldosterone-producing adenomas [1,78]. Please see Chap. 9 for details regarding the evaluation of adrenal cancer.

Hypertension and hypokalemia secondary to exogenous mineralocorticoid is extremely rare, but is well described. Offending drugs include licorice; 9-alpha-fluoroprednisolone, which is found in nasal sprays and topical preparations; and known mineralocorticoids such as desoxycortisone acetate (DOCA) and 9-alpha-fluorocortisone [8,21,23,61,65].

Pathophysiology

The etiology and pathogenesis of the hypertension in patients with primary aldosteronism has been extensively studied, but there is far from universal agreement on the interpretation of the results.

Adrenocortical adenomas arise within the zona glomerulosa. Most are less than 2 cm. About 60% are in the left adrenal. On microscopy these cells may be of four types: glomerulosa cells, reticularis cells, and large and small hybrid cells [21]. These cells produce aldosterone in vivo and in in vitro preparations. What prompts the growth of these adenomas is unknown, but adenomas are sometimes found in the presence of glomerulosa hyperplasia, as if a stimulating factor were present.

The cause of the hypertension in these patients relates to the metabolic effects of aldosterone. Under normal conditions aldosterone is secreted by the adrenal gland in response to stimulation by angiotensin II. This is produced by the action of renin on angiotensinogen, which yields angiotensin I; this is then acted upon by angiotensin-converting enzyme to produce angiotensin II (Fig. 7.1). Renin is secreted by the juxtaglomerular cells of the kidney in response to lowered pressure in the afferent arteriole, beta receptor stimulation at the juxtaglomerular cell, or diminished sodium or chloride at the macula densa. Aldosterone acts at the distal tubule to promote sodium reabsorption in exchange for potassium and hydrogen ion. In the normal feedback loop sodium retention results in increased blood pressure and hence suppression of renin [70]. With an adrenal tumor, aldosterone secretion is independent of renin and does not shut off when renin levels are suppressed by the hypertension presumably produced by sodium retention. This results in continued sodium for potassium exchange, and the clinical features of hypertension, hypokalemia, and alkalosis. See Fig. 7.1 for a diagrammatic representation of the renin-angiotensin axis in primary aldosteronism.

Aldosterone is also responsive to adrenocorticotropic hormone (ACTH) and to potassium. ACTH has a short-lived stimulatory effect on aldosterone secretion in normal man, such that with continued ACTH infusion aldosterone levels peak in 1 h and then return to baseline [50]. Hyperkalemia stimulates aldosterone secretion and hypokalemia suppresses it in normal man [16,41]. Both of these factors have been shown to play some role in the control of aldosterone secretion in adenomas [39,49,77].

Logically the hypertension in patients with adenomas should result from volume expansion. Attempts at measurement of exchangeable sodium and plasma volume have not always revealed these to be increased. Studies done following normalization of blood pressure with spironolactone and subsequent withdrawal have shown an initial increase in exchangeable sodium, plasma volume and cardiac output, without an increase in peripheral resistance. Later, however, exchangeable sodium decreases, although not to normal, and vascular resistance increases [21,52,81]. In one study some patients were even found to be hypovolemic [10]. In spite of these confusing changes in volume and resistance, patients almost invariably have a satisfactory blood pressure response to lowering volume and sodium, but have little response to agents which affect the autonomic nervous system [11].

The independence of aldosterone from angiotensin II influence and its relationship to ACTH can be observed in the diurnal pattern of aldosterone in these patients. In normal or essential hypertensive man, aldosterone increases from early morning to midday, in correlation with the rise in renin with upright posture. Thereafter aldosterone declines in parallel with cortisol. In patients with adenomas, aldosterone parallels cortisol throughout the day, so that aldosterone declines from its peak in early morning and is lower at noon [42,73]. Suppression of ACTH with dexamethasone ablates the diurnal variation, but does not lower the mean level [21].

Idiopathic hyperaldosteronism, or bilateral hyperplasia, while appearing nearly identical clinically and biochemically, has an entirely different pathophysiology, and one even less well understood. Pathologically the adrenal glands show diffuse or focal nodular zona glomerulosa hyperplasia. Microscopically no abnormalities can be seen in cell morphology [21].

These patients demonstrate both high aldosterone and low renin, as do patients with adenomas, but aldosterone secretion is not independent of renin and angiotensin II. Infusions of angiotensin II have demonstrated increased adrenal sensitivity compared with normal persons, and more like that seen in essential hypertension, while patients with adenomas have shown a normal or no response [61,80,87]. Infusion of saralasin, an angiotensin II analog which is both a blocker and a partial agonist, demonstrates the difference between

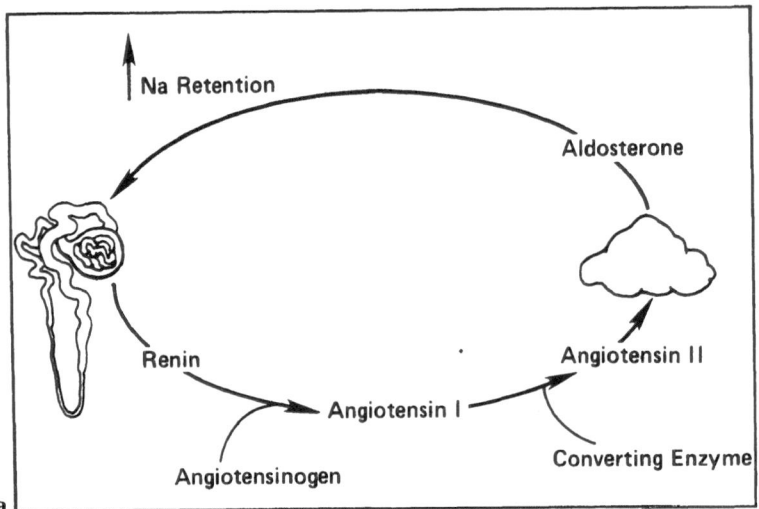

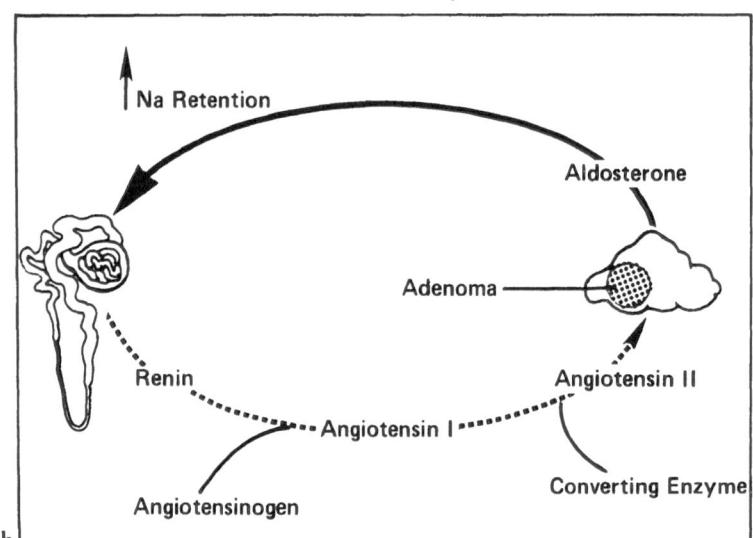

Fig. 7.1a. The renin-angiotensin/aldosterone axis in normal physiology. A complete feedback loop is formed so that the effects of renin secretion inhibit further secretion. See text for details. b. The renin-angiotensin/ aldosterone axis in primary aldosteronism. The feedback loop is interrupted because aldosterone secretion persists. See text for details.

adenomas and hyperplasia. In patients with bilateral hyperplasia angiotensin II levels are low; infusion of saralasin results in a rise in aldosterone—a response similar to that seen in normal volunteers on high salt (and low angiotensin II levels). In patients with adenomas saralasin has no effect on aldosterone, demonstrating the independence of aldosterone secretion from angiotensin [13].

To say that the pathogenesis of hyperaldosteronism in these patients is this increased sensitivity to angiotensin II would be premature, because other data exist to suggest other possibilities. Very recent studies have found the presence of an aldosterone-stimulating factor in urine of normal patients, and have found increased levels in these patients [14]. The origin of this factor is unknown, but is thought to be of pituitary origin, and perhaps in some way related to the pro-ACTH molecule pro-opiomelanocortin [22,34,38,74]. Other investigators have found no link between plasma levels or in vitro activity of pro-opiomelanocortin derivatives and aldosterone secretion [71]. Another study has found that the serotonin inhibitor cyproheptadine will lower aldosterone in idiopathic hyperplasia, but not in adenoma patients [35]. This suggests a role for either neurotransmitters or a pituitary factor controlled by neurotransmitters in the control of aldosterone secretion.

At present both possibilities carry equal weight; only further studies will explain the relationship of angiotensin II and aldosterone-stimulating factor in bilateral hyperplasia.

The cause of the hypertension in these patients is even more confusing. Measurements of sodium and plasma volume have not found these to be increased. Similarly response to diuretic has not been as consistent as in patients with adenomas. Current theory suggests that idiopathic hyperaldosteronism more resembles essential hypertension than aldosterone-producing adenoma, and is part of the continuum of low renin type essential hypertension [21,52,61,63].

Glucocorticoid-responsive hyperaldosteronism is a rare entity which resembles both the adrenal adenoma and idiopathic hyperplasia in various ways. Pathologically the hyperplasia seen is similar to that in idiopathic hyperplasia. This disease tends to occur in families and shows an autosomal dominant form of inheritance [21,24]. Diurnal variation of aldosterone is similar to that in adenomas and it parallels the cortisol changes [25]. When these patients are placed on glucocorticoid in doses sufficient to suppress ACTH for 2 weeks, the hypertension and hyperaldosteronism resolve [28,69]. This does not occur in the other causes of aldosterone excess. As mentioned previously, aldosterone responds only transiently to ACTH in normal persons and patients with adenomas, as if ACTH releases stored aldosterone, but does not promote its synthesis. Studies have shown that the enzyme steps through desoxycorticosterone do respond to ACTH in normals, but that subsequent steps do not [5]. For reasons unexplained, in these patients, ACTH does control and stimulate aldosterone secretion. Whether this is a receptor abnormality in these cells cannot currently be answered.

Adrenocortical carcinomas producing hyperaldosteronism are extremely rare. The literature consists of a few case reports. These tumors are large at the time of discovery. Differentiation from benign tumors is based on size and metastases, as in other adrenal carcinomas, since histologic features do not clearly characterize the malignant nature of these tumors. These tumors may make pure aldosterone, or a mixture of products. Hypertension and hypokalemia are due to the high levels of mineralocorticoid which may be aldosterone plus others. Removal of the tumor, if possible, will cure the hypertension [1,31,78,82].

Evaluation

Once the diagnosis of aldosterone excess is suspected, the next step is to confirm the diagnosis, and then attempt to decide which among the possible causes is most likely. Therefore, evaluation involves two steps: (1) confirmation of high, nonsuppressible aldosterone levels in association with nonstimulable renin levels, the combination of which makes the diagnosis of primary aldosteronism, and (2) differentiation between unilateral adrenal disease, which is almost always an adrenal adenoma, and bilateral disease, which is almost always idiopathic hyperaldosteronism. While one must keep in mind the possibility of adrenal carcinoma and glucocorticoid-suppressible causes of aldosterone excess, these are so rare that routine testing for these need not be carried out. In the following discussion, the tests available will be discussed by dividing them into these two categories of confirmation of aldosterone excess and differentiation of unilateral from bilateral disease.

Biochemical Evaluation

As mentioned above the first step is to confirm the presence of elevated aldosterone and suppressed renin levels. Aldosterone can be measured in both urine and blood, but must be assessed under controlled conditions. Patients should be off all antihypertensive medications which can affect renin or aldosterone (this includes almost all) for a period of 2 weeks. Depending on the level of the blood pressure this may not always be possible. Patients on spironolactone, a specific mineralocorticoid antagonist, may need to be off even longer, because suppression of aldosterone effect may result in a sustained normalization of renin. Potassium must also be normalized because, as described previously, hypokalemia may lower aldosterone levels into the normal range [40].

Once these prior conditions are established, aldosterone is then measured before and after volume loading. This can be accomplished in several ways. These include high-sodium diet [83], DOCA administration plus high-salt diet over 5 days [72,79], and saline infusion [79,76]. Most centers employ the latter approach, for the sake of time, although all have been found to be reliable. The saline infusion is conducted by measurement of plasma aldosterone in the patient after 1 h in the supine position. The patient is then given 500 ml normal saline/h over 4 h, at which time aldosterone is measured again. This procedure is well tolerated and rarely results in a significant increase in blood pressure, but obviously cannot be carried out in patients with heart failure. Also potassium must be measured and replaced, because the sodium load often results in potassium wasting and hypokalemia. If plasma aldosterone is less than 8.5–10 ng% after infusion, this essentially rules out aldosterone excess [79,87].

The presence of elevated aldosterone alone does not confirm the diagnosis, because high renin and angiotensin II can also cause hyperaldosteronism and hypokalemia. To measure renin, as with aldosterone, standardized conditions must be employed. Several approaches may be used. The two most common are the renin-sodium profile, in which an upright renin and a 24-h urine sodium value are used to compare the patient with normal persons [51], and the furosemide stimulation test in which renin and aldosterone are measured after the patient has been supine for at least 1 h, and then after the patient has received 40 mg intravenously or 80 mg orally and then has ambulated for 2–4 h [79,87]. We employ the furosemide stimulation test because of the ease of administration and the lack of need for urine collection.

Both the furosemide stimulation test and the saline infusion can be carried out on an outpatient basis in 1 day. We routinely bring the patient to our study center and in the morning perform the furosemide stimulation test, then feed the patient lunch. Following this the patient undergoes the saline infusion in the afternoon.

In most patients renin values after stimulation are less than 2 ng/ml per minute [85]. Occasionally patients are described with higher renins, but these have usually received diuretic therapy prior to study. In all cases it is important to know the normal range employed by the laboratory, since renin is not directly measured, but is assayed by how much angiotensin I is generated over time from the patient's own angiotensinogen. Therefore, depending on assay conditions, the value reported will vary.

Other newer approaches have been employed as screening tests for the diagnosis of hyperaldosteronism. In our laboratory we measure an integrated value for the aldosterone-renin ratio by collecting blood slowly with a constant withdrawal pump over 6 h. Patients with aldosterone excess have a ratio of greater than 100 [88]. Others have also looked at aldosterone-renin ratios [58].

Other tests have relied on the very low angiotensin II levels for diagnostic testing. Administration of captopril, the correcting enzyme inhibitor, lowers aldosterone levels in normal and

hypertensive man by lowering angiotensin II levels. In primary aldosteronism, either unilateral or bilateral, aldosterone levels do not fall below 15 ng% 2 h after administering 25 mg captopril orally [59]. Since, as I have said, aldosterone is dependent on angiotensin II in bilateral hyperplasia, it is surprising that captopril does not differentiate between adenomas and hyperplasia. Further testing may prove that this test is also useful in this discrimination.

Once the presence of primary aldosteronism is confirmed, other biochemical tests can be undertaken to differentiate among the various causes. The simplest of these is the anomalous response of aldosterone to upright posture seen in adenomas. As described previously, since aldosterone secretion is independent of angiotensin II, but partly responsive to ACTH, aldosterone levels will be highest in the morning. Since furosemide tests are always performed in the morning, one usually sees a rise in aldosterone from early morning to noon. In idiopathic hyperaldosteronism aldosterone has been shown to be hypersensitive to angiotensin II; this explains the observation that aldosterone levels rise from morning to noon in idiopathic hyperaldosteronism, but fall in patients with adenomas [6,55]. Therefore, the aldosterones measured during the furosemide test can also help differentiate between adenoma and hyperplasia. Unfortunately, there are false positives and negatives; therefore, an anomalous aldosterone response to posture is suggestive, but not diagnostic, of adrenal adenoma, and a rise in aldosterone with posture plus furosemide does not exclude an adenoma. In addition, glucocorticoid-suppressible hyperaldosteronism also shows a fall in aldosterone, since aldosterone is dependent on ACTH [25].

Another useful test to help differentiate is the measurement of 18-hydroxy-corticosterone. This steroid is the final precursor in the synthesis of aldosterone. This has been shown to be elevated almost invariably in adenomas, but not in hyperplasia [7,49]. Unfortunately, at present this is a research tool because the assay is not generally available.

Saralasin, as described earlier, may also help separate adenoma from hyperplasia, but is also at present a research tool.

To rule out glucocorticoid-suppressible hyperaldosteronism, one can administer dexamethasone 1–2 mg/day over 2–4 weeks and measure the response of aldosterone and blood pressure. In this condition all parameters will normalize over this period [25].

To test for the presence of adrenal carcinoma, urinary 17-hydroxysteroids and 17-ketosteroids should be obtained, since these tumors often make other steroids as well. The final diagnosis, however, may rest with surgical removal.

Localization

Although biochemical testing will usually give an indication of the presence of unilateral versus bilateral disease, the final proof remains in anatomic differentiation. Also even if one can be sure of the presence of an adenoma, it is still necessary to identify which adrenal is involved. Many approaches have been taken to localize the site of adrenal involvement, and many are still employed, indicating that each is less than perfect.

Older approaches including intravenous pyelogram, retroperitoneal insufflation with air, and even ultrasound have not been shown to be useful unless tumors are large, which these are not. Currently used imaging approaches are adrenal venography, nuclear imaging, and CT scanning. Venography has been used for the longest period, and has been successful in identifying adenomas about 70% of the time. Unfortunately, the complication rate of retroperitoneal hemorrhage causing severe pain or adrenal hemorrhage is significant, making this approach less than ideal [84,85].

Nuclear imaging with [^{131}I]6B-idiomethyl-19-norcholesterol (NP-59) in the hands of the investigators who first described this procedure and selected others has been very successful in localizing or lateralizing disease, with success exceeding 80% [4,27,30,36,37]. If this technique were universally available or more reproducible, it would be the procedure of choice. Unfortunately, other investigators have been unable to duplicate the successes first described [84], and most nuclear medicine facilities cannot perform the test. In addition, the procedure can take as long as 2 weeks, with repeated scans being taken, and exposes the patient to significant radiation. Therefore, this remains an imaging tool with limited utility.

Computed tomography scanning is now available universally. Its success rate in identifying aldosterone-producing adenomas versus bilateral hyperplasia is not as one would have hoped. To begin with, most aldosteronomas are less than 2 cm, and many are less than 1 cm. The reported success rate in identifying adenomas is 40%–90% [18,30,54,86]. One reason for the discrepancy from series to series is the improvement in CT scan equipment in recent years. Bilateral hyperplasia is also poorly identified and often under- or overdiagnosed by CT scan [18]. In addition, macronodular hyperplasia may be misdiagnosed by CT as a single adenoma. This technique has promise, especially as scanning improves. Because of its noninvasive nature (including the lack of need for contrast media for imaging the adrenal), a CT scan should still be performed. The role of nuclear magnetic resonance imaging remains to be defined.

The procedure of choice remains bilateral adrenal venous sampling with measurement of aldosterone for localization of aldosterone production. This approach is more than 90% accurate when carried out successfully [55,56,85]. Because of the variability of adrenal secretion some investigators suggest measuring adrenal effluent after administration of ACTH, thereby maximizing aldosterone and cortisol levels [85]. Others have just used cortisol:aldosterone ratios for the same purpose.

The major problem with adrenal venous sampling is in catheter positioning. The left adrenal vein, which most of the time enters the left renal vein, is easily catheterized. The right adrenal vein enters the vena cava directly the majority of the time, but can on occcasion take other paths. This vein is also small and can be confused with lumbar veins. Some contrast medium must be used to identify it as arising from the adrenal. Therefore, there is some risk of adrenal or retroperitoneal hemorrhage. And in spite of the best effort of experienced angiographers, the right adrenal vein may still elude catheterization. The frequency with which this occurs will vary depending on the experience of the radiologist, but in the hands of the best may still exceed 15%. We have reported the measurement of epinephrine levels along with cortisol and aldosterone, because levels greater than 1000 pg/ml can only be found in the adrenal vein. This insures that the sample is taken from an adrenal vein [53].

In spite of all these techniques there may still be patients in whom an adenoma is suspected, but which cannot be identified preoperatively. Therefore, there remains a place for explorative surgery. See Fig. 7.2 for a diagrammatic representation of the workup for primary aldosteronism.

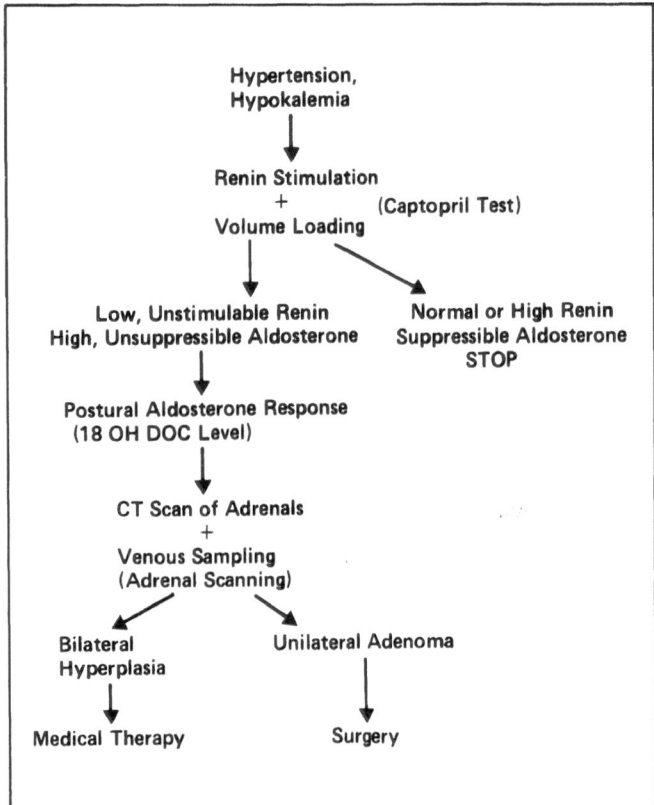

Fig. 7.2. Flow diagram of the workup of primary aldosteronism. Details are discussed in the text. After selecting patients for study, tests which confirm low renin and high aldosterone are performed. If positive, tests for differentiation between adenoma and hyperplasia, and localization procedures are performed. Depending on results, medical or surgical therapy is performed.

Therapy

Treatment of primary aldosteronism was thought to be quite simple when this syndrome was first described. Surgical removal of one or both adrenals was thought to be curative. Subsequently, it has been shown that removal of an aldosterone-producing adenoma results in cure of hypertension in 50%–70% of cases, with improvement in blood pressure in almost all the rest [2,29,30,43,60]. In patients with bilateral hyperplasia, surgery has cured the hypertension in less than 30%, and infrequently improved it, and so surgery is not indicated if bilateral disease is present [30,43]. In this situation medication is required. In addition, medication can be used in patients with adrenal adenoma preoperatively or if the patient is not a surgical candidate.

Medical Therapy

Medical therapy for primary aldosteronism needs to be directed to the precise cause of the aldosterone excess. For glucocorticoid-suppressible hyperaldosteronism, as mentioned previously, dexamethasone in a dose of 1–2 mg/day is both diagnostic and therapeutic. There is no other therapy required or indicated.

For adrenal carcinoma when surgery cannot be performed, therapy would be as in other patients with adrenal carcinoma (see Chap. 9). Patients may be treated with hormone synthesis inhibitors such as aminoglutethemide or antitumor drugs such as mitotane, or both. Most likely the patients will also require spironolactone to prevent hypokalemia and help control blood pressure.

For patients with adrenal adenoma, spironolactone has been thought to be specific therapy. This drug has been shown both to block mineralocorticoid receptors and to diminish aldosterone synthesis [3,43]. It was originally described that spironolactone was only effective in patients with adenomas, and that if blood pressure normalized this confirmed the diagnosis of adenoma. More recent studies have shown that spironolactone lowers blood pressure in patients with low renin hypertension, and in idiopathic hyperaldosteronism which may be a subset of low renin hypertension [3,9]. Thus, the response itself is not useful for making the diagnosis, but is dependent on its effect on fluid volume; for example, spironolactone's antihypertensive effect can be overridden by sodium administration [9,44].

Nonetheless, the clinical impression persists that spirinolactone alone is more likely to be successful in patients with adenomas. The dose required varies from 50 to 600 mg/day [26]. Once controlled, blood pressure does not escape control over long periods of therapy [3].

Spironolactone has significant side effects which may preclude use in many patients. Gynecomastia and impotence in men are very common in doses of 100 mg/day or greater, and can even occur on lesser doses. Epigastric discomfort is also common. Raynaud's phenomenon, lassitude, and hepatitis have also been described [21,75].

Other diuretics have also been used with success. These include the other potassium-sparing diuretics—a triamterene-hydrochlorothiazide combination, and amiloride. Since the presumed pathogenesis of the hypertension and hypokalemia is volume expansion and potassium wasting, drugs which promote sodium wasting and potassium retention should be successful. The few studies done confirm that these agents are effective [24,32].

The most interesting new medical therapy for aldosterone excess is the class of drugs which inhibit calcium channel transport. It has been shown that aldosterone secretion is calcium dependent, and calcium depletion or blockade lowers aldosterone secretion in vitro. The calcium channel blocker nifedipine has been shown to lower blood pressure, raise potassium, and lower aldosterone, over a 4-week period. The possibility of this approach for long-term therapy is of great interest, but of unproven value. Also of interest and surprise is that this drug was equally effective in patients with both adenoma and hyperplasia [66].

As described previously, surgery is not indicated in bilaterial hyperplasia, although surgical cures of as high as 38% have been described [2]. Medical therapy should begin with potassium-sparing diuretics. Other agents may be required, as described for essential hypertension. One report has described the beneficial effect of the converting enzyme inhibitor enalapril. In this study blood pressure, potassium, renin, and aldosterone were normalized in three of four patients. The fourth had macronodular hyperplasia and behaved more like a patient with an adenoma [33]. The beneficial

response in this study also helps confirm the importance of angiotensin II in stimulation of the high aldosterone levels in this condition.

Surgical Therapy

For the patients in whom an adrenal adenoma has been identified, surgical removal is indicated. The speed with which this is undertaken depends only on the suspicion of malignancy. Small adenomas are almost invariably benign. Therefore, tumor size will give some indication of the need for more immediate surgery. If the adenoma is small, pretreatment with spironolactone should be undertaken until blood pressure and potassium balance have normalized [27]. This may require from a few days to several weeks. Such treatment may also speed recovery of the suppressed zona glomerulosa of the contralateral adrenal.

The agreed upon surgical approach is a flank incision through the 11th intercostal space. See Chap. 13 for details of this and other surgical approaches.

Surgical therapy is curative in from 66% to 90% of patients with single adenomas, depending on the series described [30]. Essentially all patients are improved by surgery, if not cured. Surgical risk is low except in one older series, and given the high incidence of side effects with medications, surgery remains the treatment of choice.

Postoperatively, these patients may require exogenous mineralocorticoid to maintain sodium and potassium balance because of the suppressed remaining adrenal gland. This therapy with DOCA parenterally or 9-alpha-fluorocortisone can then be tapered as tolerated over the next several weeks. Usually by 4 weeks the suppressed adrenal has recovered, and renin and aldosterone will return to normal [47].

In summary, surgical exploration is indicated for unilateral adrenal disease, but not bilateral disease. If a definite identification of a suspected adenoma cannot be made, but is strongly suspected, a blind exploration of both adrenals may still be indicated. The surgical approach for this procedure may either be a laparotomy or bilateral flank incision, depending on the preference of the surgeon.

References

1. Arteaga E, Biglieri E, Kater C et al. (1984) Aldosterone-producing adrenocortical carcinoma—preoperative recognition and course in three cases. Ann Intern Med 101:316–321

2. Auda S, Brennan M, Gill J (1980) Evolution of the surgical management of primary aldosteronism. Ann Surg 191:1–7

3. Beevers D, Brown J, Ferriss J et al. (1973) The use of spironolactone in the diagnosis and the treatment of hypertension associated with mineralocorticoid excess. Am Heart J 86:404–414

4. Beierwaltes W, Sisson J, Shapiro B (1984) Diagnosis of adrenal tumors with radionuclide imaging. Spec Top Endocrinol Metab 6:1–54

5. Biglieri E, Schambelan M, Slaton Jr P (1969) Effect of adrenocorticotropin on desoxycorticosterone, corticosterone and aldosterone excretion. J Clin Endocrinol Metab 29:1090–1101

6. Biglieri E, Schambelan M, Brust N et al. (1974) Plasma aldosterone concentration—further characterization of aldosterone-producing adenomas. Circ Res 34, 35 [Suppl I]:183–189

7. Biglieri E, Schambelan M, Herai J et al. (1979) The significance of elevated levels of plasma 18-hydroxycorticosterone in patients with primary aldosteronism. J Clin Endocrinol Metab 49:87–91

8. Blachley J, Knochel J (1980) Tobacco chewer's hypokalemia: licorice revisited. N Engl J Med 302:784–785

9. Bravo E, Dustan H, Tarazi R (1973) Spironolactone as a nonspecific treatment for primary aldosteronism. Circulation 48:491–498

10. Bravo EL, Tarazi RC, Dustan et al. (1983) The changing spectrum of primary aldosteronism. Am J Med 74:641–651

11. Bravo E, Tarazi R, Dustan H et al. (1985) The sympathetic nervous system and hypertension in primary aldosteronism. Hypertension 7:90–96

12. Brown G, Douglas J, Bravo E (1980) Angiotensin II receptors and in vitro aldosterone responses of aldosterone-producing adenomas, adjacent nontumorous tissue, and normal human adrenal glomerulosa. J Clin Endocrinol Metab 51:718–723

13. Brown R, Kem D, Hogan M et al. (1984) Evaluation of a test using saralasin to differentiate primary aldosteronism due to an aldosterone-producing adenoma from idiopathic hyperaldosteronism. Metabolism 33:734–738

14. Carey R, Sen S, Dolan L et al. (1984) Idiopathic hyperaldosteronism—a possible role for aldosterone-stimulating factor. New Engl J Med 311:94–100

15. Conn J (1955) Primary aldosteronism: a new clinical syndrome. J Lab Clin Med 45:6–17

16. Cooke CR, Horvath JS, Moore MA et al. (1973) Modulation of plasma aldosterone concentration by plasma potassium in anephric man in the absence of a change in potassium balance. J Clin Invest 52:3028–3032

17. Davis W, Newsome H, Wright L et al. (1967) Bilateral adrenal hyperplasia as a cause of primary aldosteronism with hypertension, hypokalemia and suppressed renin activity. Am J Med 42:642–647

18. Dunnick N, Doppman J, Gill J et al. (1982) Localization of functional adrenal tumors by computed tomography and venous sampling. Radiology 142:429–433

19. Espiner E, Donald R (1980) Aldosterone regulation in primary aldosteronism influence of salt balance posture and ACTH. Clinical Endocrinology 12:277–286

20. Ferriss J, Beevers D, Brown J et al. (1978) Clinical, biochemical and pathological features of low-renin ("primary") hyperaldosteronism. Am Heart J 95:375–388

21. Ferris J, Brown J, Fraser R et al. (1981) Primary hyperaldosteronism. Clin Endocrinol Metab 10:419–52

22. Franco-Saenz R, Mulrow P, Kim K (1984) Idiopathic aldosteronism: a possible disease of the intermediate lobe of the pituitary. JAMA 251:2555–2558

23. Funder J, Adam W, Mantero F et al. (1979) The etiology of a syndrome of factitious mineralocorticoid excess: a steroid containing nasal spray. J Clin Endocrinol Metab 49:842–846

24. Ganguly A, Grim C, Weinberger M (1981) Anomalous postural aldosterone response in glucocorticoid-suppressible hyperaldosteronism. N Engl J Med 305:991–994

25. Ganguly A, Grim C, Bergstein J et al. (1981) Genetic and pathophysiologic studies of a new kindred with glucocorticoid suppressible hyperaldosteronism manifest in three generations. J Clin Endocrinol Metab 53:1040–1046

26. Ganguly A, Weinberger M (1981) Triamterene-thiazide combination: alternative therapy for primary aldosteronism. Clin Pharmacol Ther 30:246–250

27. Ganguly A, Donohue J (1983) Primary aldosteronism: pathophysiology, diagnosis and treatment. J Urol 129:241–247

28. Gill J, Bartter F (1981) Overproduction of sodium-retaining steroids by the zona glomerulosa is adrenocorticotropin-dependent and mediates hypertension in dexamethasone suppressible aldosteronism. J Clin Endocrinol Metab 53:331–337

29. Granberg P, Adamson V, Cohn K et al. (1982) The management of patients with primary aldosteronism. World J Surg 6:757–764

30. Grant C, Carpenter P, van Heerden J et al. (1984) Primary aldosteronism. Arch Surg 119:585–590

31. Greathouse D, McDermott M, Kidd G et al. (1984) Pure primary hyperaldosteronism due to adrenal cortical carcinoma. Am J Med 76:1132–1136

32. Griffing G, Cole A, Aurecchia S et al. (1982) Amiloride in primary hyperaldosteronism. Clin Pharmacol Ther 31:56–61

33. Griffing G, Melby J (1985) The therapeutic effect of a new angiotensin-converting enzyme inhibitor, enalapril maleate in idiopathic hyperaldosteronism. J Clin Hypertension 3:265–276

34. Griffing G, McIntosh T, Berelowitz B et al. (1985) Plasma B-endorphin levels in primary aldosteronism. J Clin Endocrinol Metab 60:315–319

35. Gross M, Grekin R, Gniadek T et al. (1981) Suppression of aldosterone by cyproheptadine in idiopathic aldosteronism. New Engl J Med 305:181–185

36. Gross M, Shapiro B, Grekin R et al. (1983) The relationship of adrenal gland iodomethylnorcholesterol uptake of zona glomerulosa function in primary aldosteronism. J Clin Endocrinol Metab 57:477–481

37. Gross M, Shapiro B, Freitas J (1985) Limited significance of asymmetric adrenal visualization on dexamethasone suppression scintigraphy. J Nucl Med 26:43–48

38. Gullner HG, Nicholson W, Gill J et al. (1983) Plasma immunoreactive proopiolipomelanocortin-derived peptides in patients with primary hyperaldosteronism, idiopathic hyperaldosteronism with bilateral adrenal hyperplasia, and dexamethasone-suppressible hyperaldosteronism. J Clin Endocrinol Metab 56:853–855

39. Guthrie G (1981) Multiple plasma steroid responses to graded ACTH infusions in patients with primary aldosteronism. J Lab Clin Med 98:364–373

40. Herf SM, Teates DC, Tegtmeyer CJ et al. (1979) Identification and differentiation of surgically correctable hypertension to primary aldosteronism. Am J Med 67:397–402

41. Himathongkam T, Dluhy R, Williams G (1975) Potassium-

aldosterone-renin interrelationships. J Clin Endocrinol Metab 41: 153–159

42. Hoefnagels W, Drayer J, Smals A et al. (1980) Nocturnal, daytime, and postural changes of plasma aldosterone before and during dexamethasone in adenomatous and idiopathic aldosteronism. J Clin Endocrinol Metab 51:1330–1338

43. Hunt T, Roizen M, Tyrrell J et al. (1984) Current achievements and challenges in adrenal surgery. Br J Surg 71:983–985

44. Ichikawa S, Tajima Y, Sakamaki T et al. (1984) Effect of spironolactone on fluid volumes and adrenal steroids in primary aldosteronism 48:1184–1196

45. Kater C, Biglieri E, Schambelan M et al. (1983) Studies of impaired aldosterone response to spironolactone-induced renin and potassium elevations in adenomatous but not hyperplastic primary aldosteronism. Hypertension 5[Suppl V:V]115–121

46. Katz F (1967) Primary aldosteronism with suppressed plasma renin activity due to bilateral nodular adrenocortical hyperplasia. Ann Intern Med 67:1035–1042

47. Kawasaki T, Uezono K, Ueno M et al. (1980) Influence of unilateral adrenalectomy on renin-angiotensin-aldosterone system in primary aldosteronism. Jpn Heart J 21:681–692

48. Kem D, Weinberger M, Higgins J et al. (1978) Plasma aldosterone response to ACTH in primary aldosteronism and in patients with low renin hypertension. J Clin Endocrinol Metab 46:552–560

49. Kem D, Tang K, Hanson C et al. (1985) The prediction of anatomical morphology of primary aldosteronism using serum 18-hydroxycorticosterone levels. J Clin Endocrinol Metab 60:67–73

50. Kowarski A, DeLacerada L, Migeon C (1975) Integrated concentration of plasma aldosterone in normal subjects: correlation with cortisol. J Clin Endocrinol Metab 40:205–210

51. Laragh JH (1973) Vasoconstriction-volume analysis for understanding and treating hypertension: the use of renin and aldosterone profiles. Am J Med 55:261–273

52. Lasaridis A, Brown J, Davies D et al. (1984) Arterial blood pressure and plasma and body electrolytes in idiopathic hyperaldosteronism: a comparison with primary hyperaldosteronism (Conn's Syndrome) and essential hypertension. J Hypertension 2:329–336

53. Levinson PD, Zadik Z, Hamilton BP et al. (1982) Adrenal vein epinephrine levels: a useful aid in venous sampling for primary aldosteronism. Ann Intern Med 97:690–693

54. Linde R, Coulam C, Battino R et al. (1979) Localization of aldosterone-producing adenoma by computed tomography. J Clin Endocrinol Metab 49:642–645

55. Luetscher J, Gaunguly A, Melada G et al. (1974) Preoperative differentiation of adrenal adenoma from idiopathic adrenal hyperplasia in primary aldosteronism. Circ Res 34,35 [Suppl I]:175–182

56. Lund J, Nielsen MD, Giese J et al. (1980) Localization of aldosterone-producing tumours in primary aldosteronism by adrenal and renal vein catheterization. Acta Med Scand 207:345–351

57. Lund J, Nielsen MD, Giese J (1981) Prevalence of primary aldosteronism. Acta Med Scand [Suppl]646:54–57

58. Lund J, Nielsen M, Giese J (1981) Simple screening procedure for the diagnosis of primary aldosteronism. Acta Med Scand 210:393–396

59. Lyons D, Kem D, Brown R et al. (1983) Single dose captopril as a diagnostic test for primary aldosteronism. J Clin Endocrinol Metab 57:892–896

60. Mackett M, Crane M, Smith L (1981) Surgical management of aldosterone-producing adrenal adenomas. Am J Surg 142:89–95

61. Mantero F, Armanini D, Opocher G et al. (1981) Miner-

alocorticoid hypertension due to a nasal spray containing 9-alpha-fluoroprednisolone. Am J Med 71:352–357

62. Mantero F, Fallo F, Opocher G et al. (1981) Effect of angiotensin II and converting enzyme inhibitor (captopril) on blood pressure plasma renin activity and aldosterone in primary aldosteronism. Clin Sci 61:298s–293s

63. McAreavey D, Murray G, Lever A et al. (1983) Similarity of idiopathic aldosteronism and essential hypertension—a statistical comparison. Hypertension 5:116–121

64. Menon M, Mersey J (1980) Primary aldosteronism—a review. Urological Survey 30:95–99

65. Montoliu J, Botey A, Trilla A et al. (1984) Pseudoprimary aldosteronism from the topical application of 9-alpha-fluorprednisolone to the skin. Clin Nephrol 22:262–266

66. Nadler J, Hsueh W, Horton R (1985) Therapeutic effect of calcium channel blockade in primary aldosteronism. J Clin Endocrinol Metab 60:896–899

67. New M, Peterson R (1967) A new form of congenital adrenal hyperplasia. J Clin Endocrinol Metab 27:300–305

68. Nishimiya T, Kikuchi K, Oimatsu H et al. (1984) A case of normotensive primary aldosteronism—comparison with 13 previously experienced cases with hypertension. Endocrinol Japon 31:159–164

69. Oberfield S, Levine L, Stoner E et al. (1981) Adrenal glomerulosa function in patients with dexamethasone-suppressible hyperaldosteronism. J Clin Endocrinol Metab 53:158–164

70. Oparil S, Haber E (1974) The renin angiotensin system. N Engl J Med 291:389–401

71. Racz K, Varga I, Glaz E et al. (1982) Met-enkephalin inhibits mineralocorticoid production in isolated human aldosteronoma cells. J Clin Endocrinol Metab 54:656–660

72. Rodriguez J, Lopez J, Biglieri E (1981) DOCA test for aldosteronism: its usefulness and implications. Hypertension 3 [Suppl ii]:102–106

73. Schambelan M, Brust N, Chang B et al. (1976) Circadian rhythm and effect of posture on plasma aldosterone concentration in primary aldosteronism. J Clin Endocrinol Metab 43:115–131

74. Schiffrin E, Chretien M, Seidah N et al. (1983) Response of human aldosteronoma cells in culture to the n-terminal glycopeptide of pro-opiomelanocortin an ^{3}-MSH. Horm Metabol Res 15:181–184

75. Shiroto H, Ando H, Ebitani I et al. (1980) Normotensive primary aldosteronism. Am J Med 69:603–606

76. Shuck J, Shen S, Owensby L et al. (1981) Spironolactone hepatitis in primary hyperaldosteronism. Ann Intern Med 95:708–710

77. Slaton PE Jr, Schambelan M, Biglieri EG (1969) Stimulation and suppression of aldosterone secretion in patients with an aldosterone producing adenoma. J Clin Endocrinol Metab 29:239–250

78. Slee P, Schaberg A, van Brummelen P (1983) Carcinoma of the adrenal cortex causing primary hyperaldosteronism. Cancer 51:2341–2345

79. Streeten DHP, Tomycz N, Anderson GH Jr (1979) Reliability of screening methods for the diagnosis of primary aldosteronism. Am J Med 67:403–413

80. Sutherland D, Ruse J, Laidlaw J (1966) Hypertension, increased aldosterone secretion and low plasma renin activity relieved by dexamethasone. Can Med Assoc J 95: 1109–1120

81. Tarazi R, Ibrahim M, Bravo E et al. (1973) Hemodynamic characteristics of primary aldosteronism. N Engl J Med 289:1330–1335

82. Telner A (1983) Adrenal cortical carcinoma: an unusual cause of hyperaldosteronism. Can Med Assoc J 129:731–732

83. Vaughan N, Slater J, Lightman S et al. (1981) The diagnosis

of primary aldosteronism. Lancet II:120–125

84. Vetter H, Brecht G, Fischer M (1980) Lateralization procedures in primary aldosteronism. Klin Wochenschr 58:1135–1141

85. Weinberger MH, Grim CE, Hollifield JW et al. (1979) Primary aldosteronism. Diagnosis, localization, and treatment. Ann Intern Med 90:386–395

86. White E, Schambelan M, Rost C et al. (1980) Use of computed tomography in diagnosing the cause of primary aldosteronism. N Engl J Med 303:1503–1507

87. Wisgerhof M, Brown R, Hogan M et al. (1981) The plasma aldosterone response to angiotensin II infusion in aldosterone-producing adenoma and idiopathic hyperaldosteronism. J Clin Endocrinol Metab 52:195–198

88. Zadik Z, Levin P, Hamilton B, Kowarski A (1985) Detection of primary aldosteronism by the six hour integrated aldosterone/renin ratio. Hypertension (in press)

89. Zipser RD, Speckart PF (1978) "Normotensive" primary aldosteronism. Ann Intern Med 88:655–656

Chapter 8

Cushing's Syndrome

P. A. Levin

Introduction

Cushing's syndrome is caused by excessive adrenal production of cortisol or excess administration of glucocorticoid steroids. Manifestations of Cushing's syndrome may involve nearly all organ systems of the body. There are several etiologies of endogenous cortisol overproduction leading to Cushing's syndrome (Fig. 8.1). Pituitary-dependent Cushing's syndrome (adrenocorticotropic hormone (ACTH)-secreting pituitary tumor) is the most frequent type, accounting for about two-thirds of the cases [13]. This is known as Cushing's disease. The increased secretion of ACTH leads to bilateral adrenal hyper-

plasia and high cortisol production. However, the high plasma cortisol level fails to suppress further ACTH release by the pituitary, indicating inappropriate autonomous pituitary function. These pituitary tumors are generally microadenomas (less than 10 mm in diameter) [12]. About 10% of patients may have pituitary corticotropic hyperplasia as a cause. Typical pathologic findings of a Cushing's syndrome-producing pituitary adenoma include basophilic nodular masses with PAS-positive cells.

The second most common endogenous cause of Cushing's syndrome involves a primary adrenal cortex tumor, either an adenoma or carcinoma [11]. These adrenal sources of Cushing's syndrome account for approximately 20% of cases. Benign

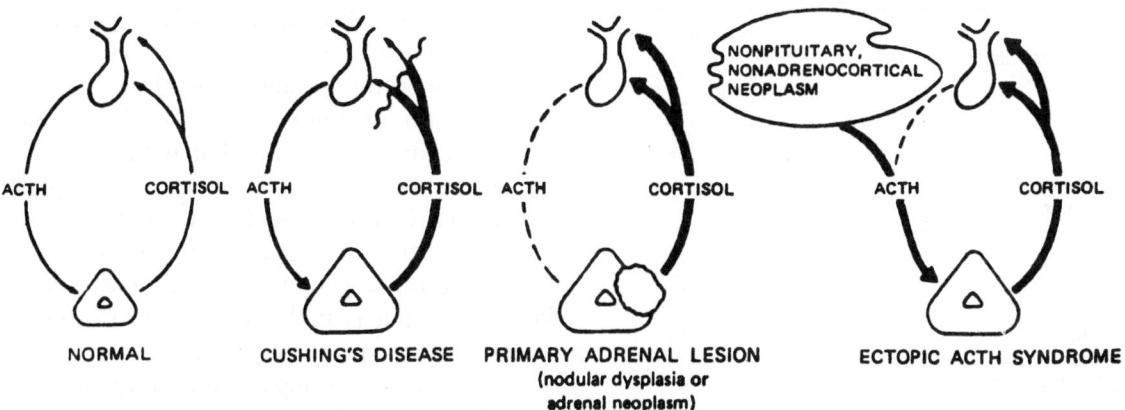

Fig. 8.1. Etiologies of Cushing's syndrome. [11]

adrenal adenomas are relatively small tumors of less than 100 g in most cases. They autonomously produce excess cortisol and thus are not under pituitary control.

Ectopic ACTH production by nonpituitary tumors represents another cause of Cushing's syndrome. Oat cell carcinoma of the lung is the most common tumor involved [21]. A recently reported rare cause of Cushing's syndrome is ectopic secretion of corticotropin-releasing factor (CRF) from a tumor [8].

Clinical Manifestations of Cushing's Syndrome

The clinical manifestations of cortisol excess are often gradual in onset so that months to several years may elapse before the full-blown clinical picture of Cushing's syndrome emerges (Table 8.1). Obesity is probably the most common manifestation [23] and an increase in central truncal fat out of proportion to extremity fat is typical. Supraclavicular fat pads and facial rounding are typical; however, massive obesity is unusual. Obtaining previous photographs of the patient is helpful in assessing whether these physical findings are new.

Numerous skin changes should be closely looked for. Patients' skin may become very thin and this is especially evident on younger patients. Purple red striae, particularly when over 1 cm wide, are typical [13]. They often occur over the lower abdomen and are more likely to be significant when found along arms, inner thigh axillary areas, and buttocks.

Table 8.1. Clinical features of Cushing's syndrome. [1,23,25,27]

	Frequency (%)
Obesity or weight gain	88
Moon facies	75
Hypertension	74
Purple striae	66
Hirsutism	65
Abnormal glucose tolerance	65
Muscle weakness	61
Menstrual disorders (usually amenorrhea)	60
Plethora	60
Acne	45
Bruising	42
Mental changes	42
Osteoporosis	40
Edema of lower extremities	39
Pigmentation	21
Hypokalemic alkalosis	17

These can be confused with the striae of marked obesity but are usually wider, redder, and associated with other skin changes when due to Cushing's syndrome. Easy bruisibility is another typical finding to look for. Also, increasing darkening of the skin occurs in many patients with pituitary ACTH-dependent Cushing's disease. Hyperpigmentation will not be present in primary adrenal causes of Cushing's syndrome.

Mild hirsutism and acne are also often found in Cushing's syndrome mainly due to adrenal androgen overproduction [25]. When increased body hair is accompanied by other signs of virilization an adrenal tumor must be considered. Hypertension is another very common finding. It is generally mild and without eye disease or renal complications. Muscle weakness with difficulty in rising from the squatting position can be found. This proximal myopathy is in part due to protein catabolism from the steroid effects. Impaired glucose tolerance occurs in many Cushing's patients. Hyperglycemia is usually mild and ketoacidosis is quite rare. Psychiatric manifestations are fairly common and include agitated depression and anxiety and psychosis [17]. Osteoporosis represents another fairly common complication [27]. Low back pain and spinal compression fractures may occur. One factor may be a decrease in circulating 1,25 vitamin D levels found to occur with excess corticosteroids. Another factor is cortisol's stimulation of calcium resorption from bone. Aseptic necrosis of the femoral head may also occur.

Hirsutism often occurs as a feature of Cushing's syndrome with a frequency of about 60% [11]. The hirsutism is typically only moderately severe. It is associated with acne in about 40% of cases and amenorrhea in 50%. When true virilization in addition to hirsutism is present, Cushing's syndrome due to adrenal carcinoma must be considered a possible etiology [13].

Routine laboratory studies may show changes consistent with Cushing's syndrome. The white blood count may be elevated but with a relative lymphopenia. Eosinophils are decreased and polycythemia may be present and related to the degree of androgen elevation. A diabetic glucose tolerance test may be present secondary to insulin resistance. Mild hypokalemia is fairly common in Cushing's syndrome. More severe hypokalemia with rapid onset may indicate an ectopic tumor source of Cushings syndrome, especially in patients over 50 years of age [2].

Diagnostic Studies for Cushing's Syndrome

The general diagnostic approach for Cushing's syndrome is first to demonstrate that hypercortisolism exists and then perform the differential diagnostic studies to localize its source.

Demonstration of Hypercortisolism

A number of different approaches have been shown to be valuable in establishing the diagnosis of Cushing's syndrome. One of the most commonly used screening tests is the overnight dexamethasone suppression test [10]. In this test 1 mg dexamethasone is given orally at 11:00 p.m. followed by measurement of the plasma cortisol at 8:00 a.m. the next morning. A plasma cortisol level of less than 5 μg/dl suggests additional studies for Cushing's syndrome should be performed [22]. A 24-h urinary collection for free cortisol and 17-hydroxycorticosteroids may also be performed, with a value over 100 μg/24 h for free cortisol being suspicious for Cushing's syndrome and 17-hydroxycorticosteroids over 15 mg/24 h also being suggestive of Cushing's syndrome [7]. A limitation of 17-hydroxycorticosteroids is that they may be increased in obesity per se without Cushing's syndrome, giving a false-positive test. However, plasma cortisol and urinary free cortisol should not be falsely increased in obesity [10]. Recently, a 6-h integrated plasma cortisol test performed in the early evening has been demonstrated to display a high degree of sensitivity in the diagnosis of Cushing's syndrome [28]. In this procedure an average evening plasma cortisol level is obtained using a continuous blood withdrawal pump (Cormed Co.) for the 6-h period. By this procedure, an average evening plasma level over 10 μg/dl may be considered diagnostic for Cushing's syndrome (Fig. 8.2). This method of diagnosis has been especially useful when other standard urine or plasma studies have shown equivocal or conflicting values. Another diagnostic test to confirm Cushing's syndrome, the low-dose dexamethasone suppression test, is also traditionally performed. In this test the patient is given 0.5 mg dexamethasone orally every 6 h for a total of 2 days. Suppression of urinary 17-hydroxycorticosteroids to < 4 μg/dl or urinary free cortisol to less than 25 μg/24 h essen-

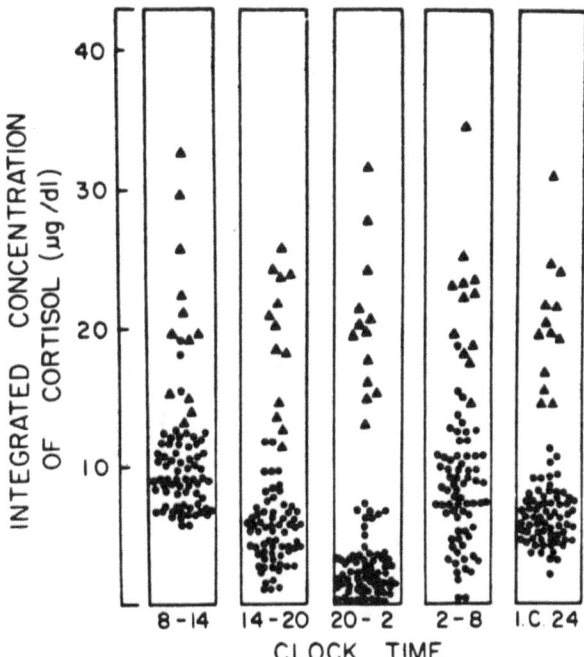

Fig. 8.2. Comparison of integrated concentrations of plasma cortisol in 68 normal persons (*circles*) and 13 patients with surgically proven Cushing's syndrome (*triangles*). [28]

tially rules out Cushing's syndrome [20]. Failure to suppress establishes the diagnosis and necessitates performance of a high-dose dexamethasone suppression test and other studies to localize the cause of Cushing's syndrome.

Localization of Cushing's Syndrome

Localization of the cause of Cushing's syndrome is the next stage in evaluation after hypercortisolism has been demonstrated. The high-dose dexamethasone test can differentiate between adrenal and pituitary causes [20]. In this test the patient is given 2 mg dexamethasone orally every 6 h for 2 consecutive days. Suppression of urinary 17-ketosteroids to less than 3 mg/24 h or to less than 50% of baseline suggests a pituitary tumor as the cause. However, failure to suppress is considered diagnostic of hypercortisolism due to adrenal adenoma, adrenal carcinoma, or possibly ectopic ACTH production [10]. When suppression testing is equivocal, the metapyrone test may assist diagnostically. Metapyrone inhibits the 11-hydroxylase enzyme blocking formation of cortisol. This cortisol drop normally leads to a feedback elevation of ACTH from the pituitary. In addition, the urinary excretion of

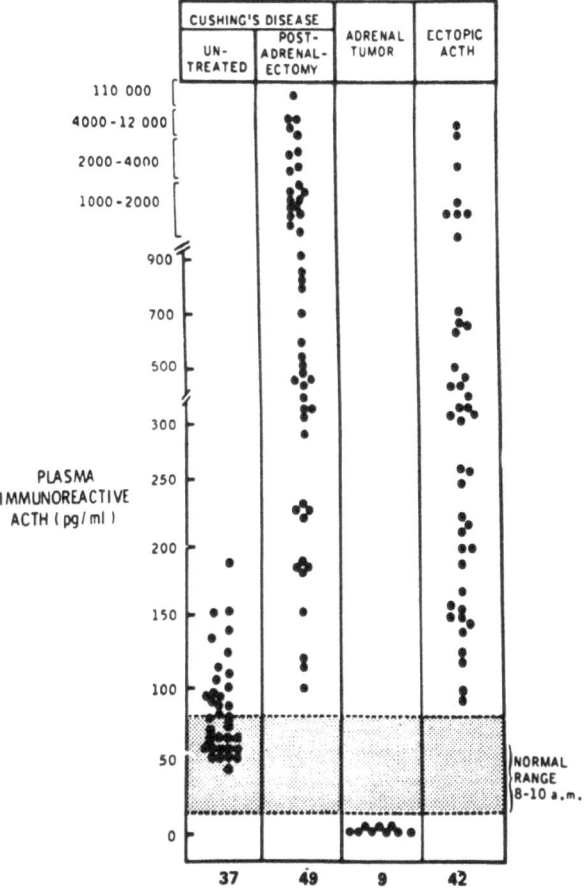

Fig. 8.3. Plasma ACTH levels in Cushing's syndrome. [4]

17-hydroxycorticosteroids is generally increased at least twofold over baseline. A normal or excessive urinary 17-hydroxycorticosteroid response to metapyrone is supportive of the diagnosis of pituitary Cushing's disease [11]. Failure to respond to metapyrone is more suggestive of Cushing's syndrome due to adrenal adenoma or carcinoma. Metapyrone is administered orally at a dose of 750 mg every 4 h for 24 h to produce a steroidogenic block. Some nausea may be a side effect of this medication. Urine samples are collected at baseline, the day of medication, and the day after. Elevated 11-deoxycortisol is usually measured to confirm adequate block.

Determination of plasma ACTH can be useful in the differential diagnosis of Cushing's syndrome (Fig. 8.3). A level greater than 500 pg/ml would favor ectopic ACTH release from a tumor, whereas levels of less than 20 pg/ml suggest adrenal carcinoma or adenoma [4]. The role of corticotropin-releasing factor (CRF) in the differential diagnosis is currently being studied.

When a person with Cushing's symptoms also has virilization or severe hirsutism, androgens should be measured. Elevated levels of dihydro-epiandrosterone (DHEA), DHEA-S, androstenedione, and urinary 17-ketocorticosteroids are suggestive of possible adrenal carcinoma. Typical DHEA levels may be over 1000 ng/ml, DHEA-S over 600 µg/dl, and 17-ketocorticosteroid excretion over 30 mg/24 h [3]. The adrenal CT scan is highly effective in localizing an adenoma or carcinoma diagnosed by suppression studies. CT evaluations for malignant invasion of other structures, large tumor size over 5 cm, tumor necrosis, and calcification will also help distinguish adrenal carcinoma from adenoma [16]. Bilaterally increased adrenal size is observed in some cases of Cushing's disease. However, normal adrenal size by CT is not an uncommon finding. An increased adrenal size may occur in both pituitary Cushing's disease and ectopic ACTH secretion.

A computed tomographic scan of the lung, mediastinum, and pancreas may also identify an ectopic source of ACTH. A CT scan of the pituitary while demonstrating a pituitary adenoma in a number of patients with Cushing's disease may be normal about 40% of the time. Therefore, a normal pituitary CT scan does not rule out an ACTH-secreting adenoma.

Cushing's syndrome due to adrenal adenoma is not usually associated with hirsutism and in fact often is associated with low or low normal values of plasma DHEA, DHEA-S, and urinary 17-ketosteroids excretion [14]. These cortisol-producing adenomas tend to suppress pituitary release of ACTH, thereby causing atrophy of the contralateral adrenal gland. The overall effect is a decrease in circulating levels of ACTH, associated with increased urinary excretion of 17-hydroxycorticosteroids but a decrease in urinary excretion of 17-ketocorticosteroids.

Diagnostic Pitfalls

A number of pitfalls must be avoided in making the diagnosis of Cushing's syndrome. Depression can be associated with failure of the overnight dexamethasone test to suppress and yield a false-positive screen [9]. Dilantin therapy can also lead to a lack of dexamethasone suppression [18]. Another important pitfall can occur in patients taking estrogens. This estrogen therapy may increase cortisol binding, producing elevated total plasma cortisol values, thereby falsely suggesting lack of dexamethasone suppression [15]. Obtaining a 24-h urinary free cortisol measurement may aid in resolving the question of estrogen effect as free cortisol is unaffected by estrogen-induced changes in cortisol binding. Alcoholism also can produce a clinical pseudo-Cushing's syndrome picture in some patients [24]. Other diagnostic dilemmas should also be considered. Some cases of long-standing pituitary Cushing's syndrome have been reported which can mimic an adrenal adenoma cause of Cushing's syndrome in numerous ways. These patients who have macronodular adrenal hyperplasia may fail the high-dose dexamethasone suppression test even though they may have elevated ACTH and sella enlargement [26]. CT scan may show a nodular form of adrenal hyperplasia. These patients generally are more successfully treated by bilateral adrenalectomy rather than transsphenoidal hypophysectomy.

Obesity may also give the physical picture of Cushing's syndrome to some extent as well as elevated urine 17-hydroxycorticosteroids. However, plasma cortisol and urinary free cortisol are unaffected by obesity and these assays are preferred in screening obese patients for Cushing's syndrome [1].

Finally, rare patients showing suppression of serum cortisol and urinary corticosteroids in response to low-dose dexamethasone testing may have Cushing's syndrome but give a false-negative test due to delayed clearance of dexamethasone [19].

Treatment

Transsphenoidal pituitary surgery for pituitary adenomas has emerged as the treatment of choice for most cases of Cushing's syndrome caused by pituitary excess of ACTH. Recent large studies have shown initial cure rates of 80% for pituitary Cushing's syndrome adenomas not extending outside the sella [5]. With suprasellar extension initial cure rates are only 50% or less. Complications have generally been mild, with transient diabetes insipidus the most common. Patients that have an initial cure with transsphenoidal surgery will demonstrate low cortisol levels within 3–4 days after surgery. Patients must be given intravenous hydrocortisone during surgery and replacement hydrocortisone or prednisone after surgery. We typically check patients for a cure by measuring baseline cortisol off hydrocortisone a week after surgery. In cured patients morning plasma cortisol will be less than $5 \mu g/dl$ or urinary free cortisol under $20 \mu g/24 h$ [6].

In patients with extrasellar or invasive tumor extension a cure may not be obtained. In these patients bilateral adrenalectomy may be needed for cure. Women desiring future pregnancy may also be candidates for bilateral adrenalectomy rather than transsphenoidal surgery.

Additional therapeutic options for pituitary Cushing's syndrome include pituitary irradiation. Other therapies tried with limited success include use of the serotonin antagonist cyproheptadine or the dopamine antagonist bromocriptine. When a benign adrenal adenoma is the cause of Cushing's syndrome, unilateral adrenalectomy of the tumor is the therapy. It should be remembered that cortisol-secreting adrenal tumors suppress pituitary ACTH levels so that the contralateral adrenal will be atrophic. Therefore, during and after adrenal surgery the patient may have adrenal insufficiency and maintenance steroids must be administered until laboratory studies show adrenal function has returned toward normal.

Primary therapy for adrenal carcinomas causing Cushing's syndrome is surgical resection. However, in only about 10% of cases is the tumor confined to the adrenal gland. Surgical resection may lead to moderately long-term control but rarely cure of the disease. Treatment of metastases has been by the adrenolytic o,p'-DDD (Mitotane) in a dose of 2–6 g/day and by the enzymatic blocker aminoglutethimide with up to 70% reduction in steroids [11]. Radiotherapy has been used in some series with limited success. Five-year survival has been in the range of 30% according to current studies. When adrenalectomy is selected as therapy for Cushing's syndrome, consideration must be given to the postoperative occurrence of Nelson's syndrome. This syndrome describes the development of a pituitary adenoma secreting ACTH and melanin-stimulating hormone (MSH) following adrenalectomy. It occurs in about 10% of adrenalectomy patients and is associated with development of intense hyperpigmentation. These adenomas can be fairly aggressive, with frequent sella enlargement and extrasellar involvement including development of visual field defects. Blood ACTH levels are found to be extremely elevated. Some studies have suggested that pituitary irradiation may decrease the incidence of Nelson's syndrome [6]. However, proper postoperative steroid replacement and regular checks for hyperpigmentation and sella enlargement play the most important role in decreasing the chance of developing a severe Nelson's syndrome.

References

1. Aron D, Tyrrell J, Fitzgerald P et al. (1981) Cushing's syndrome: problems in diagnosis. Medicine 60:25–35
2. Azzapardi J, Williams E (1968) Pathology of nonendocrine tumors associated with Cushing's syndrome. Cancer 22:274–286
3. Bertagna C, Orth D (1981) Clinical and laboratory findings and results of therapy in 58 patients with adrenocortical tumors. Am J Med 71:855–875
4. Besser G, Edwards C (1972) Cushing's syndrome. Clin Endocrin Metab 1:451–458
5. Boggan J, Tyrrell J, WIlson C (1983) Transsphenoidal microsurgical management of Cushing's disease. J Neurosurg 59:195–200
6. Burch W (1985) Cushing's disease. Arch Int Med 145:1106–1111
7. Burke C, Beardowell C (1973) Cushing's syndrome: an evaluation of the clinical usefulness of urinary free cortisol and other urinary steroid measurements in diagnosis. Quart J Med 42:175–294
8. Carey R, Varma S, Drake C (1984) Ectopic secretion of corticotropin releasing factor as a cause of Cushing's syndrome. N Eng J Med 311:13
9. Carroll B, Curtis G, Mendola J (1976) Neuroendocrine regulation in depression. Arch Gen Psychiatry 33:1039–1048
10. Crapo L (1979) Cushing's syndrome: a review of diagnostic tests. Metabolism 28:955–975
11. Cutler GB (1985) A review of endocrinology: diagnosis and treatment. FAES, Bethesda, Maryland, p 521
12. Daughaday W (1984) Cushing's disease and basophilic microadenomas. N Eng J Med 310:919
13. Felig P, Baxter J, Broadus A et al. (1981) Adrenal cortex, in endocrinology and metabolism. McGraw Hill, New York, pp 385–496
14. Gabrilone J, Freidberg E, Nicholis G (1983) Peripheral blood steroid levels in Cushing's syndrome due to adrenocortical carcinoma or adenoma. Urology 22:576–579
15. Grekin R (1980) The adrenal gland in endocrinology. Mazzaferri E (ed). Medical Examination Publishing Co., New York, pp 293–359
16. Hussain S, Belldegrun A, Seltzer S et al. (1985) Differentiation of malignant from benign adrenal masses. AJR 144:61–65
17. Jubiz W, Meikle A, Levinson R (1970) Effects of diphenylhydantoin on the metabolism of dexamethasone. N Eng J Med 283:11–15
18. Jubiz W (1978) The adrenals in endocrinology. McGraw-Hill, New York, pp 81–90
19 Kapcala LP, Hamilton SM, Meikle AW (1984) Cushing's disease with 'normal suppression' due to decreased dexamethasone clearance. Arch Intern Med 144:636–637
20. Liddle G (1960) Tests of pituitary-adrenal suppressibility in the diagnosis of Cushing's syndrome. JCEM 20:1539–1560
21. Liddle G, Nicholson W, Island D et al. (1969) Clinical and laboratory studies of ectopic humoral syndromes. Recent Prog Horm Res 2E:283
22. Mezby J (1971) Assessment of adrenocortical function. N Eng J Med 285:735–742
23. Plotz C, Knowlton A, Ragan C (1952) The natural history of Cushing's syndrome. Am J Med 13:597
24. Rees L, Besser G, Jeffcoate W (1977) Alcohol induced pseudo-Cushing's syndrome. Lancet 1:726–728
25. Ross E, Marshall-Jones P, Friedman M (1966) Cushing's syndrome: diagnostic criteria. Quart J Med 35:149–160
26. Smals A, Pieters G, Haelst U et al. (1984) Macronodular adrenocortical hyperplasia in long-standing Cushing's disease. JCEM 58:25–31
27. Soffer L, Ianncerone A, Gabrilone J (1966) Cushing's syndrome: a study of 50 patients. Am J Med 30: 129–146
28. Zadik Z, DeLacerda L, Kowarski A (1982) Evaluation of the 6 hour integrated concentration of cortisol as a diagnostic procedure for Cushing's syndrome. J Clin Endocrin Metab 54:1072–1074

Chapter 9

Carcinoma

A. Zabbo, R. A. Straffon, and J. E. Montie

Introduction

Primary malignancies of the adrenal gland include those arising from the adrenal medulla (neuroblastoma and malignant pheochromocytoma, discussed elsewhere in this text), and those from the adrenal cortex (adrenocortical carcinoma). Adrenocortical carcinoma may originate from cells in any of the three layers of the normal adrenal cortex. As such these cancers are capable of producing a variety of steroid precursors, end products, and metabolites which give rise to clinical syndromes and laboratory findings of excessive steroid secretion. Any of the functional adrenal steroids may be produced in excess including androgens, estrogens, glucocorticoids, or mineralocorticoids. The signs and symptoms of steroid excess may be the presenting findings in these patients. In addition, many adrenocortical carcinomas are clinically nonfunctional and in these patients the presenting symptoms will be related to the primary mass or to metastatic disease.

Adrenocortical carcinoma is so rare that no single individual or institution will generate a large experience with this carcinoma. The literature is replete with many case reports of odd manifestations of this disease. The reported series are of two types. Single institution reviews of moderate size have been reported but these span over 2 or more decades. The largest of these series, for example, is that of

M.D. Anderson Hospital. Even this large cancer referral center saw only 77 cases over a 30-year period [36]. The other type of series is multi-institutional reviews in which the various manifestations, treatments, and outcomes are catalogued. In either case, interpretation of results is difficult due to variances in diagnostic and therapeutic modalities applied over time or among institutions.

Leading to further difficulties in interpretation of the literature is the variable natural history of this disease [6]. Early series held that patients presenting with metastatic disease met with quick demise. While this in general is true multiple case reports of long-term survival even in the presence of metastatic disease have recently appeared. In addition, patients have been noted to have disease-free intervals as long as 10–12 years before recurrent local or metastatic disease appears [35]. This has led some authors to the impression that the disease progresses rapidly [19] while others feel that this cancer is slow in its capacity for local extension and metastatic capability [29].

Epidemiology

In discussing the epidemiology of adrenocortical carcinoma it is important to note the differences between information derived from literature reports and that derived from cancer registries. Review of the literature reports would lead to the conclusion that this cancer is twice as prevalent among women than men. However, information from the cancer registries indicates a slightly higher incidence among men than women [26]. The reporting bias of the literature results from the easier detection of virilizing tumors and those that cause Cushing's syndrome among women. Indeed among reported series of "nonfunctional" tumors, there are twice as many men as women [33].

From cancer registry data the incidence of adrenocortical carcinoma is approximately two per million population per year [26]. The disease has been reported to occur in all age groups from congenital [4] to geriatric, with clustering of the reported cases in the 4th–6th decade of life [21,26,36]. Again, probably resulting from easier clinical detection, women have been reported to contract this disease about 1 decade earlier in life on average than men [32].

No race predilection for this cancer has been described nor have any environmental factors been implicated. No clear genetic association has been established for this cancer.

Among children adrenocortical carcinoma represents 6% of childhood adrenal cancers, making it far less common than neuroblastoma but slightly more common than pheochromocytomas in this age group [30].

Children with hemihypertrophy or Beckwith-Wiedemann syndrome have been noted to be at increased risk for this malignancy [50]. These groups have also been noted to have a high incidence of adrenal adenomas and it is suggested that this may be a premalignant lesion. However, adrenal adenomas must have a very slight malignant potential as they are relatively common in autopsy series while adrenocortical carcinoma is very rare. Nevertheless, it would be important to screen these high-incidence groups with periodic intravenous urograms, ultrasound of the adrenals, or computed tomography of the adrenals. It will be necessary in these cases then to try to differentiate between lesions that would be adrenocortical adenoma versus adrenocortical carcinoma (see below).

There have been several reports of patients with congenital adrenal hyperplasia later developing adrenocortical carcinoma. No clear calculated risk for this association has been established [5,38].

Clinical Presentation

A variety of endocrine manifestations can result from steroid excess produced by adrenocortical carcinomas. It must be remembered that adrenocortical carcinoma is so rare that other causes of these endocrinopathies will be more common. The exception to this statement is that among children with Cushing's syndrome or virilization adrenocortical carcinoma is the most common cause [55].

Cushing's syndrome is the most common endocrinologic manifestation of adrenocortical carcinoma [8]. Of course pituitary adenoma and adrenal adenoma are the more likely causes of this syndrome [43]. One clue that may lead to increased clinical suspicion of carcinoma is that carcinomas have been noted to have "mixed" syndromes of glucocorticoid and androgen excess while bilateral adrenal hyperplasia and adenomas more commonly produce single steroid syndromes, such as Cushing's syndrome [23]. Thus the hirsutism produced with Cushing's syndrome should be distinguished from other signs of virilization caused by excess androgens.

Virilization in women and girls or precocious puberty in boys by excessive androgen secretion is the most easily recognizable syndrome associated with adrenocortical carcinoma. Growth acceleration may be the most striking feature in children [56]. Other causes of virilization include exogenous steroids, adrenal adenomas, and ovarian and testicular tumors. Ovarian tumors generally produce testosterone while adrenal tumors produce other androgens such as dehydroepiandrosterone or androstenedione. These intermediates may be converted to testosterone peripherally. An occasional adrenal adenoma may produce testosterone as its primary metabolic metabolite [45].

Feminization of a child or adult male may result from estrogen synthesis by the tumor [14]. Thus adrenocortical carcinoma should be included in the differential diagnosis of gynecomastia in the male but will be rare compared with other causes.

There have been multiple reports of primary aldosteronism due to mineralocorticoid secretion by adrenocortical carcinomas [1,3,16,42,48]. It is conjectured that in some of these cases aldosterone may be secondary to compression of the renal artery by the tumor causing renin-induced secondary aldosteronism. Again the majority of primary aldosteronism cases are due to benign adenomas. Other endocrinopathies including hypoglycemia [34] and inappropriate antidiuretic hormone [12] have been reported in association with adrenocortical carcinoma.

Among the group of patients with nonfunctional tumors will be included adult men with androgen-secreting tumors. No clinical effect will be noted in adult men from such excess androgens. These patients will present with local symptoms of pain or tenderness from the mass. Occasionally, fever, associated with tumor necrosis and a large mass, will be noted [17]. Other generalized complaints such as weakness secondary to anemia, indigestion, or myalgias may be noted. Hypertension secondary to steroid excess or from compression of the renal artery might also be noted. These tumors sometimes reach enormous size and detection of the mass on physical exam may be the presenting sign. Signs and symptoms of metastatic disease are too often the presenting features of both functional and nonfunctional tumors.

Often noted in the literature is the delay in time from onset of symptoms to diagnosis [26,30]. The insidious nature of endocrinologically induced changes in appearance which are readily recognizable to the physician may go unrecognized by the patient and family. In the past the delay in diagnosis has to some extent been associated with prolonged endocrinologic evaluation. With the newer imaging modalities being more readily available and employed in such patients it is anticipated that this delay in diagnosis will decrease.

Endocrinologic Evaluation

The endocrine evaluation of adrenal function and hyperfunction has been described in Chap. 4 of this volume. Also the differential diagnosis of various endocrine manifestations that may be associated with adrenocortical masses has been presented previously. Only the features that suggest differentiation of adrenocortical carcinoma from other causes of endocrinopathy will be reviewed here.

Adrenocortical carcinomas are generally considered to be inefficient in their production of steroids. This explains why these tumors commonly reach such a large size before clinical symptoms develop. This is in contradistinction to functional adrenal adenomas whose production of steroids is so efficient that even in the presence of marked clinical symptoms localization of the adenoma can be elusive. Thus in any patients with a palpable mass and signs of steroid excess, adrenocortical carcinoma should be suspected.

In general, discovery of large quantities of steroid end product or metabolites far in excess of normal ranges is associated with carcinoma [31]. Adrenal carcinomas are usually associated with high levels of urinary 17-ketosteroids. Twenty-four-hour urinary 17-ketosteroids in excess of 20 mg/g creatinine are indicative of carcinoma [6]. Seventeen-hydroxycorticosteroids and 17-ketogenic steroids may also be elevated. As with adenomas, dexamethasone suppression tests will be negative. Stimulation with ACTH results in increased steroid production frequently from adenomas, rarely from carcinomas.

Extensive endocrinologic workup may be necessary to show that "nonfunctional" carcinomas are actually producing steroid metabolites. Pregnenolone metabolites may be demonstrated on 24-h urine collections. Even in the face of normal steroid excretion, suppression tests may show the autonomous nature of steroid excretion by the tumors [33]. Again it should be emphasized that extensive endocrinologic workup should not significantly delay surgical intervention in those patients with suggestive features of adrenocortical carcinoma (see below).

Radiologic Evaluation

The time-honored method of demonstrating adrenal masses is the intravenous urogram. Displacement of the upper pole of either kidney downward or laterally is a sign of an adrenal mass. Tomography may demonstrate the mass more readily. The inferior displacement of the upper pole of the kidney seen on lateral or oblique projections from the intravenous urogram may also lead to a diagnosis of an adrenal mass. Calcification in the area of the adrenal mass on the plain film may be present with carcinoma but may also be associated with other benign adrenal pathology.

Arteriography and venography were formerly major diagnostic techniques to distinguish adrenal masses. Venography is still helpful in some cases of small adrenal masses not seen on other studies to localize the source of excess steroid production. Tumors not large enough to be seen on currently available imaging studies are likely to be adenomas and not carcinomas. Arteriography is helpful more in determining the anatomy in preparation for operative approach to the tumors than for diagnosis. Imaging of the renal arteries is important as resection of these tumors usually requires concomitant nephrectomy. The features on arteriography of adrenocortical carcinoma are those of hypervascularity with neovascularity but less AV shunting than is seen with renal carcinomas. Arteriography may occasionally be useful to differentiate an adrenal tumor from an upper pole renal tumor that is not distinguishable on other imaging techniques.

Adrenocortical carcinomas are capable of invading the venous system and inferior venacavography is recommended prior to surgical removal of any large adrenal mass or when the kidney on the ipsilateral side is nonfunctional.

Formerly, retroperitoneal pneumography with gas being injected in the presacral area was used to outline the kidneys and adrenals. This technique has been totally replaced with the newer imaging modalities of computed tomography and ultrasound [11]. These techniques will show solid density masses which may have nonhomogeneous areas associated with tumor necrosis.

With the widespread use of CT and ultrasound a new diagnostic dilemma has arisen, that of the incidental adrenal mass. A recent review has shown that adrenal masses will be detectable in 0.6% of abdominal CT scans [15]. With improved scanners, this rate might increase even further as autopsy series show an incidence of 1.5%–8.5% of adrenal nodules, mostly adenomas < 1 cm [6]. Since most of these small adrenal masses are of no clinical consequence, detection could lead to a large number of unnecessary operations. This is well documented in recent reports of surgery done for such incidental adrenal masses [5,40].

The differential diagnoses of adrenal masses are as follows:
Ganglioneuroma
Neuroblastoma
Pheochromocytoma (benign and malignant)
Adrenal cyst
Adrenal hemorrhage (fresh or organized)
Adrenocortical carcinoma

Adrenocortical adenoma
Myelolipoma
Adenolipoma
Metastases

The tumors of the adrenal medulla will generally be diagnosed by clinical symptoms and biochemical testing for catecholamines and their metabolites. The remaining differential diagnosis is among adrenocortical masses. Adrenal cysts may have a characteristic appearance on computed tomography and fine needle aspiration of clear fluid could confirm the benign nature of such a lesion. If bloody fluid is obtained on percutaneous aspiration then the mass must be treated as a potential malignancy. However, even in this case, only a small percentage will actually be malignant adrenal masses.

Functional adrenal masses should be removed in most cases and full endocrinologic testing including stimulation and suppression tests for the glucocorticoids and mineralocorticoids will select functional tumors. The remaining question to be answered concerning nonfunctional adrenal masses is: "Is this mass malignant?" If not, then no surgical therapy need be undertaken. The recent analysis and review of this problem by Copeland suggests guidelines for handling this dilemma [10]. In his extrapolation, Copeland showed that over 4000 operations would be needed among adrenal masses over 1.5 cm in diameter to remove one carcinoma. This percentage increases significantly when a 6-cm limit for operation is considered. Thus surgical removal of all nonfunctional masses > 6 cm should be undertaken. Among masses < 6 cm cystic lesions should be handled as mentioned previously. Thus full endocrinologic testing should be undertaken to rule out either functional adrenal medullary or cortical tumor. This should include suppression testing even in the presence of normal steroid levels as occasional carcinomas will be found with normal steroid levels that do not suppress. Any tumor demonstrating excess steroid secretion should be removed. Follow-up CT scans at 2, 6, and 18 months should demonstrate any mass progressing in size and these intervals are recommended based on estimates of the doubling time of adrenocortical carcinoma.

Fine needle aspiration of adrenal masses for cytologic evaluation has been reported in several cases and small series [22,35]. Because of the rarity of this tumor and difficulty in determining malignancy on morphologic characteristics it is not anticipated that needle aspiration will lead to significant progress in this disease. Needle aspiration can be very helpful in diagnosing the presence of metastatic disease [18].

Staging

The most widely applied staging system is that suggested by MacFarlane and revised by Sullivan [49]. The other accepted system is the TNM system that is compared in Table 9.1. Most patients will present with stage 3 and 4 tumors and thus survival is limited.

To complete the clinical staging, it is necessary to realize the patterns of metastatis. Metastases to the liver and lungs are most common, with less-frequent distant metastases being to lymph nodes, bone, brain, and other soft tissues. Local extension into the kidney or other adjacent viscera is common as well as regional lymph node involvement. The recommended metastatic workup then includes chest X-rays with tomography as indicated. A CT scan of the adrenals done for diagnosis would also demonstrate potential local extension and intra-abdominal metastases. Bone scans can probably be reserved for those patients with symptoms of bony pain or elevated alkaline phosphatase.

Special nuclear scans designed to visualize adrenal tissue have been reported as demonstrating sites of metastases. These, however, have not been widely applied and their value is unconfirmed [13,44].

Therapy

Surgical removal of all disease is the only reliable therapy for adrenocortical carcinoma. The surgical approaches to the adrenal gland are described in Chap. 13. For suspected adrenocortical carcinoma a transabdominal or thoracoabdominal approach is used to obtain the wide exposure necessary for resection of these sometimes large tumors and access to the remainder of the abdomen for accurate operative staging.

Perioperative steroid replacement should be routine especially if a functioning carcinoma is being removed as the controlateral adrenal gland is likely to have been suppressed. Postoperative steroid replacement should be directed by the results of functional testing.

Occasionally adrenalectomy only is possible but usually these tumors are so large that nephroadrenalectomy will be necessary. These tumors may also invade the kidney directly and as such the presence and function of the contralateral kidney must be assessed preoperatively. Local extension to surrounding structures may be present and patients should be routinely prepared for potential bowel resection. Because surgical resection is the only reliable therapy, extensive local resection of the disease including splenectomy, partial hepatectomy, or pancreatectomy is advisable if it appears that all local disease can be resected. Several authors have noted that significant palliation of endocrinopathies can be achieved with resection of large masses even when residual disease is left behind [8]. Residual or recurrent endocrine syndromes could be treated with steroid synthesis inhibitors such as metyrapone or aminoglutethimide.

Table 9.1. Comparison of staging systems for adenocortical carcinoma

Numerical stage	Primary tumor	Lymph nodes	Local extension	Metastases	TNM stage
1	< 5 cm	Negative	Negative	Negative	T1 N0 M0
2	> 5 cm	Negative	Negative	Negative	T2 N0 M0
3	Any size	Negative	Positive	Negative	T3 N0 M0
	Any size	Positive	Negative	Negative	T1–2 N1 M0
	Any size	Positive	Positive	Negative	T3 N1 M0
4	Any size	Positive/ negative	Positive/ negative	Positive	– – M1

Possible extension of adrenocortical carcinoma into the venous system should be recognized preoperatively and extraction of the tumor thrombus from the vena cava or resection of the vena cava may be necessary. If complete evaluation demonstrates only solitary resectable metastases, it should be addressed with aggressive surgery. Several cases of resection of locally recurrent disease and recurrent distant disease requiring multiple laparotomy or thoracotomy have been described [2,39,47]. In most cases such events will likely lead to quick demise of patients but again as surgery offers the only form of therapy with reliable results aggressive removal of resectable disease in properly selected patients may be rewarding. Adjuvants to surgery when the resection is not complete have met with some response but have not been found to be curative [36]. Only a few reports of the effectiveness of radiation therapy are available. Some authors have claimed good response [17,32], while others have been disappointed [9]. Radiation therapy should be considered unproven at the current time but it is not unreasonable to treat residual local disease or symptomatic metastases.

Chemotherapy has likewise been disappointing. Mitotane (o,p'-DDD) was derived from the pesticide industry. Initial reports of a 30% clinical response rate and up to 69% decrease in steroid production led to the early hope that this would be an effective agent [26]. Although there have been reports of occasional complete responses [7,30], other series have shown no definite survival benefits from the use of this agent [19]. Recent reports of therapeutic monitoring of drug levels to insure that high levels of the drug have been achieved for a significant period have led to somewhat better results [53]. Such high levels would result in a marked gastrointestinal toxicity as well as reversible neuromuscular side effects. It remains to be seen if these reports of delivering high levels of o,p'-DDD as detectable by serum level monitoring will result in a significant percentage of responses.

Other forms of chemotherapy, usually including *cis*-platinum, have given small response rates and suggest that coordinated trials of multidrug chemotherapy, possibly including o,p'-DDD, may lead to further improvement in treatment [20,51].

Prognosis

Several studies have attempted to draw correlations between the histology of the primary adrenocortical tumors and their malignant potential. In general the features associated with malignancy are pleomorphism of the nuclei, frequent mitotic figures, and vascular or capsular invasion [24,25]. Other authors have stated that multiple factorial analysis of the histologic and clinical features of the tumors leads to a more accurate predictor of malignancy [37,46,53,54].

Despite all these studies of the nature of the primary tumor, stage at the time of diagnosis is probably the most important factor in determining prognosis. Only those patients with stage I and II tumors have been found to achieve predictable disease-free survival. In reported series, women seem to have a better prognosis than men and functional tumors a better prognosis than nonfunctional tumors, but none of these correlations are separated from stage at the time of diagnosis [41]. As most patients will present with stage III and IV tumors, the overall 5-year survival in most series ranges from 10% to 25% [28, 36].

Outlook

The only reliable way to improve long-term survival would be with detection of the tumors at an earlier stage and prompt surgical removal. There is little likelihood that patients with this disease will be diagnosed earlier even with the newer imaging modalities as the nature of the clinical symptoms of this disease is such that they present when the patient has advanced stage. Thus effective adjuvant therapy will be necessary if significant impact is to be made on survival. Possibly earlier institution of o,p'-DDD therapy with therapeutic monitoring may lead to improved responses. As no single institution will generate enough experience with this disease, progress will be likely only through coordinated efforts among multiple institutions.

References

1. Alterman SL, Dominguez C, Lopez-Gomez A et al. (1969) Primary adrenocortical carcinoma causing aldosteronism. Cancer 24:602–609
2. Appelqvist P, Kostiainen S (1983) Multiple thoracotomy combined with chemotherapy in metastatic adrenal cortical carcinoma: a case report and review of the literature. J Surg Onc 24:1–4
3. Arteaga E, Biglieri EG, Kater CE et al. (1984) Aldosterone-producing adrenocortical carcinoma. Ann Intern Med 101:316–321
4. Artigas JLR, Niclewicz ED, Silva ADPG et al. (1976) Congenital adrenal cortical carcinoma. J Ped Surg 11:247–252
5. Bauman A, Bauman CG (1982) Virilizing adrenocortical carcinoma. Development in a patient with salt-losing congenital adrenal hyperplasia. JAMA 248:3140–3141
6. Bertagna C, Orth DN (1981) Clinical and laboratory findings and results of therapy in 58 patients with adrenocortical tumors admitted to a single medical center (1951 to 1978). Am J Med 71:855–875
7. Boven E, Vermorken JB, van Slooten H et al. (1984) Complete response of metastasized adrenal cortical carcinoma with op'DDD. Case report and literature review. Cancer 53:26–29
8. Brennan MF, Saxe A (1983) Adrenal neoplasms. In: Copeland EM (ed) Surgical oncology, John Wiley and Sons, New York, pp 423–449
9. Bulger AR, Correa RJ (1977) Experience with adrenal cortical carcinoma. Urology 10:12–18
10. Copeland PM (1984) The incidentally discovered adrenal mass. Ann Surg 199:116–122
11. Daneman A, Chan HSL, Martin J (1983) Adrenal carcinoma and adenoma in children: a review of 17 patients. Pediatr Radiol 13:11–18
12. Falchuk KR (1973) Case report. Inappropriate antidiuretic hormone-like syndrome associated with an adrenocortical carcinoma. Am J Med Sci 266:393–395
13. Forman BH, Antar MA, Touloukian RJ et al. (1974) Localization of a metastatic adrenal carcinoma using ^{131}I-19-iodocholesterol. J Nuc Med 15:332–334
14. Gabrilove JL, Sharma DC, Woltiz HH et al. (1965) Feminizing adrenocortical tumors in the male. A review of 52 cases including a case report. Medicine 44:37–79
15. Glazer HS, Weyman PJ, Sagel SS et al. (1982) Non-functioning adrenal masses: incidental discovery on computed tomography. AJR 139:81–85
16. Greathouse DJ, McDermott MT, Kidd GS et al. (1984) Pure primary hyperaldosteronism due to adrenal cortical carcinoma. Am J Med 76:1132–1136
17. Greenberg PH, Marks C (1978) Adrenal cortical carcinoma: a presentation of 22 cases and a review of the literature. Am Surg 44:81–85
18. Gross BH, Goldberg HI, Moss AA et al. (1983) CT demonstration and guided aspiration of unusual adrenal metastases. J Comput Assist Tomogr 7:98–101
19. Hajjar RA, Hickey RC, Samaan NA (1975) Adrenal cortical carcinoma. A study of 32 patients. Cancer 35:549–554
20. Haq MM, Legha SS, Samaan NA et al. (1980) Cytotoxic chemotherapy in adrenal cortical carcinoma. Cancer Treat Rep 64(8):909–913
21. Harrison JH, Mahoney EM, Bennett AH (1973) Tumors of the adrenal cortex. Cancer 32:1227–1235
22. Heaston DK, Handel DB, Ashton PR et al. (1982) Narrow gauge needle aspiration of solid adrenal masses. AJR 138:1143–1148
23. Heinbecker P, O'Neal LW, Ackerman LV (1957) Functioning and nonfunctioning adrenal cortical tumors. Surg Gyn Obst 105:21–33
24. Hogan TF, Gilchrist W, Westring DW et al. (1980) A clinical and pathological study of adrenocortical carcinoma. Cancer 45:2880–2883
25. Hough AJ, Hollifield JW, Page DL et al. (1979) Prognostic factors in adrenal cortical tumors. A mathematical analysis of clinical and morphologic data. Am J Clin Path 72:390–399
26. Hutter AM, Kayhoe DE (1966) Adrenal cortical carcinoma. Clinical features of 138 patients. Am J Med 41:572–580
27. Hutter AM, Kayhoe DE (1966) Adrenal cortical carcinoma. Results of treatment with op'DDD in 138 patients. Am J Med 41:581–592
28. Huvos AG, Hajdu SI, Brasfield RD et al. (1970) Adrenal cortical carcinoma. Clinicopathologic study of 34 cases. Cancer 25:354–361
29. Javadpour N (1983) Adrenal neoplasms. In: Javadpour N (ed) Principles and management of urologic cancer, 2nd edn. Williams and Wilkins, Baltimore, pp 560–580
30. Kay R, Schumacher OP, Tank ES (1983) Adrenocortical carcinoma in children. J Urol 130:1130–1132
31. Kelly WF, Barnes AJ, Cassar J et al. (1979) Cushing's syndrome due to adrenocortical carcinoma—a comprehensive clinical and biochemical study of patients treated by surgery and chemotherapy. Acta Endocr 91:305–318
32. King DR, Lack EE (1979) Adrenal cortical carcinoma. A clinical and pathological study of 49 cases. Cancer 44:239–244
33. Lewinsky BS, Grigor KM, Symington T, et al. (1974) The clinical and pathologic features of "non-hormonal" adrenocortical tumors. Cancer 33:778–790
34. Lipsett MB, Hetz R, Ross GT (1963) Clinical and pathophysiologic aspects of adrenocortical carcinoma. Am J Med 35:374–383
35. Montali G, Solbiati L, Bossi MC et al. (1984) Sonographically guided fine-needle aspiration biopsy of adrenal masses. AJR 143:1081–1084
36. Nader S, Hickey RC, Sellin RV et al. (1983) Adrenal cortical carcinoma. A study of 77 cases. Cancer 52:707–711
37. O'Hare MJ, Monaghan P, Neville AM (1979) The pathology of adrenocortical neoplasia: a correlated structural and functional approach to the diagnosis of malignant disease. Human Path 10:137–154
38. Pang S, Becker D, Cotelingam J et al. (1981) Adrenocortical tumor in a patient with congenital adrenal hyperplasia due to 21-hydroxylase deficiency. Pediatrics 68: 242–246
39. Potter DA, Strott CA, Javadpour N et al. (1984) Prolonged survival following six pulmonary resections for metastatic adrenal cortical carcinoma: a case report. J Surg Oncol 25:273–277
40. Prinz RA, Brooks MH, Churchill R et al. (1982) Incidental asymptomatic adrenal masses detected by computed tomographic scanning. Is operation required? JAMA 248:701–704
41. Richie JP, Gittes RF (1980) Carcinoma of the adrenal cortex. Cancer 45:1957–1964
42. Sakashita S, Kashiwagi A, Maru A et al. (1984) Primary aldosteronism due to adrenal cortical carcinoma. J Urol 132:959–961
43. Scott HW, Foster JH, Liddle G et al. (1965) Cushing's syndrome due to adrenocortical tumor: 11-year review of 15 patients. Ann Surg 162:505–516
44. Seabold JE, Haynie TP, DeAsis DN et al. (1977) Detection of metastatic adrenal carcinoma using ^{131}I-6-B-iodomethyl-19-norcholesterol. J Clin Endocrinol Metab 45: 788–796
45. Schteingart DE, Woodbury MC, Tsao HS et al. (1979) Virilizing syndrome associated with an adrenal cortical

adenoma secreting predominantly testosterone. Am J Med 67:140–146

46. Schteingart DE, Oberman HA, Friedman BA et al. (1968) Adrenal cortical neoplasms producing Cushing's syndrome. A clinicopathologic study. Cancer 22:1005–1013

47. Shaw KM, Peters JL, Fisher C et al. (1979) Prolonged survival with adrenal cortical carcinoma. Postgrad Med J 85:765–767

48. Stone NN, Janoski A, Muakkassa W et al. (1984) Mineralocorticoid excess secondary to adrenal cortical carcinoma. J Urol 132: 962–965

49. Sullivan M, Boileau M, Hodges CV (1978) Adrenal cortical carcinoma. J Urol 120:660–665

50. Tank ES, Kay R (1980) Neoplasms associated with hemihypertrophy, Beckwith-Wiedemann syndrome and aniridia. J Urol 124:266–268

51. van Slooten H, van Oosterom AT (1983) CAP (cyclophosphamide, doxorubicin, and cisplatin) regimen in adrenal cortical carcinoma. Cancer Treat Rep 67:377–379

52. van Slooten H, Moolenaar J, Van Seters AP et al. (1984) The treatment of adrenocortical carcinoma with op'DDD: prognostic implications of serum level monitoring. Eur J Cancer Clin Oncol 20:470–530

53. van Slooten H, Schaberg A, Smeenk D et al. (1985) Morphologic characteristics of benign and malignant adrenocortical tumors. Cancer 55:766–773

54. Weiss LM (1984) Comparative histologic study of 43 metastasizing and nonmetastasizing adrenocortical tumors. Am J Surg Pathol 8:163–169

55. Young JD, Karmi SA (1978) Diagnosis and management of adrenal tumors. In: Skinner DG, Dekernion JB (eds) Genitourinary cancer. Saunders, Philadelphia, pp 166–178

56. Zaitoon MM, Mackie GG (1978) Adrenal cortical tumors in children. Urology 12:645–649

Chapter 10

Pheochromocytoma

B. P. M. Hamilton

Introduction

A pheochromocytoma is a chromaffin cell tumor which has the ability to synthesize and secrete catecholamines, and these in turn produce symptoms in the afflicted patient. The catecholamine secretion, rather than the underlying neoplasm, renders a pheochromocytoma clinically important and dangerous, yet a potentially curable form of secondary hypertension. The chromaffin cell which gives rise to a pheochromocytoma derives its name from its ability to synthesize and store catecholamines, and therefore stain brown on treatment with chromium salts. These cells are found mainly in the adrenal medulla, but also appear along the ganglia and paraganglia of the sympathetic chain and organs of Zuckerkandl located anteriorly at the bifurcation of the aorta. Chromaffin cells are derived from the primitive neural crest and share with other neural crest cell lines the ability to take up amine precursors and decarboxylate them, giving rise to the acronym APUD cells (amine precursor uptake and decarboxylation) [64,69]. This relationship of APUD cells explains the presence of pheochromocytoma as one part of familial dystrophies of APUD cells, as in multiple endocrine adenomas type II (MEA-II) [6]. Sympathogonia, the primordial stem cells arising from the neural crest, migrate out of the central nervous system and differentiate into ganglion cells, neuro-

blasts, or chromaffin cells [14]. Tumors may arise from each of these cell lines, namely neuroblastoma, ganglioneuroma, and pheochromocytoma.

Eighty to ninety percent of pheochromocytomas are in one or both adrenal glands but they may be located anywhere along the sympathetic chain and rarely in aberrant sites. Extraadrenal pheochromocytomas may also be called paragangliomas [62]. They arise most frequently from the organ of Zuckerkandl and in the urinary bladder. Those arising from specialized chemoreceptor tissue in the carotid body, glomus jugulare, and aortic body have been separately classified as chemodectomas, but are in fact true paragangliomas and may be functional, secreting norepinephrine.

About 10% of pheochromocytomas are malignant. The criterion for this is the presence of distant metastases, in paraaortic lymph nodes predominantly but also in liver, lungs, and bone. Malignancy cannot be determined by histology alone and benign tumors may invade the pheochromocytoma capsule [56]. About 10% of pheochromocytomas are also bilateral. In the case of familial pheochromocytomas, however, where there is a generalized dystrophy of chromaffin tissue as in MEA-II, pheochromocytomas may commonly occur bilaterally even though one side may present years before the other [13]. This form of familial pheochromocytoma has been shown to have a precursor stage of adrenal medullary hyperplasia which is also associated with catecholamine overproduction [10,11].

Incidence

Pheochromocytomas are rare. They have been found in babies a few months old and in nonagenarians. In autopsy series they have been reported in 0–0.25% of cases. In the Mayo Clinic experience, 54 pheochromocytomas were found at autopsy between 1928 and 1977. Of these, only 13 had been diagnosed in life and of the 41 undiagnosed, death was related to the presence of the pheochromocytoma in 30 [79]. In the general hypertensive population, pheochromocytomas probably occur in about 1 out of every 500 patients [34]. It is clear, therefore, that screening of every hypertensive patient would not be cost-effective. With the discovery of undiagnosed and unsuspected pheochromocytomas at autopsy, and the increasing use of imaging procedures which may demonstrate unsuspected adrenal masses, the question of a possible nonsecreting pheochromocytoma arises. This would explain the occasional report of a pheochromocytoma with normal catecholamine levels in the blood and urine and a normal response to provocative and suppressive testing. In this regard, 621 CT scans of the adrenal area in oncological patients were recently reviewed. Thirty-seven adrenal masses were detected, 25 of which represented metastases. Only one was an unexpected pheochromocytoma [61]. We have recently seen a patient who presented with normal blood pressure and a large adrenal mass. Preoperatively all testing for a pheochromocytoma was negative and the patient underwent exploratory surgery uneventfully without alpha or beta adrenergic blockade. The mass was a pheochromocytoma with large areas of necrosis and hemorrhage. On electron microscopy typical catecholamine secretory granules were noted. It is probable that this was a nonsecreting pheochromocytoma.

Clinical Features

The classical clinical feature of a pheochromocytoma is a paroxysmal hypertensive crisis. This is of course extremely dramatic, and if observed or described will immediately raise the possibility of an underlying pheochromocytoma. In an analysis of 507 cases, however, it only occurred in about

Table 10.1. Common symptoms and signs of pheochromocytoma in adults and differences in children. Data derived from [44] (507 cases), [86] (100 cases), and [82] (95 children)

	% of cases
Hypertension	>90
Sustained	30 (children 90)
Sustained with crises	30
Paroxysmal	30
Headache	80
Sweating	70
Palpitations	65 (children 30)
Pallor	45
Nausea ± vomiting	40 (children 70)
Nervousness	35
Fundoscopic changes	30 (children 70)
Weight loss	25 (children 45)
Epigastric or chest pain	20

one-third. Sixty percent had sustained hypertension and about half of these had super-added crises. Roughly 10% had no hypertension [43] (Table 10.1).

The paroxysm is a manifestation of acute catecholamine release from the tumor. Headache occurs in about 80% of patients, and excessive sweating, palpitations, and a feeling of apprehension are also common. The patient may experience chest, abdominal, or back pain and sometimes parasthesiae in the arms. The face may be blanched and after the attack may flush somewhat. The paroxysm of hypertension may lead to secondary angina, myocardial infarction, and pulmonary edema. Paroxysms or crises may be precipitated by certain maneuvers which disturb the abdominal contents, such as exercise, bending, urination or defecation, palpation of the abdomen, or taking an enema. This may be a particular hazard with the enlarging uterus during pregnancy. Paroxysms may also occur with medically related events, for instance, with the injection of histamine for gastric analysis, at the induction of anesthesia, following the administration of an opiate, with tricyclic antidepressants [1], with adrenal glucocorticoids [18] or adrenocorticotropic hormone (ACTH), and with the angiotensin receptor blocker saralasin [23]. In some patients, a particular stimulus precipitates the event; in others no particular stimulus can be defined. Paroxysms vary frequently in duration and severity and may occur many times a day or as seldom as every few months. With these paroxysmal symptoms patients are frequently thought to have a psychoneurotic problem.

Pheochromocytomas occur more frequently in thin people or are associated with weight loss and, occasionally, fever is present. A true cardiomyopathy or myocarditis unexplained by the high blood pressure alone, and apparently due to the toxic effects of high levels of catecholamines on the myocardium, is a problem with pheochromocytomas which remain untreated for a long period. On occasions, patients may have clear evidence of a pheochromocytoma with high catecholamine levels and yet have few or no symptoms. Such patients, however, are not protected from the grave risk of a hypertensive crisis with such procedures as arteriography, anesthesia, and surgery.

On physical examination, orthostatic hypotension may be a prominent finding and in the presence of hypertension is a strong clue to a possible pheochromocytoma. The orthostasis has been attributed to reduced intravascular volume resulting from chronic vasoconstriction [77], but is probably more related to reduced sensitivity of baroreceptors and adrenergic reflexes because of the high circulating catecholamine levels and a down-regulation of adrenergic receptors [42,78]. The features of a familial syndrome which is associated with pheochromocytoma may be present and these should be carefully checked for, namely, thyroid enlargement and mucosal neuromas of the lids and tongue in MEA-II and III [48,88] and evidence of the neuroectodermal dysplasias (vide infra) [35] (Table 10.2).

Routine laboratory tests may be abnormal. A high hematocrit has again been related to reduced intravascular plasma volume but in some pheochromocytomas there is a true ectopic production of erythropoietin and an increased red cell mass. An elevated white blood cell count without a shift to the left is consistent with demargination of white cells secondary to generalized vasoconstriction. The plasma glucose may also be elevated. This is usually of mild degree and reflects a suppression of insulin secretion by catecholamines and stimulated hepatic glucose output.

End Organ Damage and Complications

Evidence of accelerated hypertension is frequently detected in the ocular fundi. This appears to be more frequent than in essential hypertension and severe fundal changes are particularly noted in children with pheochromocytoma [45]. Surprisingly, renal damage does not run parallel with this and tends to be minimal even with advanced retinopathy [65]. A variety of electrocardiographic changes have been reported and ECG changes occurring during a paroxysm and reverting to normal afterwards are particularly suggestive of a pheochromocytoma. Many deaths are unexpected and sudden with pheochromocytoma and appear to be related to catecholamine-induced damage to the cardiac conduction system in some cases. Myocardial infarction occurs with increased frequency and opiates given for chest pain may precipitate a pheochromocytoma paroxysm. Acute pulmonary edema may be a consequence of the paroxysm or associated cardiac damage, and occlusion of small pulmonary arteries by chronic fibrosis and acute platelet aggregates has been noted at autopsy [46]. As mentioned above, pheochromocytoma cardiomyopathy is a distinct entity apparently related to the long-term toxic effects of catecholamines on the myocardium. There appears to be a definite association between pheochromocytoma and cholelithiasis, as yet unexplained. A paroxysm can be associated with either a thrombotic or hemorrhagic stroke. Renovascular hypertension has been reported. In one of our cases this was due to surgical damage to the renal artery at the time of tumor removal. In other cases it has been ascribed to compression of the renal artery by the tumor. The secondary hyperaldosteronism from renal artery stenosis may produce hypokalemia and when this occurs the other possibility to be considered would be ectopic ACTH production from the pheochromocytoma [54]. Adrenal insufficiency has been reported preoperatively in patients on rare occasions and may occur after tumor removal if the ectopic ACTH syndrome is present. Hemorrhagic necrosis in a pheochromocytoma may be a disastrous event. This can mimic an acute abdomen or a cardiovascular catastrophe and calls for prompt removal of the tumor. In one series, this event appeared to be related to phentolamine administration [86].

Biochemistry

Pheochromocytomas are of particular medical interest because they secrete catecholamines. A catecholamine, by definition, is an amine containing a 3,4-dihydroxyphenyl (catechol) nucleus. Catecholamines include epinephrine, norepinephrine, and dopamine and are synthesized from tyrosine as indicated in Fig. 10.1. The source of tyrosine is dietary intake but tyrosine may also be formed from phenylalanine in the liver. The major catecholamine produced in the adrenal medulla is epinephrine while norepinephrine is released from sympathetic postganglionic neuron axon terminals. The neurons of the central nervous system release dopamine, epinephrine, and norepinephrine. Tyrosine hydroxylase, which promotes the hydroxylation of tyrosine to form dopa, is the rate-limiting enzyme in catecholamine biosynthesis. By feedback tyrosine hydroxylase is inhibited with the synthesis of catecholamines and its synthesis is increased with prolonged stimulation of the adrenergic nervous system. The adrenal medulla also contains the enzyme phenylethanolamine N-methyl transferase (PNMT). This catalyzes the N-methylation of norepinephrine to epinephrine, the final product of

catecholamine biosynthesis. PNMT is induced by glucocorticoids and these are in high concentration in the adrenal medulla which receives portal venous blood from the adrenal cortex. This requirement for glucocorticoids in the synthesis of epinephrine probably explains why norepinephrine is the dominant catecholamine synthesized by extraadrenal pheochromocytomas where a high concentration of glucocorticoids is lacking.

Cryer has shown with infusion experiments that it is necessary to achieve a plasma level of norepinephrine in the 1500–2000 pg/ml range to achieve a hemodynamic response [17]. Only rarely are these levels reached under physiological conditions. It seems, therefore, that norepinephrine functions primarily as a local synaptic neurotransmitter. With epinephrine a hemodynamic response is achieved at levels of 50–100 pg/ml. These are levels which are frequently seen under stressful situations. Epinephrine, therefore, appears to be the mediator of the stress reaction.

Both norepinephrine and epinephrine exert their effects through alpha and beta adrenergic receptors and it is the nature of the receptor on a particular organ which dictates the particular organ response to catecholamine stimulation [82]. Alpha adrenergic receptors are present in the peripheral arterioles and stimulation of these leads to vasoconstriction. Beta adrenergic receptors have been subdivided into beta 1 and beta 2 subtypes. Beta 1 receptors are present in the heart, and stimulation leads to increased heart rate and contractility. They are also the receptors in the juxtaglomerular apparatus of the kidney. Beta 2 receptors are present in the bronchi and the peripheral arterioles as well as in some parenchymal organs like the liver and the pancreas. It is considered that beta 1 receptors are largely stimulated through postganglionic adrenergic nerve fibers, whereas beta 2 receptors are stimulated by the hormone epinephrine carried in the bloodstream. Major therapeutic advances have been made in recent years with the development of both alpha and beta receptor blocking agents. These will be discussed later. A relationship exists between catecholamine levels and the population of receptors. Catecholamine depletion leads to an increased population of receptors, and thus an increased sensitivity to any catecholamine stimulation present. On the other hand catecholamine excess, as in pheochromocytoma, leads to a reduced population of receptors and thus catecholamine insensitivity.

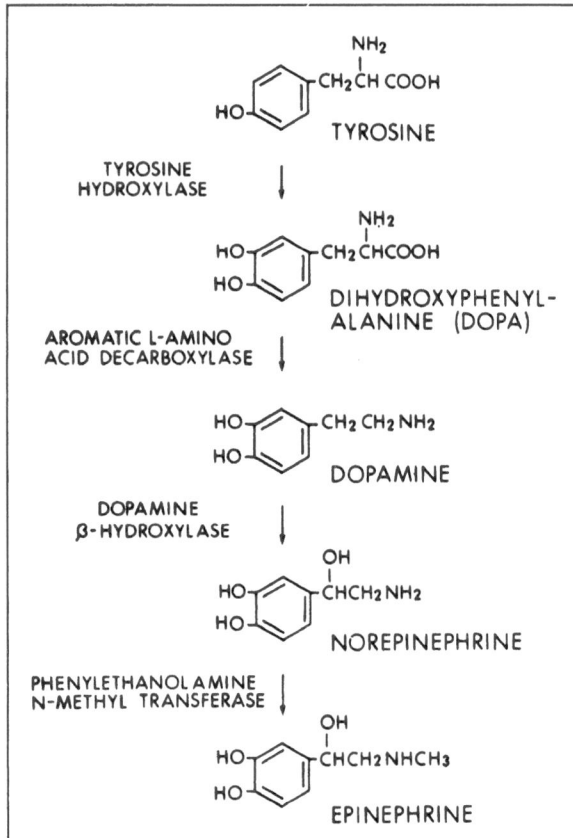

Fig. 10.1 Catecholamine biosynthesis. [Reproduced with permission from Felig et al. (1981) Endocrinology and Metabolism. McGraw-Hill, New York].

Catecholamines are degraded by two principal enzyme systems (Fig. 10.2): catechol-O-methyl transferase (COMT) and monoamineoxidase (MAO). In the presence of COMT and the methyl-donor S-adenosylmethionine, norepinephrine and epinephrine are converted to their respective 3-O-methyl derivatives, normetanephrine (NMN) and metanephrine (MN). These in turn may be converted in the presence of MAO via an aldehyde intermediate and aldehyde oxidase to 3-methoxy-4-hydroxymandelic acid. This is the major end product of norepinephrine and epinephrine degradation and is usually known as vanillylmandelic acid (VMA). An alternative degradation pathway may also occur where norepinephrine and epinephrine are converted initially in the presence of MAO to 3,4-dihydroxymandelaldehyde, which, again through the intermediary aldehyde oxidase step, is finally converted in the presence of COMT to VMA. Dopamine undergoes a similar degradation pathway, except that the metabolites of dopamine lack the hydroxyl group which is present on the beta-carbon of norepinephrine and epinephrine. The end product of this degradation is homovanillic acid (HVA), which corresponds to VMA from norepinephrine and epinephrine.

In contrast to the intermittent nature of the clinical symptoms, most pheochromocytomas probably secrete catecholamines continuously. The amount of secretion, however, fluctuates widely. Paroxysms are presumably due to a sudden acute surge in catecholamine secretion. It has been shown that

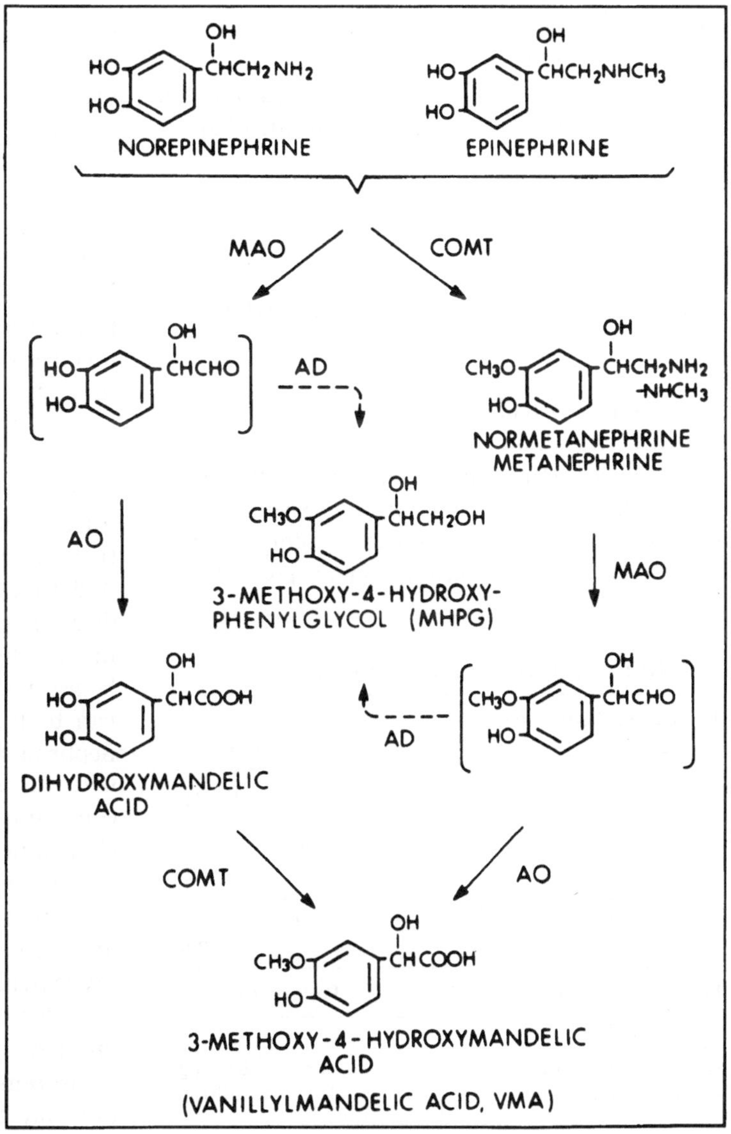

Fig. 10.2 Catecholamine degradation. *COMT,* catecholamine-0-methyl transferase; *MAO,* monoamine oxidase; *AO,* aldehyde oxidase; *AD,* alcohol dehydrogenase.

small pheochromocytomas tend to secrete intact epinephrine and norepinephrine and thus produce symptoms, while larger tumors tend to release large quantities of biologically inactive catecholamine metabolites [16]. The symptomatology may be therefore much less pronounced. Most pheochromocytomas produce excessive quantities of both norepinephrine and epinephrine. It has been claimed that epinephrine production points to a location in the adrenal medulla but epinephrine secretion has been associated with extraadrenal pheochromocytomas. Predominant or isolated epinephrine secretion is rare and may produce a distinctive clinical picture [63] (vide infra). Feldman [30] has shown that most pheochromocytomas contain dopamine but secrete very little of it. Two cases have been reported where dopa and dopamine secretion occurred together with that of epinephrine and norepinephrine. These patients were normotensive and it was suggested that the hypotensive action of dopa and dopamine counteracted the hypertensive effects of norepinephrine [53].

Diagnosis of Pheochromocytoma

The diagnosis of a pheochromocytoma is made with the demonstration of elevated levels of catecholamines or their metabolites in the blood and urine (Table 10.2). To embark on expensive localization procedures, or even exploratory surgery, because of clinical suspicion alone, is poor medical

Table 10.2. Catecholamines and metabolites

Twenty-four hour urine	Upper limit of normal range	
Free catecholamines		100 μg
Epinephrine	20 μg	
Norepinephrine	80 μg	
Metanephrines		1.3 mg
Metanephrine	0.4 mg	
Normetanephrine	0.9 mg	
VMA (vanillylmandelic acid)		6.5 mg
Plasma catecholamines	Positive test	
Baseline	> 950 pg/ml	
Glucagon stimulation	3 × or > 2000 pg/ml	
Clonidine suppression	> 500 pg/ml	

practice. One carefully collected acid-preserved 24-h urine specimen, assayed for VMA, total metanephrines, or total free catecholamines, constitutes an excellent, highly reliable, screening test. If drug interference and the problems of 24-h urine collection are excluded, the reliability of these tests approaches 95%; but different centers may place their reliance on different tests. VMA is probably measured most commonly. Older VMA assays were based on a reaction between the phenolic acid group and various diazo dyes and the resulting colored compound formed was measured in a colorimeter. This was a nonspecific reaction with many interfering factors, including bananas, coffee, and vanilla [34]. A much more reliable assay involves the conversion of VMA to vanillin, which can then be measured directly with a spectrophotometer [67]. Certain drugs may interfere: monoamineoxidase inhibitors lower VMA and at the same time raise metanephrine excretion. Nalidixic acid may increase and clofibrate may decrease VMA excretion. A clue to the specificity of the VMA test is the normal range given by the laboratory. A range of 10–15 mg/24 h indicates the old colorimetric test. An upper limit of 6.8 mg implies a much more reliable spectrophotometric assay. Metanephrines are more consistently elevated in pheochromocytomas than VMA. Again, the assay involves the conversion to vanillin, which is measured by spectrophotometry. The upper limit of normal in the method described by Pisano is 1.3 mg/24 h [66]. There seems to be less interference with this assay than with VMA. X-ray contrast media, as from an intravenous pyelogram (IVP), may decrease metanephrine levels for up to 3 days after the X-ray. Chlorpromazine, benzodiazepines, and MAO inhibitors may all increase metanephrine levels. Free catecholamines can also be assayed in the urine [15] and in addition these can be fractionated into norepinephrine and epinephrine moieties. The usual assay is fluorometric with the measurement of the highly fluorescent compounds obtained by the oxidation of catecholamines to trihydroxyindole derivatives. Tetracyclines, quinidine, and chlorhydrate can interfere with the analysis and certain drugs alter the levels in vivo. Methyldopa (forming alphamethylnorepinephrine), isoproterenol, theophylline, and prochlorperazine can all raise, while clonidine and fenfluramine lower, free catecholamines. The measurement of urinary-free catecholamines is probably less reliable than either VMA or metanephrines, but has definite utility. When the specimen is fractionated, an elevated epinephrine level combined with an elevated norepinephrine level points to an adrenal pheochromocytoma as opposed to an extraadrenal location. An isolated elevation of epinephrine may facilitate the diagnosis of a pheochromocytoma which has a specific set of symptoms and signs. We have found the epinephrine fraction to be the most useful index in screening for familial pheochromocytoma as part of MEA-II [39]. In the rare patient with periodic paroxysms where the urinary catecholamine metabolites are normal between episodes, a timed urine collection for the 4 h following the paroxysm assayed for free catecholamines may be most helpful in making the diagnosis. Determination of catecholamine metabolites in this situation is less likely to indicate the rapid and significant changes in catecholamine excretion. Although 24-h urine collections are desirable, it has been shown that where these cannot be obtained accurately, overnight collections and bracketed 2- to 4-h collections provide comparable results [47]. In this situation, the concentrations of catecholamines or metabolites are expressed per milligram of creatinine.

In most patients with pheochromocytoma all three urine tests are positive. Out of the 64 documented patients studied by Sjoerdsma et al. [77], there were only two assay results within the normal range. However, there is no doubt that some patients may have positive results for one assay and not for the other. For instance, the Cleveland Clinic Group [7] have reported in 43 patients with surgically confirmed pheochromocytomas that 25 had falsely negative VMA assays, and 9 falsely negative metanephrine assays. In one patient an elevated metanephrine level was the only detectable biochemical abnormality. Confirming the excellence of the metanephrine assay, Gitlow reported in 1970 his experience with 92 pheochromocytoma patients and 9500 controls. False-negative assays were obtained in 4% with the metanephrine assay, 21% with free catecholamines, and 29% with VMA [34].

Plasma catecholamines are measured routinely by catechol-O-methyl transferase radioenzymatic assay [26]. Liquid chromatography with electrochemical detection is also available in certain centers [36]. Any source of exogenous catecholamines such as nose drops or weight-reducing pills and alphamethyldopa raise plasma catecholamine levels and clonidine suppresses them under physiologic conditions. Definite precautions should be taken when the blood sample for plasma catecholamines is obtained. To avoid a falsely elevated level from the stress of the needle insertion, the patient is required to lie supine in a quiet area after a needle attached to a heparin lock is inserted. The sample is obtained painlessly 30 min later. The red cells should be separated from the plasma within 5 min because they take up catecholamines very quickly and may produce a falsely low plasma level.

Bravo and Gifford [7] have reported their experience with 64 patients with documented pheochromocytoma collected over a 5-year period. Only four of those patients had plasma catecholamine values that fell within the 95% confidence limits for patients with essential hypertension—i.e., under 950 pg/ml. None of the pheochromocytoma patients had values that fell within the normal range for age- and sex-matched normotensive controls. In three other series [17,27,33] of 13, 15, and 13 patients respectively, only two patients had plasma catecholamine levels which were less than 1000 pg/ml. Cryer had previously shown that plasma norepinephrine concentrations in excess of 2000 pg/ml were required to produce biological effects. It was not surprising, therefore, that the levels found in pheochromocytoma patients considerably exceeded that figure in most instances. The mean plasma catecholamine level in one series was 5600 pg/ml and 11 100 pg/ml in another. Other workers have reported a significant incidence of false-negative results and recommend that urinary tests be retained as screening procedures. In 15 patients documented by urine tests, Plouin [68] had false-negative results on three occasions. Manger and Gifford [57] report that patients with sustained hypertension in their experience invariably had elevated plasma catecholamine levels whereas 37.5% with paroxysmal hypertension had normal plasma catecholamines when their blood pressures were also normal.

Plasma catecholamine determinations appear to be useful in providing further validation of urinary tests and in catching a burst of catecholamine secretion during a paroxysm. As with fractionated urinary catecholamines an elevated plasma epinephrine is highly suggestive of an adrenal location for the pheochromocytoma. The measurement of plasma catecholamines is also highly useful in provocative tests and in selective venous catheterization as a localizing procedure (vide infra).

Recently a biochemical assay has been reported measuring increased platelet catecholamine levels.

This appears to be a sensitive and reliable indicator of pheochromocytoma, but false-negative results occur and this test is not routinely available [90].

The extent to which the screening tests described above should be used in the search for possible cases of pheochromocytoma is controversial. If they were applied to every hypertensive and using Gitlow's estimate that the prevalence of pheochromocytomas is 0.5% among the hypertensive population [34], then four out of every five positive urinary metanephrine determinations would be, in fact, false positives. A false positive would lead to the necessity for repeat tests and other investigations, vastly increasing the cost. It is, therefore, expedient to rely heavily on clinical suspicion based on history and physical examination, in electing to screen patients for pheochromocytomas.

Pharmacological Testing

A number of pharmacological tests for the diagnosis of pheochromocytoma have been used over the years, both provocative (inducing a hypertensive response) and suppressive (inducing a fall in blood pressure). Earlier tests have become virtually obsolete because of their danger and high incidence of both false-negative and false-positive results, but recently there has been a resurgence of interest in pharmacological testing, utilizing not only blood pressure response but also changes in plasma catecholamines. These have been particularly useful in patients studied in between paroxysms when the usual urinary screening tests are normal, but there remains a suspicion that a pheochromocytoma is present.

Provocative Tests

Intravenous histamine (10–25 mg of the base), tyramine (1–2 mg), and glucagon (0.5 mg, then 1.0 mg if no response to smaller dose) have all been used. Of these the glucagon test [7,74], because it has fewer side effects, is the only one used to any extent. In a positive test suggestive of a pheochromocytoma, there is a rise in blood pressure of 20/15 mmHg in excess of the rise seen with a cold pressor test. Blood drawn at the peak of the blood pressure rise after the glucagon [51] should dem-

onstrate a clear rise of at least threefold in plasma catecholamines or an increase to over 2000 pg/ml.

Suppression Tests

The hypotensive response to intravenous phentolamine (regitine test) was formerly widely used in the diagnosis of pheochromocytoma. After test doses of 0.5 and 1 mg with no fall in blood pressure, a dose of 5 mg is usually given and a blood pressure fall of greater than 35/25 mmHg is considered a positive Test. This test has had a high incidence of both false-positive and false-negative results and even with the small test dose, profound hypotension may occur.

Two new suppression tests are now in use which are much more diagnostically reliable and much safer. Pentolinium is a preganglionic blocking agent. It has been shown that, when given intravenously in a dose of 2.5 mg, it will suppress physiologically elevated plasma catecholamines but will have no effect on the elevated level associated with an autonomously functioning pheochromocytoma. In the series reported by Brown et al. [9], the test was correct in separating 18 patients with a pheochromocytoma from 20 patients who had intermittently elevated plasma pheochromocytomas for other reasons. Pentolinium may cause acute urinary retention and is no longer available in the United States.

Clonidine is an alpha-2 adrenergic agonist which will also suppress the release of catecholamines from nerve terminals and thus the elevated levels associated with any activation of the sympathetic nervous system, but will have no effect on the autonomous production from pheochromocytomas. Clonidine (0.3 mg) is given by mouth and the plasma catecholamines are measured at baseline and at the 3-h point [8]. In patients without pheochromocytoma, the plasma catecholamine value should fall below 500 pg/ml [52]. In the experience of Bravo, applying this test to 32 patients with pheochromocytomas, only one patient gave a false-negative result. Since clonidine has a central effect in lowering blood pressure, both pheochromocytoma patients and other hypertensives may have a hypotensive response. This could be a problem in patients concurrently taking beta adrenergic blocking agents or who are volume depleted and occasionally results in marked bradycardia, a reduction in cardiac output, and severe hypotension. Bravo et al. describe pitfalls to be avoided with the clonidine test [7]. Beta adrenergic blocking agents may prevent the ability of clonidine to suppress catecholamines in nonpheochromocytoma patients because they interfere with the hepatic clearance of catecholamines. Investigators should be wary of radioimmunoassays that measure both free and conjugated catecholamines since false-positive results may be obtained. This is because conjugated catecholamines have a long half-life especially in renal failure patients.

However, even with the radioenzymatic determination of free plasma catecholamines false-negative and false-positive tests have been reported and further experience with the clonidine suppression test is obviously required. At this time, however, it appears to be the best and safest pharmacological test available when a patient is hypertensive. Glucagon can be substituted if the patient is normotensive at the time of testing.

Localization

When the presence of a pheochromocytoma has been confirmed by biochemical tests it is necessary to localize the tumor or tumors. No localizing procedure, however, should be performed until such a diagnosis has been made. Currently, the abdominal CT scan is the best test available [32]. It is non-invasive and is capable of detecting tumors 1 cm in diameter or greater. It is estimated that its overall accuracy in the diagnosis of pheochromocytoma is between 90% and 95%. Ultrasonography is less accurate and IVP with or without tomograms of the suprarenal areas is outmoded except where more modern procedures are unavailable. An IVP can be performed if the surgeon wishes to be reassured that two functioning kidneys are present, but application of blocks for compression films may precipitate a hypertensive crisis. Unfortunately, CT scanning does not carry the same high degree of accuracy in the detection of tumors outside the renal-adrenal area. In this situation, sampling of venous blood at many sites from the neck to the pelvis may indicate the site of venous drainage from a pheochromocytoma by a sudden surge in catecholamine concentration [3]. Such "hot spots" detected by venous sampling may be further studied by arteriography or CT scanning in order to dem-

onstrate a tumor. However, the radiologist should avoid performing venography at the same time as venous sampling as this has been reported to produce rupture of adrenals and pheochromocytomas [24].

Arteriography, with the advent of CT scanning, is less often needed, but provides a valuable alternative and may provide additional information concerning the anatomy of the blood supply of the tumor, especially when it is near the hilum of the kidney or close to the great vessels. Arteriography is an invasive procedure which may precipitate a hypertensive crisis even in a normotensive patient who has never previously been known to have a paroxysm. It is therefore essential that patients be prepared before this procedure with alpha adrenergic blocking agents as discussed later.

Radiocholesterol scanning for pheochromocytomas has been largely abandoned, but a new scanning technique using [131I]meta-iodobenzylguanidine (MIBG) is extremely promising [75]. This radionuclide is an analog of norepinephrine and is specifically concentrated in adrenergic vesicles. The normal adrenal medulla is not visible, but most tumors of all sizes, in the adrenals and elsewhere, both benign and malignant, are located easily. Tumors too small to be seen by CT scan and even adrenal medullary hyperplasia have been visualized [85]. The MIBG scan may have particular utility in demonstrating that a mass revealed by CT scanning is adrenergic in origin although carcinoids and possibly other APUD tumors are also visualized. The flowchart in Fig. 10.3 summarizes the application of the diagnostic and localization techniques described.

Treatment

Surgical excision remains the only satisfactory method of treating pheochromocytomas. However, the preoperative and intraoperative period can be associated with large swings in blood pressure and malignant arrhythmias. Postoperatively profound hypotension may occur. Therefore, careful medical coverage (Table 10.3, p. 132) is mandatory with skilled, experienced anesthesia and surgery.

Although not practiced routinely in all centers, we begin alpha adrenergic blockade with phenoxy-

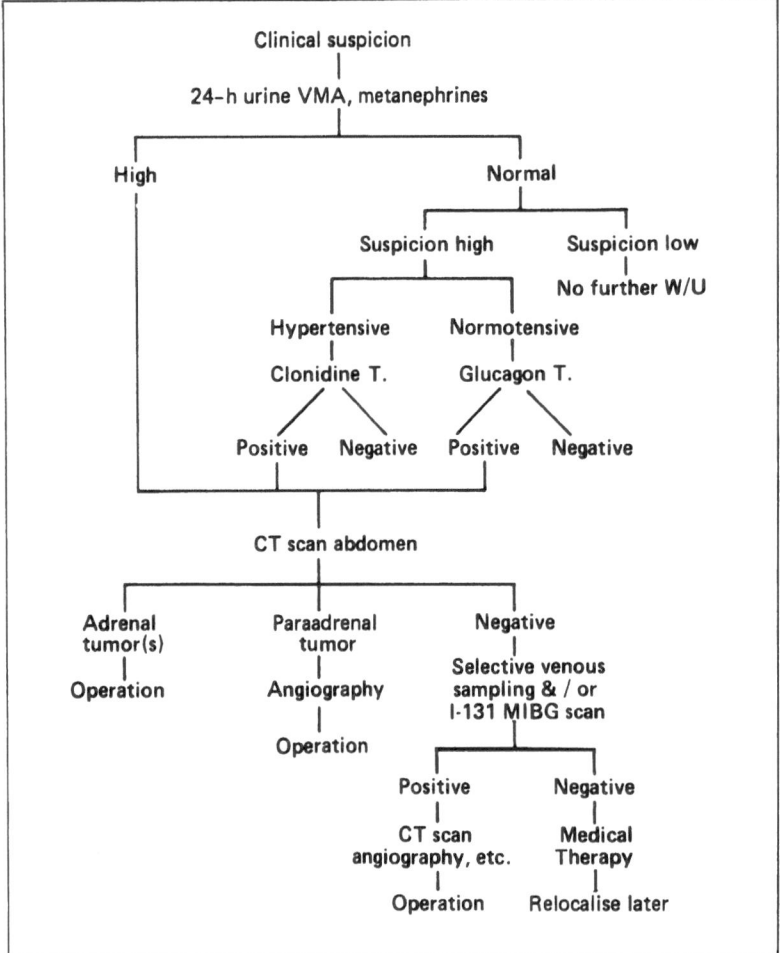

Fig. 10.3 Flowchart for investigation of a possible pheochromocytoma.

benzamine, 10 mg orally, twice daily, as soon as possible and increase the dose slowly up to a maximum of 20 mg, four times a day to obtain smooth blood pressure control. The patient is then protected through the remainder of the preoperative period and during any further evaluation procedures such as arteriography. The alpha blockade also provides relatively stable blood pressure control through the induction of anesthesia and the conduct of the surgery. In addition, pheochromocytoma patients are frequently volume depleted because of continued peripheral vasoconstriction. The alpha blockade, by relieving this vasoconstriction, allows blood volume to be restored preoperatively. The catastrophic postoperative hypotension that was formerly a major surgical problem is thus avoided. To facilitate blood volume expansion we give intravenous fluids over the preoperative period and in some centers two to three units of whole blood are given 12–18 h before

the operation [20]. These measures, plus careful operative hemostasis and blood replacement, all help to counter postoperative hypotension. The alpha blockade may also promote "up regulation" of alpha adrenergic receptors. The patient, therefore, becomes sensitive again to physiological levels of catecholamines, adrenergic reflexes are restored, and the patient postoperatively is again able to respond to the stimulus of hypotension with peripheral vasoconstriction and increased cardiac output.

Beta adrenergic blockade is not used routinely in many centers preoperatively [7] but is appropriate if there is tachycardia present (which can be aggravated by alpha blockade) or if there is a cardiac arrhythmia. We begin with propranolol, 10 mg three times a day and, increase the dose gradually up to 40 mg three times a day. If thought necessary, beta blockade should only be introduced after adequate alpha blockade has been achieved. Otherwise a paradoxical pressor response may occur [71]. As an alternative to phenoxybenzamine, prazosin (2–5 mg, twice daily), an alpha 1 adrenergic blocker [60], or labetalol [70] (a combined alpha and beta adrenergic blocker) can be used. The use of both agents has been reported in the literature, but the experience is not great and the alpha blockade provided does not seem to be as potent or as reliable. Also, anomalous pressor responses to labetalol have occurred possibly because this is predominantly a beta blocker [28].

In view of the much improved control of blood pressure which alpha blockade provides, it may seem surprising that it is not used routinely in all centers. Some groups argue that the stabilization of blood pressure achieved with alpha blockade robs the surgeon during the operation of valuable information obtained from observing changes in blood pressure [57]. For instance, in the absence of alpha blockade a surgeon may observe a rise in blood pressure when the tumor is palpated, a fall in blood pressure when the tumor is completely removed, or the persistence of high blood pressure when further tumors remain. It is also claimed that alpha blockade may lead to enhancement of the hypotensive effects of thiopental (Pentothal) during induction, may increase venous oozing, and may lead to greater hypotension with hemorrhage because of loss of reflex vasoconstriction. The argument for no alpha blockade may be valid with an extremely experienced team looking for a tumor that is difficult to locate or where multiple tumors are suspected. However, modern localization techniques, including CT scanning, MIBG scanning, and selective venous catheterization for plasma catecholamine levels, make this approach less often necessary.

If a hypertensive crisis occurs before the patient can be taken to surgery, then more acute control of blood pressure is required. The patient is nursed in the head upright position and given the alpha adrenergic blocker phentolamine intravenously 2–5 mg every 5 min until the blood pressure is controlled. The effect of phentolamine is transient and it may be necessary to set up a constant infusion of phentolamine or otherwise of sodium nitroprusside. A solution containing 100 mg of either drug in 500 ml 5% dextrose can be prepared and infused at a rate adequate to control the blood pressure. With prolonged nitroprusside infusions or in the presence of renal failure, it is necessary to monitor blood thiocyanate levels because concentrations in excess of 10 mg/dl may produce toxic psychosis.

If serious tachycardia or arrhythmias develop, propranolol may also be given intravenously 1–2 mg over a 5- to 10-min period. Once the crisis is controlled the pheochromocytoma patient can be switched to oral preoperative medication as described above.

Operative Management

Despite the preoperative measures described above, alpha blockade is often not complete and surgery in patients with pheochromocytomas is associated with marked swings in blood pressure and hypotension after tumor removal. Tachycardia and cardiac arrhythmias are also common. The key to successful surgery is continuous monitoring and display of the ECG, and intraarterial and central venous or pulmonary capillary wedge pressure (Swan-Ganz catheter). The wedge pressure is a better guide to volume replacement than the central venous pressure, but the insertion of a Swan-Ganz catheter may trigger arrhythmias in these patients. The following agents should be drawn up and made ready for immediate administration: intravenous phentolamine—both bolus and infusion; nitroprusside—for infusion (these two agents are for a sudden rise in blood pressure); intravenous propranolol—for tachycardia; lidocaine—for arrhythmias; and intravenous norepinephrine (Levophed) available for possible postoperative hypotension (Table 10.3).

Blood should be replaced quantitatively as it is lost and plasma or 5% albumin is given in whatever quantity needed to combat hypotension after the tumor has been removed.

Blood pressure and volume control is probably more important than the choice of anesthetic agent. However, the halogenated hydrocarbons have been used successfully, halothane initially and more recently methoxyflurane, isoflurane, and enflurane (Ethrane) [21]. These reduce significantly the pressor action of catecholamines but like cyclopropane may potentiate catecholamine-induced arrhythmias. Hence, the need for constant vigilance on the part of both surgeon and anesthesiologist and the immediate availability of propranolol and lidocaine. In some centers, neuroleptanalgesia (droperidol, and phenoperidine or Fentanyl) is gaining popularity as it is claimed that greater stability of blood pressure is obtained and the danger of arrhythmias is reduced [81].

Table 10.3. Drugs in the medical management of pheochromocytoma

1. Alpha adrenergic blockers
   Acute: Phentolamine 2–5 mg i.v.
   Chronic: Phenoxybenzamine (dibenzyline) 10–20 mg
              t.i.d. to q.i.d.
              Prazosin (Minipress) 1–5 mg b.i.d.
2. Beta adrenergic blockers (*after* alpha blockade)
   Acute   Propranolol 1–2 mg i.v.
              Labetalol (alpha + beta) 20–40 mg i.v.
   Chronic: Propranolol 10–40– mg q.i.d.
              or other ß-blocker
              Labetalol 200–600 mg b.i.d.
3. Catecholamine synthesis inhibitor
              Alpha-methyl *p*-tyrosine (metyrosine) 250 mg
              to 1 g b.i.d.
4. Hypertensive crisis
              Phentolamine (regitine) i.v. 2–5 mg (bolus) or
              100 mg in 500 ml normal saline (infusion)
              Nitroprusside 50 mg in 500 ml normal saline
              (infusion)
5. Hypotension
              Norepinephrine (Levophed) infusion
6. Arrhythmias
              Lidocaine 50–100 mg i.v. (20–50 mg/min)
              Propranolol 0.5–2 mg i.v.

The anterior transperitoneal surgical approach is now considered mandatory for an intraabdominal pheochromocytoma as these tumors may be multiple and extraadrenal [88]. The operation must be performed delicately, with good access, and the patient "dissected away from the tumor" [31]. The strategy involves immediate ligation of tumor blood vessels, removal of the identified tumor, and thorough exploration for additional tumors in both adrenals and at all sites at which abdominal paraganglia may be found. Early ligation of tumor venous drainage should prevent seeding of malignant cells [4]. If a pheochromocytoma cannot be totally resected, it is still worthwhile debulking as much as possible to reduce catecholamine release by the residual tumor to a minimum. If a single adrenal tumor is found, the entire gland is removed. If bilateral tumors are present, it is advisable, if possible, to leave some adrenocortical tissue intact in order to avoid lifelong dependence on steroid replacement therapy. Because of the high incidence of coexisting cholelithiasis, the gallbladder should be examined during exploration and removed if necessary [57].

After tumor removal and in the postoperative period, as already mentioned, hypotension may be a serious complicating problem. Many factors may be involved: continued blood loss at operative sites with inadequate replacement, down regulation of adrenergic receptors, and insensitivity of adrenergic reflexes because of prior catecholamine excess, and alpha and beta adrenergic blockade (e.g., with phenoxybenzamine and propranolol), which would have a similar effect. The rigorous monitoring during surgery should be continued in this postoperative period, until the patient is stable. Because of the acquired insensitivity to catecholamines, intravenous norepinephrine (Levophed) for the hypotension has produced poor results and led to the term "irreversible shock." Adequate attention to blood volume replacement with whole blood and plasma makes the administration of norepinephrine less necessary. Hypertension may also occur as a result of fluid overload, residual pheochromocytoma tissue, or inadvertent ligation of the renal artery [57]. If this occurs, urine collections for catecholamines are collected after the fourth postoperative day and analyzed before reexploration is contemplated. Severe hypoglycemia may also occur. Presumably, the sudden reduction in catecholamines inhibits the glycogenolysis process and may enhance insulin secretion [2].

Prognosis

With benign tumors, the 5-year survival rate is 96% and 75% of patients are rendered normotensive. In the Mayo Clinic series of 77 patients operated on in the 1970s the operative mortality was 5% and the 5-year survival 88% [37]. In the minority of patients who remain hypertensive there is no evidence of residual tumor and the cause for the hypertension is uncertain.

Although surgeons and physicians involved in the surgical care of pheochromocytomas recognize that operations now go much smoother with modern preoperative preparation, convincing data concerning the change in operative mortality related to this improved preparation are hard to find. In the Hammersmith experience, 3 of 17 patients died before modern preoperative measures were adopted, while only 1 of 41 undergoing a total of 45 operations suffered an operative death after that time [88].

Patients with sporadic tumors should be followed for about 2 years and should have urine collections at least once a year to rule out late recurrence. In familial cases, the follow-up period must be much longer and other components of the familial syndrome must be considered (see below).

Subtypes of Pheochromocytoma

Pheochromocytoma of the Urinary Bladder

The bladder is a rare site for an extraadrenal pheochromocytoma and represents less than 1% of all cases and less than 0.1% of all bladder tumors. Nevertheless, more than 100 cases have been reported. Most tumors are small and intramural and about 90% are benign. The majority present between the ages of 10 and 20 years [19].

The characteristic symptoms are headache and/or syncope on micturition or when the bladder is distended [59]. There may be also symptoms related to any bladder tumor, namely, hematuria and frequency. Tumors at the base of the bladder may be palpated rectally, and the diagnosis is confirmed by cystoscopy and biopsy. The majority of patients reported have been cured by operation, which is usually a partial cystectomy. Many of the malignant pheochromocytomas manifest as local recurrence, but some have metastasized widely. About 20% of patients die within 1 year and 60% within 5 years [88].

Pheochromocytoma During Pregnancy

Pregnancy and the pressure of a gravid uterus on the posterior abdominal wall may aggravate the symptoms of a pheochromocytoma and expose occult tumors. Although it is a much less common cause of hypertension in pregnancy than preeclamptic toxemia, a pheochromocytoma is important to exclude and if not recognized before delivery is associated with a maternal mortality of about 40% and an infant mortality of about 50%. In early pregnancy, removal of the tumor has been recommended, whereas in the later months, patients may be treated with adrenergic blocking agents as indicated until close to term [25]. However, Manger and Gifford [57] in their review prefer to remove a pheochromocytoma in pregnancy as soon as it is discovered regardless of the duration of pregnancy. If pregnancy is carried to term, cesarean section is recommended with tumor removal at the same

time. In this way the patient is not exposed to the stress of a vaginal delivery.

Pheochromocytoma in Children

Pheochromocytoma has been reported in children even less than 1 year of age. The majority of these cases are familial and the tumors multiple and often extraadrenal. The hypertension is usually persistent and may be very severe with grade 3 or 4 retinopathy [45,80]. The Riley-Day syndrome (familial dysautonomia) can mimic pheochromocytoma in childhood and, in addition, may be associated with increased excretion of homovanillic acid (HVA) in the urine.

Pheochromocytoma with Predominant or Isolated Epinephrine Secretion

Occasionally, pheochromocytomas have been described which secrete predominantly epinephrine rather than norepinephrine [62,63]. The clinical features may be somewhat different from those recognized with a classical pheochromocytoma. The patient may be normotensive and have bouts of orthostatic hypotension more profound than is usually seen [40] presumably due to beta 2 stimulated vasodilatation in the peripheral arterioles by epinephrine. In addition, metabolic features such as weight loss and hyperglycemia may be prominent.

Pseudo- or Nonpheochromocytoma

Only a small fraction, probably less than 10%, of those patients screened for a pheochromocytoma turn out to have this tumor. This is because the symptoms which arouse suspicion are nonspecific and can be caused by a number of other conditions. Clinical confusion arises frequently in neurotic patients with hyperkinetic circulations and in perimenopausal or postmenopausal women with highly labile blood pressure. Bouts of angina may give rise to sudden paroxysms of high blood pressure, probably the result of an adrenergic reflex stimulated from a reduction in coronary blood flow. Excessive catecholamine release also explains the hypertensive crises which occur in patients taking monoamineoxidase inhibitors who then ingest tyramine-containing cheeses or wine. Hypoglycemia may produce a pheochromocytoma-like picture, also due to stimulated adrenergic reflexes and catecholamine release. Neurogenic hypertension related to various central nervous system lesions such as tumors, strokes, and trauma can also confuse the diagnosis. Kuchel [50] has suggested that some patients with "pseudo-pheochromocytomas" have a decreased rate of inactivation of catecholamines leading to increased free levels in the circulation. Perhaps the most frequent cause for misdiagnosis is the use of inaccurate, nonspecific urinary assays for VMA and the presence of substances and medications which interfere with laboratory assays.

Familial Pheochromocytoma

The familial occurrence of pheochromocytoma has been recognized since the 1940s. In many of these families it is now clear that the pheochromocytoma is part of a syndrome associated with the inheritance of other endocrine abnormalities or as part of a neuroectodermal dysplasia (phakomatosis). Inheritance is by an autosomal dominant trait with a high degree of penetrance. Of the 29 families with familial pheochromocytoma reviewed in 1968, it occurred as an isolated phenomenon in 16 families [83]. But it is hard to estimate at this point whether a simple form of familial pheochromocytoma exists.

The clinical features of familial pheochromocytoma are similar to the sporadic nonfami-

Table 10.4. Familial pheochromocytoma syndromes (autosomal dominant)

A. Multiple endocrine adenomas (MEA)	
(pheochromocytoma incidence 75% or more)	
MEA-I	Hyperparathyroidism
(Werner's)	Islet cell tumors of pancreas
	Pituitary tumors
MEA-II	Pheochromocytoma
(Sipple's)	Medullary carcinoma of the thyroid
	Hyperparathyroidism
MEA-III	Pheochromocytoma
(Mucosal	Medullary carcinoma of the thyroid
neuromas	Mucosal neuromas
syndrome)	Ganglioneuromatosis of gut
B. Neuroectodermal dysplasias	
(pheochromocytoma incidence 5%–10%)	
(phakomatoses)	
Multiple neurofibromatosis	
(von Recklinghausen's)	
Tuberous sclerosis	
Encephalotrigeminal angiomatosis	
(Sturge–Weber)	
von Hippel–Lindau's disease	

lial cases except that they occur in younger people and are bilateral in most cases, even though one tumor may present years before the other. The question has also been raised that malignancy may be more common in familial pheochromocytoma. In one kindred, 4 of 19 cases had either local recurrence or metastases, which is about twice the expected incidence of malignancy. From analyses of other kindred, however, malignancy seems distinctly uncommon.

The familial endocrine neoplastic syndromes, multiple endocrine adenomas type I (MEA-I) and type II (MEA-II) (also known as multiple endocrine neoplasia types I and II [MEN-I and MEN-II]) and the phakomatoses are discussed separately (Table 10.4).

Neuroectodermal Dysplasias

These are a group of related disorders each with a combination of central nervous system abnormalities and skin lesions. The syndromes are strongly familial, and all have been associated with pheochromocytoma [35].

Von Recklinghausen's disease or multiple neurofibromatosis is the most common and the most commonly associated with pheochromocytoma, which is said to occur in 10%–12% of cases. The disorder is characterized by multiple neurofibromata on peripheral nerves which are visible and palpable as small cutaneous tumors. In addition, there are multiple other skin lesions including vascular nevi, hairy nevi, skin polyps, and areas of pigmentation known as café-au-lait spots. Vascular malformations of the brain, meningiomas, gliomas, and retinal tumors have all been described with this condition.

Tuberous sclerosis is characterized by special nevi of the face known as adenoma sebaceum and mental retardation. Small tumors of the brain and in the walls of the ventricles may occur and seizures are common. Brain malformations and cysts and tumors in other organs may also occur. The same patient may have both neurofibromatosis and tuberous sclerosis.

In the Sturge-Weber syndrome there is a readily visible, large facial hemangioma or port wine stain over the distribution of the trigeminal nerve. Angiomatous malformations of the brain and meninges, often in the same distribution as the skin lesion, are common and seizures are a complication.

Von Hippel-Lindau disease is the term given to the combination of angiomatosis of the retina and cystic cerebellar hemangiomas which may also occur on the spinal cord. As with tuberous sclerosis, multiple cysts and tumors may occur in other organs and some patients have also had the Sturge-Weber syndrome.

It is obviously important to consider one of these familial syndromes in the history and physical examination of a patient with a possible pheochromocytoma. In addition, patients with these syndromes who have hypertension should be strongly suspected of harboring a pheochromocytoma.

Multiple Endocrine Neoplasia Syndromes

MEA-I (MEN-I) or Wermer's syndrome was the first of these three syndromes to be delineated and like the other two, described below, appears to be a familial congenital dystrophy of APUD cells arising from the neural crest. MEA-I is characterized by adenomas of the pituitary which may be associated with hyperprolactinemia, or acromegaly, hyperparathyroidism, and islet cell tumors of the pancreas [5,88]. The latter most commonly are gastrinomas producing the Zollinger-Ellison syndrome and insulinomas producing hypoglycemia. More rarely carcinoids, glucagonomas, and VIPomas producing the pancreatic cholera or Verner-Morrison syndrome have been described. Presumably somatostatinomas will also turn up in the MEA-I syndrome in due course.

In its true form, MEA-I does not have pheochromocytoma as one of its components, and it is distinct from MEA-II, which is described below. However, multiple examples of a "crossover" syndrome with components of both MEA-I and MEA-II have been described; for example, pituitary tumors, parathyroid hyperplasia, and pheochromocytoma; islet cell tumors and pheochromocytoma; and MEA-II with the Zollinger-Ellison syndrome [41].

MEA-II or Sipple's syndrome consists of calcitonin-secreting medullary carcinoma of the thyroid, hyperparathyroidism, and pheochromocytoma. Since the advent of sensitive assays for calcitonin in the blood, medullary carcinoma of the thyroid has usually been diagnosed first in an afflicted family member [58]. However, in early family studies, pheochromocytoma was the dominant lesion and indeed accounted for 30% of the deaths in one MEA-II kindred [10]. The pheochromocytoma of MEA-II has certain distinctive features. It appears to begin as adrenal medullary hyperplasia, which is initially diffuse, then nodular, and finally neoplastic with multiple tumors in the affected glands [12]. This would appear to be analogous to the C-cell hyperplasia occurring as a preneoplastic lesion leading on to medullary carcinoma of the thyroid. Compared with a sporadic pheochromocytoma, this tumor is more likely to be asymptomatic or associated with paroxysmal hypertension and is thus more difficult to diagnose [39]. It should be carefully screened for in afflicted families, however, since if undetected it may lead to a hypertensive crisis during surgery for medullary carcinoma of the thyroid. Clearly the pheochromocytoma in these families should be dealt with first. The MEA-II pheochromocytoma, even at the adrenal medulla hyperplasia stage, is associated with increased excretion of epinephrine; and measurement of fractionated catecholamines in the urine, specifically for the epinephrine level, may be the only means of making the diagnosis [39]. Preliminary results suggest that [131I]MIBG scintigraphy can also reveal adrenal medullary hyperplasia in MEA-II [85].

In many series the incidence of pheochromocytoma in MEA-II is reported to be less than that of thyroid medullary carcinoma, but this probably reflects the sensitivity of the screening tests for each tumor, and every MEA-II patient should be strongly and continually suspected of harboring a pheochromocytoma which is likely to be bilateral.

Surgical treatment for pheochromocytoma in MEA-II is controversial to some extent, since some surgeons would advocate bilateral adrenalectomy because of the high incidence of bilateral pheochromocytomas, even though the patient is committed to lifelong steroid maintenance therapy A more conservative and probably rational approach would appear to be removal of the pheochromocytoma detected and careful follow-up at 6 monthly or yearly intervals thereafter to detect a pheochromocytoma on the contralateral side [89].

MEA (MEN) II-b or III is a variant of MEA-II in which there are also mucosal neuromas but hyperparathyroidism is rare [48]. In contrast to MEA-II, over half the cases appear to be sporadic and a similar number show the complete syndrome while about 10% have the combination of neuromas and pheochromocytomas alone. Mucosal neuromas are the hallmark of the disease and occur in all afflicted patients. Most commonly they occur in the mouth, about the lips, tongue, and buccal mucosa, giving a "lumpy bumpy" appearance. There may also be neuromas visible on the eyelids, and the corneal nerves visible by slit lamp are thickened and medullated. Ganglioneuromatosis of the gut may also be present leading to motility problems such as constipation, diarrhea, and megacolon [12]. A Marfanoid appearance with arachnodactyly is present in most patients.

The medullary carcinoma of the thyroid and pheochromocytoma are similar to those in MEA-II. It is not clear why the incidence of hyperparathyroidism is so low but this point argues against the theory that high calcitonin levels from medullary carcinoma induce the parathyroid hyperplasia in MEA-II. In some cases of the syndrome, café-au-lait spots are seen but the full-blown picture of von Recklinghausen's disease in association with this syndrome has not been reported. The management of patients with MEA-III would appear to be identical to that of MEA-II. The mucosal neuroma aspect of the clinical picture may present early in life, while the thyroid carcinoma and pheochromocytoma develop much later, and with recognition of this syndrome, prophylactic thyroidectomy has been performed in young children.

Malignant Pheochromocytoma

The usual histologic hallmarks of malignancy are of little use in making this diagnosis with respect to pheochromocytoma. To qualify as malignant a pheochromocytoma must be associated with distant metastases, but tumors within the paraganglion system whether they are secreting catecholamines or not are frequently multicentric. Therefore, a secondary deposit to qualify as a metastasis must involve sites where paraganglia are not usually found. In addition, benign pheochromocytomas may show local penetration of the capsule and gross invasion of adrenal veins or even of the vena cava without any tendency toward widespread dissemination. These latter tumors could well be regarded as malignant since they are difficult to remove in toto and are prone to local recurrence. Their management, therefore, is similar to that of malignant pheochromocytomas with distant meta-

stases. As mentioned above, the incidence of malignancy in pheochromocytomas is in the region of 10%–15% but may be less frequent in children [57] although 11 of 30 patients in the recently reported Ann Arbor series were under the age of 20 years [73]. Apart from the presence of metastases, there are no clinical or biochemical features which distinguish a malignant pheochromocytoma, but a comparatively high proportion appear to occur in extraadrenal sites. Of the 30 patients in the Ann Arbor series, 20 had metastases in bone, 4 each in liver and lymph nodes, 3 in lung, and 2 in peritoneum. Malignant pheochromocytoma appears to be a slow-growing, indolent tumor in some patients, and metastases may not appear for years after initial therapy. On the other hand, some patients rapidly develop widespread disease and die quickly.

Several surgical groups advocate radical removal of the primary lesion together with involved lymph nodes and, where necessary, a nephrectomy [55,72]. Recurrent tumors may also be removed when detected by careful follow-up. Mahoney and Harrison treated seven such cases in this fashion and five were free of disease 4–21 years after the initial treatment and the two who died survived 7 and 10 years, respectively.

Chemotherapy for malignant pheochromocytoma has been disappointing [22]. Cyclophosphamide has been the most frequently used drug alone or in combination, and this has provided some palliation in about half of the patients. Vincristine has produced similar results [72]. On the basis of the response obtained with streptozocin in other APUD tumors, we treated two patients with malignant pheochromocytomas with a streptozocin regimen, but both showed no response whatsoever either in decline in catecholamine levels or in regression of tumor [38]. Feldman [29], with a slightly different protocol, has since reported tumor regression and a decrease in VMA levels in one patient treated with streptozocin. As previously discussed [131I]MIBG is a radiopharmaceutical agent developed at the University of Michigan which is taken up by pheochromocytoma tissue and is proving to be an excellent scan both for the primary tumor and for metastatic lesions. Recently, the same substance in much higher doses has been used to treat malignant pheochromocytomas. Sisson et al. [76] obtained some objective response in two out of five patients with a reduction in tumor size and catecholamine secretion. Vetter et al. [87] reported two patients with minor improvement. Keiser et al. [49] report that only one of five patients with malignant pheochromocytomas had appreciable uptake of [^{131}I]MIBG into the tumor. In three such patients they used combination chemotherapy, which had been previously shown to be successful with metastatic neuroblastoma, a disease which has similarities to malignant pheochromocytoma. These workers used a combination of cyclophosphamide, vincristine, and dacarbazine. A virtual complete response was obtained in one patient, and a partial response in the other two. The results, therefore, are promising, but the experience is very small.

The literature on radiation therapy contains about 44 patients treated since 1960. The response of soft tissue lesions has been disappointing, but relief of bone pain has generally been achieved and in some instances progression of bone metastases has been arrested.

Even if malignant pheochromocytoma tissue cannot be totally eradicated, it is still appropriate to treat these patients medically and thus control the symptoms related to catecholamine secretion. The management involves the use of alpha and in some cases beta blockade as described above under preoperative preparation of benign pheochromocytomas (p. 130). Metyrosine may also be useful [4]. This blocks tyrosine hydroxylase, the rate-limiting enzyme in norepinephrine synthesis. It is appropriate to start with a dose of 250 mg twice a day, gradually increasing this by 250–500 mg/day to a total dose which is under 3 g/day. This appears to be satisfactory for reduction of catecholamine blood levels. The side effects are sleepiness, diarrhea, and crystalluria, but the crystalluria can be largely avoided by encouraging the patient to maintain a high liquid intake. Some surgeons even advocate the use of this agent preoperatively, which then decreases the need for alpha and beta blockers, since these can aggravate hypotension developing after the tumor has been removed.

Ectopic ACTH Syndrome

Pheochromocytoma is a relatively common cause of the ectopic ACTH syndrome and one of the few types which can be cured by operation. Theoretically, this should be a particularly severe form of pheochromocytoma since ACTH infusion can promote pheochromocytoma crisis. However, this was not the case in the 33 cases reported in 1977

[54]. As with other forms of ectopic ACTH syndrome the classical hallmarks of Cushing's syndrome may not be particularly prominent but the presence of hypokalemic alkalosis may be a strong clue. It is important to make this diagnosis preoperatively and administer steroids to the patient at the time of tumor removal, otherwise Addisonian crisis may develop postoperatively.

References

1. Achong MR, Keane PM (1981) Pheochromocytoma unmasked by desipramine therapy. Ann Intern Med 94:358–359
2. Allen CT, Imri ED (1977) Hypoglycemia as a complication of removal of a pheochromocytoma. Canad Med Assoc J 116:363–364
3. Allison DJ, Brown MJ, Jones DH et al. (1983) Role of venous sampling in locating a pheochromocytoma. Br Med J 286:1122–1124
4. Atuk NO (1983) Pheochromocytoma: diagnosis, localization and treatment. Hosp Pract 18:187–202
5. Ballard HS, Frame B, Hartsock RJ (1964) Familial multiple-endocrine adenoma-peptic ulcer complex. Medicine 43:481–516
6. Bolande RP (1974) The neurocristopathies: a unifying concept of disease arising in the neural crest maldevelopment. Human Pathol 5:409–429
7. Bravo EL, Gifford RW Jr (1984) Pheochromocytoma: diagnosis, localization and management. N Engl J Med 311:1298–1303
8. Bravo EL, Tarazi RC, Fouad FM et al. (1981) Clonidine-suppression test: a useful aid in the diagnosis of pheochromocytoma. N Engl J Med 305:623–626
9. Brown MJ, Allison DJ, Jenner DA et al. (1981) Increased sensitivity and accuracy of pheochromocytoma diagnosis achieved by use of plasma-adrenaline estimations and a pentolinium-suppression test. Lancet 1:174–177
10. Carney, JA, Go VLW, Sizemore GW (1976) Alimentary-tract ganglioneuromatosis a major component of the syndrome of multiple endocrine neoplasia Type 2b. N Engl. J Med 295:1287–1291
11. Carney JA, Sizemore, GW, Tyce GM (1975) Bilateral adrenal medullary hyperplasia in multiple endocrine neoplasia Type II: the precursor of bilateral pheochromocytoma. Mayo Clin Proc 50:3–10
12. Carney JA, Sizemore GW, Sheps SG (1976) Adrenal medullary disease in multiple endocrine neoplasia Type II: pheochromocytoma and its precursors. Am J Clin Pathol 66:279–290
13. Cerny JC, Jackson CE, Talpos GB et al. (1982) Pheochromocytoma in multiple endocrine neoplasia Type II: an example of the two hit theory of neoplasia. Surgery 92:849–852
14. Coupland RE (1965) The natural history of the chromaffin cell. Longmans, Green and Company, London
15. Crout JR (1961) Catecholamines in urine. In: Standard methods of clinical chemistry, Vol 3, Academic Press, New York, pp 62–80
16. Crout JR (1966) Pheochromocytoma. Pharmacological Rev 18:651–657
17. 1980 Cryer PE (Physiology and pathophysiology of the

human sympathoadrenal neuroendocrine system. N Engl J Med 303:436–444

18. Daggett P, Franks S (1977) Steroid responsiveness in phaeochromocytoma. Br Med J 1:84

19. Das S, Bulusu NV, Low EP (1983) Primary vesical pheochromocytoma. Urology 21:20–25

20. Dereo GA JR, Stewart BH, Tarazi RW Jr (1974) Preoperative blood transfusion and the safe surgical management of pheochromocytoma: review of 46 cases. J Urol 111:715–721

21. Desmonts JM, LeHouelleur J, Remond DP et al. (1977) Anesthetic management of patients with pheochromocytoma. Br J Anesthesia 49:991–998

22. Drasin H (1978) Treatment of malignant pheochromocytoma. W J Med 128:106–111

23. Dunn FG, DeCarvalho JGR, Kem DC et al. (1976) Pheochromocytoma crisis induced by saralasin; relation of angiotensin analogue to catecholamine release. N Engl J Med 295:605–607

24. Dunnick NR, Doppman JL, Gill JR (1982) Failure to ablate the adrenal gland by injection of contrast material. Radiology 142:67–69

25. El-Minawi MF, Paulino E, Custa M et al. (1971) Pheochromocytoma masquerading as pre-eclamptic toxemia. Am J Obstet Gynecol 109:389–395

26. Engelman K, Portnoy R, Lovenberg W (1968) A sensitive and specific double-isotope derivative method for the determination of catecholamines in biological specimens. Am J Med Sci 255:259–268

27. Engleman K, Portnoy B, Sjoersdma A (1970) Plasma catecholamine concentrations in patients with hypertension. Circulation Res 26, 27 (Suppl 1):1–141–145

28. Feek CM, Earnshaw PM (1980) Hypertensive response to labetalol in phaeochromocytoma. Br Med J 2:387

29. Feldman JM (1983) Treatment of metastatic pheochromocytoma with streptozocin. Arch Int Med 143:1799–1800

30. Feldman JM, Blalock JA, Zern RT et al. (1979) The relationship between enzyme activity and the catecholamine content and secretion of pheochromocytomas. J Clin Endocrinol Metab 49:445–451

31. Geelhoed GW (1983) Problem management in endocrine surgery. Yearbook Medical Publishers, Chicago

32. Geelhoed GW, Druy EM (1983) Adrenal radiography: problems and pitfalls in adrenal localization. World J Surg 7:209–222

33. Geffen LB, Rush RA, Louis WJ (1973) Plasma dopamine, beta hydroxylase, and noradrenaline amounts in essential hypertension. Clin Sci 44:617–620

34. Gitlow SE, Mendlowitz M, Bertani LM (1970) The biochemical techniques for detecting and establishing the presence of a pheochromocytoma. Am J Cardiol 26:270–279

35. Glushien AS, Mansuy MM, Littman DS (1953) Pheochromocytoma: its relationship to the neurocutaneous syndromes. M J Med 14:318

36. Goldstein DS, Feuerstein GF, Izzo JL Jr et al. (1981) Validity and reliability of liquid chromatography with electrochemical detection for measuring plasma levels of norepinephrine and epinephrine in man. Life Sci 28:467–475

37. Hamberger B, Russell CF, VanHeerden JA et al (1982) Adrenal surgery: trends during the 70's. Am J Surg 144:523–526

38. Hamilton BPM, Cheikh IE, Rivera LE (1977) Attempted treatment of inoperable pheochromocytoma with streptozocin. Arch Intern Med 137:762–765

39. Hamilton BP, Landsberg L, Levine RJ (1978) Measurement of urinary epinephrine in screening for pheochromocytoma in multiple endocrine neoplasia type II. Am J Med 65:1027–1032

40. Hamrin B (1962) Sustained hypotension and shock due to adrenalin-secreting pheochromocytoma. Lancet 2:123–125

41. Hansen OP, Hansen M, Hansen HH (1976) Multiple endocrine adenomatosis of mixed type. Acta Med Scand 200:327–331

42. Harden KT (1983) Agonist-induced desensitization of the beta-1-adrenergic receptor-linked adenylate cyclase. Pharmacol Rev 35:5–32

43. Herman NH, Mornex R (1964) Human tumors secreting catecholamines. MacMillan, New York

44. Hume DM (1968) Pheochromocytoma. In: Astwood EB, Cassidy CE (eds) Clinical endocrinology, vol 2. Grune and Stratton, New York, p 519

45. Hume DM (1960) Pheochromocytoma in the adult and in the child. Am J Surg 99:458–496

46. James TN (1976) De subitaneis mortibus XIX on the cause of sudden death in pheochromocytoma, with special reference to the pulmonary arteries, the cardiac conduction system, and the aggregation of platelets. Circulation 54:348–356

47. Kaplan NM, Krammer NJ, Holland OB et al. (1977) Singlevoided urine metanephrine assays in screening for pheochromocytoma. Arch Intern Med 137:190–193

48. Khairi RA, Dexter RN, Burzynski NJ (1975) Mucosal neuroma, pheochromocytoma, and medullary thyroid carcinoma: multiple endocrine neoplasia Type 3. Medicine 54:89–112

49. Keiser HR, Goldstein DS, Wade JL et al. (1985) Treatment of malignant pheochromocytoma with combination chemotherapy. Hypertension 7 (Suppl 1) 1–18—1–24

50. Kuchel O, Buu NT, Hamet P et al. (1981) Essential hypertension with low conjugated catecholamines imitates pheochromocytoma. Hypertension 3:347–355

51. Levinson PD, Hamilton BP, Mersey JH (1983a) Plasma norepinephrine and epinephrine responses to glucagon in patients with suspected pheochromocytoma. Metabolism 32:998–1001

52. Levinson PD, Lance BK, Kowarski AA (1983b) Catecholamine suppression testing in patients with pheochromocytomas and normal plasma catecholamine levels. Lancet I:1216–1217

53. Louis WJ, Doyle AE, Heath WC et al. (1972) Secretion of dopa in phaechromocytoma. Br Med J 4:325–327

54. Luton J-P, Thieblot P, Bricair E (1977) Association syndrome de Cushing-pheochromocytome. Nouv Presse Med 6:4053–4057

55. Mahoney EM, Harrison JH (1977) Malignant pheochromocytoma: clinical course and treatment. J Urol 118:225–229

56. Manger WM, Gifford RW Jr (1977) Pheochromocytoma. Springer, Berlin, Heidelberg, New York

57. Manger WM, Gifford RW Jr (1982) Hypertension secondary to pheochromocytoma. Bull NY Acad Med 58:138–158

58. Melvin KEW, Miller HH, Tashjian AH Jr (1971) Early diagnosis of medullary carcinoma of the thyroid gland by means of calcitonin assay. N Engl J Med 285:1115–1120

59. Messerli FH, Finn M, MacPhee AA (1982) Pheochromocytoma of the urinary bladder. JAMA 247:1863–1864

60. Nicholson JP Jr, Vaughn ED, Pickering TG et al. (1983) Pheochromocytoma and prazosin. Ann Intern Med 99:477–479

61. Pagani JJ, Barnardino ME (1982) Incidence and significance of serendipitous CT findings in the oncologic patient. J Comp Assist Tomog 6:268–275

62. Page LB, Copeland RB (1968) Pheochromocytoma. Disease A Month I:1–40

63. Page LB, Raker JW, Berberich FR (1969) Pheochromocytoma with predominant epinephrine secretion. Am J Med 47:648–652

64. Pearse AGE (1969) The cytochemistry and ultrastructure of polypeptide hormone-producing cells of the APUD series and the embryologic, physiologic, and pathologic implications of the concept. J Histochem Cytochem 17:303–310

65. Pickering G (1968) High blood pressure. Grune and Stratton, New York, p 543

66. Pisano JJ (1960) A simple analysis for normetanephrine and metanephrine in urine. Clin Chim Acta 5:406–414

67. Pisano JJ, Crout JR, Abraham D (1962) Determination of 3-methoxy 4-hydroxy mandelic acid in urine. Clin Chim Acta 7:285–291

68. Plouin PF, Duclos JM, Menard J et al. (1981) Biochemical tests for diagnosis of pheochromocytoma: urinary versus plasma determinations. Br Med J 282:853–854

69. Polak JM, Post FWD, Pearse AGE (1971) Fluorogenic amine tracing of neural crest derivatives forming the adrenal medulla. Gen Comp Endocrinol 16:132–136

70. Reach G, Thibonnaer M, Chevillard C et al. (1980) Effects of labetalol on blood pressure and plasma catecholamine concentrations in patients with phaeochromocytoma. Br Med J 280:1300–1301

71. Ross EJ, Prichard BN, Kaufman L et al. (1967) Preoperative and operative management of patients with pheochromocytoma. BMJ 1:191–198

72. Scott WH, Reynolds V, Green N et al. (1982) Clinical experience with malignant pheochromocytomas. Surg Gynecol Obstet 154:801–818

73. Shapiro B, Sisson JC, Lloyd R et al. (1984) Malignant pheochromocytoma: clinical, biochemical, and scintigraphic characterization. Clin Endocrinol 20:189–203

74. Sheps SG, Maher FT (1968) Histamine and glucagon tests in diagnosis of pheochromocytoma. JAMA 205:895–899

75. Sisson JC, Frager MS, Valk TW et al. (1981) Scintigraphic localization of pheochromocytoma. N Eng J Med 305:12–17

76. Sisson JC, Shapiro V, Beierwaltes WH et al. (1984) Radiopharmaceutical treatment of malignant pheochromocytoma. J Nuc Med 25:197–206

77. Sjoerdsma A, Engelman K, Waldmann TA et al. (1966) Pheochromocytoma: current concepts of diagnosis and treatment. Ann Intern Med 65:1302–1326

78. Spavely MD, Motulsky HJ, Moustafa E et al. (1982) Beta-1-adrenergic receptor subtypes in the rat renal cortex: selective regulation of beta-1 adrenergic receptors by pheochromocytoma. Circ Res 51:504–513

79. St. John-Sutton MG, Sheps SG, Lie JT (1981) Prevalence of clinically unsuspected pheochromocytoma. Mayo Clin Proc 56:354–360

80. Stackpole RH, Melicow MM, Uson AC (1963) Pheochromocytoma in childhood. J Pediatr 63:314–330

81. Stamenkovic L, Spierdijk J (1976) Anesthesia in patients with pheochromocytoma. Anesthesia 31:941–945

82. Steer ML (1977) Adrenergic receptors. Clin Endocrinol Metab 6:577–595

83. Steiner AL, Goodman AD, Powers SR (1968) Study of a kindred with pheochromocytoma medullary thryroid carcinoma, hyperparathyroidism, and Cushing's disease: multiple endocrine neoplasia Type II. Medicine 47:371–409

84. Thomas JE, Rook ED, Kvale WF (1966) The neurologist's experience with pheochromocytoma: review of 100 cases. JAMA 197:100–104

85. Valk TW, Frager MS, Gross MD et al. (1981) Spectrum of pheochromocytoma in multiple endocrine neoplasia: A scintigraphic protrayal using I[131] metaiodobenzylguanidine. Ann Intern Med 94:962–967

86. Van Way CW III, Faraci RP, Cleveland HC et al. (1976) Hemorrhagic necrosis of pheochromocytoma associated with phentolamine administration Ann Surg 184:26–30

87. Vetter H, Fisher M, Muller-Rensing R et al. (1983) I[131]-metaiodobenzylguanidine in treatment of malignant pheochromocytomas. Lancet 2: 107

88. Welbourn RB, Manolas KJ, Khan O (1984) Tumors of the neuroendocrine system. In: Current problems in surgery, vol. 21. Yearbook Medical Publishers, Chicago

89. Wells SA, Norton JA (1978) Medullary carcinoma of the thyroid and multiple endocrine neoplasia-II syndromes. In: Friesen SR (ed) Surgical endocrinology: clinical syndromes, J B Lippincott, Philadelphia

90. Zweifler AJ, Julius S (1982) Increased platelet catecholamine content in pheochromocytoma: a diagnostic test in patients with elevated plasma catecholamines. N Engl J Med 306:890–894

Chapter 11

Neuroblastoma

B. López-Ibor and A. D. Schwartz

Neuroblastomas originate from the primitive neural crest cells that normally give rise to the adrenal medulla and the sympathetic nervous system. They are the most common solid malignant tumors in infancy and are second only to brain tumors as the type of solid malignancy presenting during the first decade of life.

Incidence

Neuroblastomas occur in approximately 1 per 100 000 children per year [33]. According to the Third National Cancer Survey in the United States, they occurred in 9.6 white children and 7.0 black children per million each year from 1969 to 1971 [86]. Although they represent only 7% of all cases of childhood cancer, they result in 15% of pediatric deaths due to cancer [19].

Etiology

The etiology of neuroblastoma remains unknown. Environmental factors are suggested by the fact that the tumor is uncommon in children living in certain geographic areas such as the Burkitt's lymphoma belt in Africa [59]. An association of neuroblastoma with neurofibromatosis [85] and Hirschprung's disease [11] has been reported. A number of cases have been found in infants with the fetal hydantoin syndrome and fetal alcohol syndrome, two disorders consisting of unusual patterns of congenital anomalies which occur in children who have had in utero exposure to these drugs [23,47,70].

Numerous reports of cases of neuroblastoma occurring in more than one family member suggest that some patients may inherit the potential to develop this tumor in an autosomal dominant fashion. A two-mutation model for familial neurolastoma has been proposed [48]. According to this theory, two mutations are required for the malignant phenotype to occur. In sporadic or nonfamilial cases the two mutations occur in the somatic cell (sympathicoblast), while in familial cases the first mutation is inherited in the germ cell line and the second occurs in the somatic cell.

The hereditary cases of neuroblastoma are often associated with chromosomal abnormalities, often involving the deletion of material from chromosome 1 [9]. This is believed to predispose individuals to develop the tumor, but does not make it inevitable, presumably because a normal allele of the deleted gene remains on the intact chromosome. Among the most commonly observed chromosomal abnormalities are the double-minute sphere (dms) chromosomes and a giant marker chromosome with a long, nonbanding, homogeneously staining region

(HSR). The dms chromosomes are small, paired chromatin bodies that lack a centromere and probably originated from the breakdown of the HSR [7]. These two chromosomal anomalies are not specific for neuroblastoma but have been identified in two-thirds of the tumors studied.

evaluates not only the degree of maturation of the neuroblastic cell population, but the development of the stromal component as well [73]. This new grading system appears to offer a major contribution in predicting the prognosis of patients with this tumor.

Pathology

The histological composition of neural crest tumors may vary from a neuroblastoma, composed of primitive sympathetic nervous tissue, to a ganglioneuroma, its benign counterpart, composed of mature ganglion cells. Ganglioneuroblastomas are intermediate in the degree of differentiation, but have invasive potential and are capable of metastasizing. They are highly malignant and clinically behave like neuroblastomas.

The neuroblastoma may appear macroscopically encapsulated, but it has poorly defined margins and infiltrates the surrounding tissues. Microscopically, it is characterized by a diffuse growth of undifferentiated very primitive neuroblastic cell nests, irregularly separated by thin, fibrovascular septa. The cells may group around a tangle of young nerve fibers in rosette-like structures, an early sign of tumor differentiation.

The neuroblastoma is occasionally difficult to differentiate histologically and clinically from other childhood small round cell tumors such as the embryonal rhabdomyosarcoma, Ewing's tumor, and non-Hodgkin's lymphoma. It may even be confused with leukemia when neuroblastoma cells infiltrate and replace the normal bone marrow. Electron microscopy may be helpful in making the diagnosis in such situations, because neuroblastoma cells have cytoplasmic structures consisting of neurofilaments, neurotubules, and neurosecretory granules [54]. These granules are cytoplasmic accumulations of catecholamines. A rapid fluorescence assay for intracellular catecholamines has been reported to be positive in over 80% of cases of neuroblastoma [65].

There have been several attempts to correlate the degree of tumor differentiation or maturation with prognosis. Aside from the clearly benign cases of ganglioneuroma, these efforts have usually been unsuccessful. Recently, a new histological classification for neuroblastoma has been reported which

Clinical Features

Approximately 50% of patients with neuroblastoma are diagnosed during the first 2 years of life and over two-thirds are diagnosed before 5 years of age. Neuroblastomas have been diagnosed by sonography even before birth [43] or immediately after birth with metastases in the placenta [3]. It has been postulated that a neoplasm diagnosed during adolescence is due to an exacerbation of growth of a tumor that has been dormant since early childhood [84].

The clinical manifestations of the disease often depend upon the location of the primary tumor. The most common site of origin is within the abdomen, with 45% arising in an adrenal gland, and 24% in the retroperitoneal sympathetic ganglia. About 4% arise in the pelvis, 15%–20% in the mediastinum, and 2%–6% in the cervical region [33]. Some tumors may arise in the olfactory bulb (esthesioneuroblastoma), presenting with unilateral nasal obstruction and epistaxis.

Intraabdominal neuroblastomas are palpated as hard, nontender masses in the flank, often extending across the midline. A plain X-ray of the abdomen reveals calcification in 50%–60% of the cases which is diffuse, finely stippled, or, less commonly, amorphous and coalescent [28] (Fig. 11.1). A higher incidence of calcification in neuroblastoma is now being documented because of the common use of CT scanning [24]. Calcification within the tumor is believed to be the result of tumor necrosis.

Presacral neuroblastomas may present with urinary frequency, inability to void due to extrinsic bladder obstruction [41], or constipation due to rectal compression. Tumors in this location can usually be palpated on digital examination of the rectum. Growth of a pelvic tumor through the sacroiliac notch may result in a palpable mass in the perineal region or buttock. Metastatic tumor to the testicle from a retroperitoneal neuroblastoma has also been reported [13].

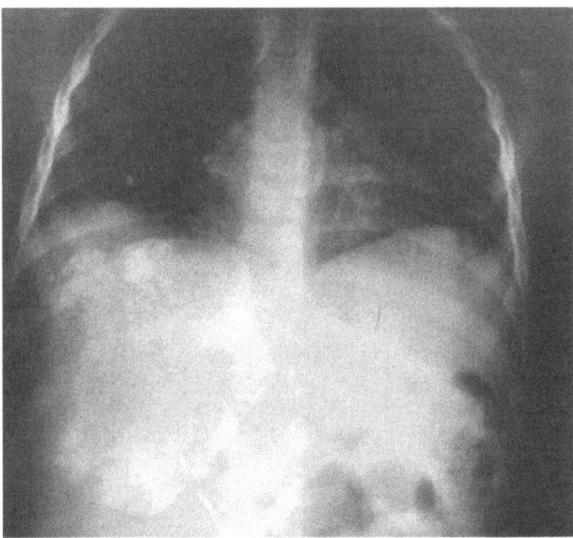

Fig. 11.1. Abdominal roentgenogram of a child with a large calcified flank mass which proved to be neuroblastoma. [Reprinted with permission from *Ped Clin N Am* 32:758 (1985)].

Neuroblastomas arising from a thoracic or abdominal paravertebral ganglion have an unusual tendency to grow through the intervertebral foramen, forming a dumbbell-shaped mass [2,80]. The intraspinal component may cause spinal cord compression. It is not unusual for the signs and symptoms of spinal cord compression to be the first indication of the presence of neuroblastoma. Prompt relief of this situation by surgery or radiation therapy is extremely important because the majority of patients with neuroblastoma having this presentation have an excellent chance of survival [80]. It is not uncommon for a patient to be cured of neuroblastoma, but be left paraplegic because of irreversible tumor damage to the spinal cord. In about 40% of the cases, the intraspinal component of the tumor may not be clinically apparent [2].

Thoracic neuroblastomas may cause dyspnea or upper respiratory tract symptoms because of airway compression. More frequently, a posterior mediastinal tumor is found incidentally when a chest X-ray is taken for reasons unrelated to the tumor (Fig. 11.2). Primary cervical tumors may present as unilateral neck masses, often associated with a Horner's syndrome (myosis, ptosis, enophthalmos, and anhydrosis). This neurological complication also may result from the surgical removal of the tumor from this ganglion.

Unfortunately, neuroblastoma often presents with symptoms due to widespread metastatic disease. In fact, disseminated disease is present in 70% of children over 1 year of age and in 40%–50% of those under 1 year of age [33]. Bone involvement by the tumor produces severe pain with or without palpable metastases. The skull and tubular bones are the most frequently involved. Skeletal roentgenograms show small lytic defects with irregular margins and periosteal reaction. [^{99m}Tc] disphosphonate bone scans may be positive weeks before the metastatic lesions can be detected by X-rays [42,78]. Both skeletal survey and bone scan appear to be complementary in detecting metastatic disease to the bone [46,55]. Bone marrow involvement is present in more than 50% of the patients [14], but the tumor cell "rosettes," considered typical of neuroblastoma, are seen only in 2% of the samples [26]. Small clumps of tumor cells are more commonly seen (Fig. 11.3).

Neuroblastoma may metastasize to the orbits, resulting in proptosis and ecchymotic discoloration of the eyelids (Fig. 11.4). The tumor may also metastasize to the skin. This is especially common during the neonatal period, when metastatic subcutaneous nodules have been reported to occur in as many as 32% of cases [69] (Fig. 11.5). The liver and lymph nodes also are common sites for metastatic disease. Intracranial dissemination may involve the meninges, but intracerebral metastases are very rare.

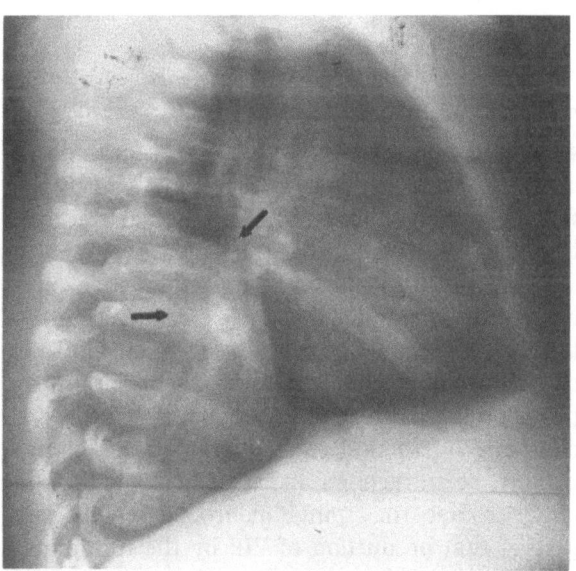

Fig. 11.2. Large posterior mediastinal neuroblastoma in a child who had the findings of spinal cord compression, but no pulmonary symptoms. Note the complete block demonstrated by myelography (*black arrow*). [Reprinted with permission from Altman AA, Schwartz AD (1983) Malignant diseases of infancy, childhood and adolescence. 2nd ed., WB Saunders Co., Philadelphia, p. 371].

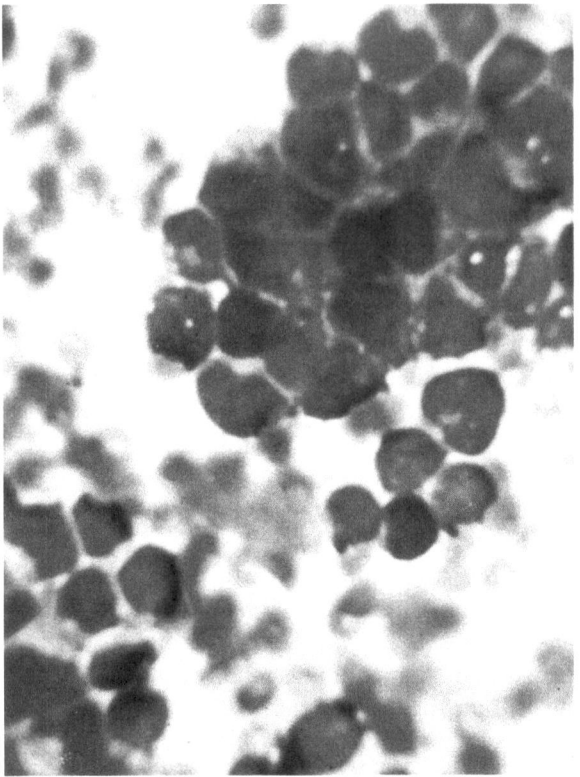

Fig. 11.3. Neuroblastoma cells found in a bone marrow aspiration. Unlike leukemic blast cells, these cells are in a cluster that share cytoplasm. [Reprinted with permission from Altman AA, Schwartz AD (1983) Malignant diseases of infancy, childhood & adolescence. 2nd ed., WB Saunders Co., Philadelphia, p. 373].

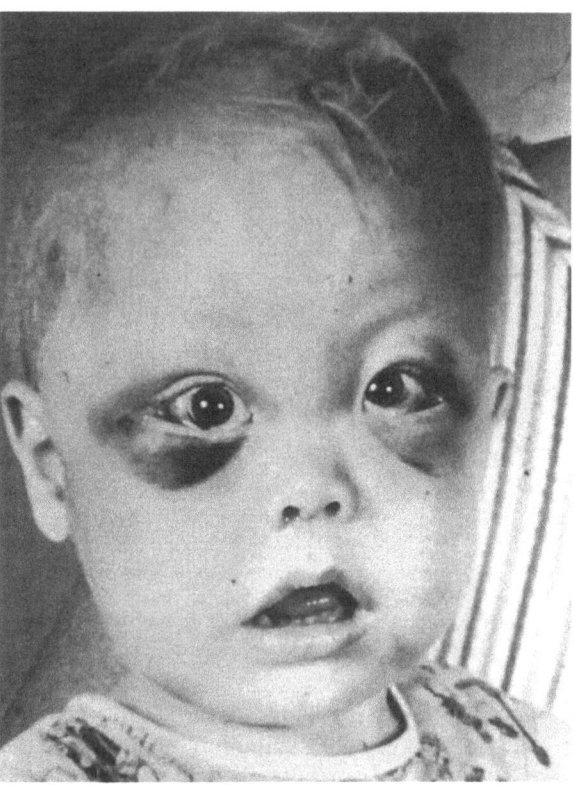

Fig. 11.4. Periorbital metastatic neuroblastoma. Note the right sixth cranial nerve paralysis secondary to increased intracranial pressure from meningeal metastases. (Courtesy of Dr. Howard Pearson, Yale-New Haven Hospital) [Reprinted with permission from Altman AA, Schwartz AD (1983) Malignant diseases of infancy, childhood & adolescence. 2nd ed., WB Saunders Co., Philadelphia, p. 373].

Occasionally, patients may present with disseminated tumor and the site of the primary tumor cannot be identified. There is usually a history of weight loss, irritability, and fever when the child has widely disseminated disease.

Two unusual clinical syndromes have been reported in association with neuroblastoma. Intractable diarrhea, due to secretion by the tumor cells of an enterohormone called vasoactive intestinal polypeptide (VIP), has been reported in 7%–9% of children with neural crest tumors [67]. This has usually been reported in association with ganglioneuromas or ganglioneuroblastomas, suggesting that production of VIP by the tumor cells is an indication of maturation of the tumor [58]. Another uncommon association with neuroblastoma is an acute myoclonic encephalopathy manifested by opsoclonus, myoclonus, and truncal ataxia [71]. It has been postulated that this is due to cerebellar damage produced by an antibody directed

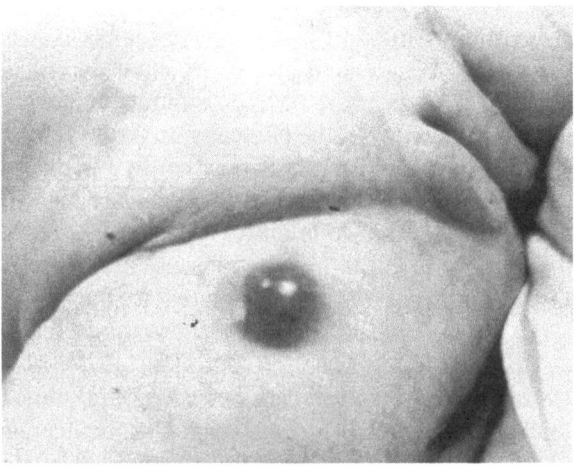

Fig. 11.5. Subcutaneous neuroblastoma nodule in a neonate. (Courtesy of Dr. Howard Pearson, Yale-New Haven Hospital) [Reprinted with permission from Altman AA, Schwartz AD (1983) Malignant diseases of infancy, childhood & adolescence. 2nd ed., WB Saunders Co., Philadelphia, p. 372].

against a neuroblastoma antigen that cross-reacts with an antigen in cerebellar cells [60]. This syndrome often disappears after removal of the tumor, but it also has occurred months after tumor removal [18].

Biochemical Features

Over 90% of patients with neuroblastoma have increased levels of catecholamines and/or their metabolites in the urine. This is believed to be due to their increased production or their defective storage within tumor cells. Vanillylmandelic acid (VMA) and homovanillic acid (HVA) are the most frequently assayed urinary catecholamines. A VMA/HVA ratio of 1.5 or greater has been shown to be associated with a more favorable outcome [75].

Urinary excretion of catecholamines should be measured prior to surgery or any other form of therapy in every child in whom the diagnosis of neuroblastoma is suspected, because serial urinary catecholamine determinations are of value in following the response to treatment. Their levels decline as the tumor mass decreases, and often increase before there is clinical evidence of relapse. Thus, periodic assays of the urinary excretion of VMA and HVA during the course of the disease should be obtained. A 24-h urine collection is the ideal method for catecholamine measurement. This may be impractical, however, in the young child. A single urine specimen may be used, and the catecholamine excretion compared with the amount of creatinine present in the sample. A rapid "spot" test for VMA [51] and a VMA test strip [53] are also useful to follow patients with a known VMA-secreting tumor. These techniques may be of limited value, especially at diagnosis, because of the considerable number of false-positive and -negative values that have been reported to occur [1,45]. A diet restricted in certain foods such as tea, coffee, fruits, or vanilla-containing products is recommended, especially when colorimetric assays or "spot tests" are used.

Other biochemical markers have been described in patients with neuroblastoma. Among those that are not specific for this type of tumor, urinary cystathionine and carcinoembryonic antigen (CEA) are the most frequently measured. Elevated serum

ferritin levels measured by counterimmunoelectrophoresis have been described in patients with neuroblastoma. Serum ferritin is derived from the tumor and correlates well with the presence of active disease. Elevated levels of serum ferritin at diagnosis return to normal with clinical remission [37]. Moreover, the ferritin levels at diagnosis appear closely related to the outcome of the patients [38]. Of interest is the observation that children with a disseminated form of tumor called stage IV-S disease have normal ferritin levels, even when their tumors are actively growing [36,37]. These young patients have an extremely good prognosis.

Increased levels of neuron-specific enolase (NSE) have been described in the serum of patients with neuroblastoma and in the tumor tissue itself [87]. NSE is an isoenzyme of the glycolytic enzyme enolase, which has been shown to be highly specific for neurons and neuroendocrine cells [68]. Serum NSE levels reflect the clinical course of the disease, with levels being high at diagnosis, decreasing during remission and increasing again at relapse [56]. In addition, this tumor marker appears to be highly specific for neuroblastoma [44,82,87].

Diagnostic Evaluation and Staging

The diagnostic studies indicated in the child with neuroblastoma will vary with the site of the primary tumor. The physical examination should include a careful and complete neurologic evaluation in search of signs of extradural tumor extension, a frequent occurrence in patients with tumors arising in the paravertebral sympathetic ganglia. Oblique views of the spine to visualize the intervertebral foramen should be obtained in every patient with a paravertebral tumor. Children with abdominal tumors require an intravenous pyelogram. This study usually shows anterolateral and inferior displacement of the kidney with little or no distortion of the pyelocalyceal system if the tumor arises in the adrenal medulla. If it arises in the paravertebral sympathetic chain, the ipsilateral ureter is often displaced laterally.

Valuable information is often obtained by ultrasonography in evaluating a patient with an abdominal or pelvic tumor. A neuroblastoma usually appears as a complex mixture of solid and cystic components [55]. Computed tomography (CT) is particularly helpful in assessing tumor location and its relationship to adjacent structures. Enlarged retroperitoneal lymph nodes and metastatic disease to the liver, bones, or other organs also can be identified. Extension of paravertebral tumor into the spinal canal is also demonstrable with the newer scanners, and is accomplished if intrathecal contrast material is administered at the time of the scan [31]. CT scanning clearly has become an essential part of the evaluation of the patient with neuroblastoma prior to surgery [24].

Evaluation for metastatic disease should include a complete skeletal survey, bone scan, liver scan, and evaluation of the bone marrow. In addition, urinary catecholamine levels should be measured in all patients, and serum ferritin and neuron-specific enolase may be of value because of their prognostic significance.

The staging system most frequently used, that proposed by Evans et al. [21], is described below:

Stage	Description
I	Tumor confined to the organ or structure of origin.
II	Tumor extending in continuity beyond the organ or structure of origin but not crossing the midline. Regional lymph nodes on the ipsilateral side may be involved.
III	Tumor extending in continuity beyond the midline. Regional lymph nodes may be involved bilaterally.
IV	Remote disease involving skeleton, parenchymatous soft tissues, or distant lymph node groups.
IV-S	Otherwise classified as having stage I or II, but with remote disease confined to one or more of the following sites: liver, skin, or bone marrow (without radiographic evidence of bone metastases on complete skeletal survey). Most patients with this stage are under 1 year of age.

For tumors arising in midline structures, penetration beyond the capsule and involvement of the lymph nodes on the same side is considered stage II. Bilateral extension of any sort is considered stage III.

A surgicopathologic staging system, different from that of the Evans system, has been used at the St. Jude Children's Research Hospital since 1967.

One advantage of this system is that it separates patients who truly have localized disease from those with disease disseminated to lymph nodes. The prognosis for children with neuroblastoma metastatic only to regional lymph nodes appears to be no different from that of patients of similar age with widely disseminated tumor [40,62]. A system combining both the Evans and St. Jude staging systems has recently been developed by one of the national pediatric oncology study groups. Hopefully, one staging system will eventually become universally accepted in order to allow various institutions and study groups to compare their data.

Prognosis

Multiple factors have been investigated in children with neuroblastoma to determine their relationship with prognosis. The extent of the disease (Evans clinical stage) and the age at the time of diagnosis appear to be independent variables that clearly correlate with disease-free survival and cure. The overall survival rate of 74% for children diagnosed between 0 and 11 months of age drops to 26% for patients diagnosed between 12 and 23 months of age, and to 12% for those diagnosed at 2 years of age or older. Patients with Evans stage I or II disease generally have a good prognosis, while few children with regional or widespread metastatic disease (stages III and IV) survive. The survival rate for children with neuroblastoma noted by Breslow and McCann in 1971 [8], which shows the relationship of both age and clinical stage to survival (Fig. 11.6), has changed little over the years. The interesting group of children with stage IV-S disease, in whom the tumor may be widely spread to the bone marrow, liver, and/or skin, have an unusually good prognosis.

The site of origin also appears to influence the chances of survival. Children with cervical, mediastinal, or pelvic tumors have a better prognosis than do those with abdominal primary tumors [20]. Lymph node involvement [40,62], elevated serum ferritin levels [36,37], elevated serum neuron specific enolase [56], and gallium uptake by the tumor [6] have all been reported to indicate a poor prognosis. The histologic classification system recently

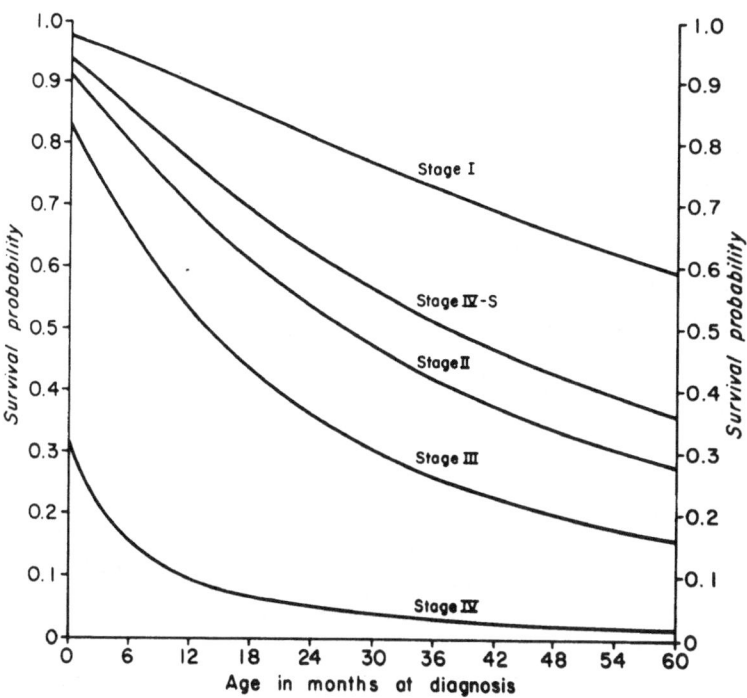

Fig. 11.6. Estimated probability of 2-year disease-free survival of children with neuroblastoma based on stage of disease and age in months at diagnosis. [Reprinted with permission from Breslow and McCann (1971) Statistical estimation of prognosis for children with neuroblastoma. *Cancer Res* 31:2098].

proposed by Shimada et al. also appears to be able to predict the prognosis [73].

Despite the fact that the neuroblastoma is a very aggressive malignancy with a mortality rate of approximately 70%, it has the highest rate of spontaneous remission of any malignant tumor. This has been noted mainly in children under 6 months of age with stage II or stage IV-S disease [19]. The incidence of spontaneous regression may, in fact, be much higher than is clinically apparent if one considers the incidence of neuroblastomas "in situ" found in infants at autopsy. These tumors are morphologically and cytologically identical to typical neuroblastomas but are microscopic in size. The incidence of these minute neuroblastomas in children under 3 months of age has been reported to be as high as 1 in 250, which is 40 times higher than the incidence of clinically diagnosed neuroblastomas [4].

Neuroblastoma may also undergo differentiation to a benign ganglioneuroma. This unusual phenomenon was first described over 50 years ago by Harvey Cushing [15]. Although spontaneous remission and maturation have been attributed, at least in part, to host immune defense mechanisms, no methods of immunotherapy have been shown to be effective in treatment.

Treatment

Therapy of neuroblastoma is often difficult to evaluate because of the unpredictable nature of the tumor and the lack of uniform criteria for defining the response to treatment. Neuroblastomas are friable, highly vascular tumors that tend to surround and invade adjacent structures. Therefore, surgery has to be meticulously planned. Surgery is only urgent when massive hemorrhage occurs into the tumor, or there is evidence of progressive spinal cord compression. Complete surgical removal of stage I and II tumors is often possible. Although it is desirable to remove the tumor en bloc, the surgeon should excise it piecemeal when vital structures such as major arteries are surrounded by the tumor, or when the neoplasm invades the spinal canal [72]. The 2-year disease-free survival for children with stage I and II disease varies from 84%, when complete resection is achieved, to 63%, when only partial resection is possible [49]. There is no evidence that further therapy improves survival, even when macroscopic disease is left behind [16,38,89].

The role of surgery in patients with stage III and IV tumors has yet to be defined. Biopsy or partial excision for diagnostic purposes is often all that can be done, but placement of metal clips to outline the remaining tumor is useful to help the radiation therapist design radiation portals and to follow the response to therapy. The sampling of lymph nodes is of value because of the prognostic significance of their involvement.

Although neuroblastomas are sensitive to radiation and chemotherapy, recurrence of the tumor in the absence of complete surgical excision is a common occurrence. If a tumor is considered unresectable, it is appropriate to attempt reduction of tumor size with chemotherapy with or without radiation therapy and later attempt surgically to remove all residual tumor. Complete resection of the primary tumor does not appear to improve survival in patients with stage IV disease [76].

The neuroblastoma is a radiosensitive tumor, but the exact role of radiation therapy in its treatment remains to be defined. It does not appear to benefit patients with stage I or II tumors even when macroscopic disease remains following surgery [16,83,89]. It is common practice to irradiate residual stage III tumor after surgery although it is not clear whether radiation improves survival in these cases [16,83]. Radiation therapy clearly plays a role in the palliative treatment of patients with bone pain.

Chemotherapy is usually the initial treatment of choice for patients with extensive local or disseminated disease at diagnosis. A variety of combinations have been used, based on their antitumor activity when used as single agents, or on their different mechanisms of action or different forms of toxicity (Table 11.1). These combinations have improved the rate of response and length of survival, but, unfortunately, the cure rate has not dramatically changed over the years.

Patients with stage IV-S tumors, especially those under 6 months of age, are a unique group of children whose tumors often regress spontaneously. The available treatment modalities for older children may have an unbearable toxicity in this young group of patients. Therefore, tissue diagnosis is usually all that is indicated. It has been recommended that the primary tumor be resected at some point during the course of the disease, because the rare patient may develop a late recurrence at the primary site [64]. Mechanical problems due to an enlarged, massively infiltrated liver that compromises the respiratory function of the patient may require small doses of radiation therapy or chemotherapy. Some authors recommend this gentle

Table 11.1. Chemotherapy combinations with activity against neuroblastomas

Combination	Response rate (includes complete and partial)	References
VCR + CTX	24%–56%	[12,22,66,77,79]
ADR + DTIC	26%	[10,52]
VCR + DTIC	10%	[12]
VCR + CTX + ADR	31%–70%	[29,61,88]
VCR + CTX + DTIC	80%	[25]
VCR + CTX + DTIC + ADR	30%–94%	[5,25,30]
VCR + CTX + DNR + CDDP	55%	[74]
VCR + ADR + NH$_2$ + CTX + CDDP + DTIC	78% (complete responses)	[27]
VCR + ADR + CDDP + VM-26 + DTIC + CTX	90% (only 10 patients)	[57]
CTX + ADR	70%	[34]
VM-26 + CDDP	68%	[39]

Abbreviations: VCR, vincristine; CTX, cytoxan; DTIC, dacarbazine; ADR, adriamycin; DNR, daunorubicin; CDDP, *cis*-platinum; NH$_2$, nitrogen mustard

treatment approach to all infants younger than 1 year of age with stage I, II, or III disease following surgery. They advocate the use of little or no radiation therapy or chemotherapy even when macroscopic tumor is left behind [63]. Others, however, disagree with this approach and treat all patients, regardless of age, according to the extent of their disease [33].

Newer experimental approaches to the treatment of patients with disseminated neuroblastoma include total body radiation, either in fractionated periodic low doses [17] or in sequential segmental doses, used along with chemotherapy [35]. Bone marrow transplantation following supralethal doses of chemotherapy and/or radiation therapy [32,50] are also under investigation. Monoclonal antibodies conjugated to magnetic microspheres have been used to remove tumor cells from bone marrow which is destined for autologous transplantation, with encouraging preliminary results [81]. Such experimental forms of therapy are not available at most medical centers.

In summary, new and innovative approaches to the treatment of neuroblastoma are clearly needed. The progress in treating disseminated disease has been disappointing when compared with the results being achieved in the treatment of other childhood malignancies.

References

1. Addanki S, Gombos RH, Hinnenkamp ER et al. (1977) Screening tests for vanillylmandelic acid. J Pediatr 90:955–957

2. Akwari OE, Payne WS, Onofrio BM et al. (1978) Dumbbell neurogenic tumors of the mediastinum. Diagnosis and management. Mayo Clin Proc 54:353–358

3. Anders D, Kindermann G, Pfeiffer U (1973) Metastasizing fetal neuroblastoma with involvement of the placenta simulating fetal erythroblastosis. J Pediatr 82:50–53

4. Beckwith JB, Perrin EV (1963) In situ neuroblastoma: a contribution to the natural history of neural crest tumors. Am J Pathol 43:1089–1104

5. Berthold F, Treuner J, Branders WE et al. (1982) Neuroblastomstudie NBL 79 der Gesellschaft für Pädiatrische onkologie-Zwischen Bericht nach 2 Jahren. Klin Paediatr 194:262–269

6. Bidani N, Kirchner PT, Maohr JW et al. (1980) Gallium scan as a prognostic indicator in neuroblastoma. Clin Nucl Med 5:450–453

7. Biedler JL, Spengler BA (1976) Metaphase chromosome anomaly: association with drug resistance and cell-specific products. Science 191:185–187

8. Breslow N, McCann B (1971) Statistical estimation of prognosis for children with neuroblastoma. Cancer Res 31:2098–2103

9. Brodeur GM, Green AA, Hayes FA (1980) Cytogenetic studies of primary human neuroblastoma. In: Evans AE (ed) Advances in neuroblastoma research. Raven, New York, pp 73–80

10. Cangir A, Morgan SK, Land VJ et al. (1976) Combination chemotherapy with adriamycin and dimethyl-triazeno-imidazole-carboxamide (DTIC) in children with metastatic solid tumors. Med Ped Oncol 2:183–190

11. Carachi R, Auldist AW, Chow CW (1982) Neuroblastoma and Hirschsprung's disease. Z Kinderchir 35:24–25

12. Carli M, Pastore G, Peilongo G (1982) The role of chemotherapy in neuroblastoma. In: Raybaud C, Clement R, Lebreuil G, et al. (eds) Pediatric oncology. International Congress Series 570. Excerpta Medica, pp 151–159

13. Casola G, Scheible W, Leopold G (1984) Neuroblastoma metastatic to the testis: ultrasonographic scanning as an aid to clinical staging. Radiology 151:475–476

14. Cozzuto C, de Bernardi B, Correlli A et al. (1979) Bone marrow biopsy in children. A study of 111 patients. Med Pediatr Oncol 6:57–64

15. Cushing H, Wolbach SB (1927) The transformation of a malignant paravertebral sympathicoblastoma into a benign ganglioneuroma. Am J Pathol 3:203–215

16. D'Angio GJ (1982) The role of radiation therapy in neuroblastoma. In: Raybaud C, Clement R, Lebreuil G, et al. (eds) Pediatric oncology. International Congress Series 570. Excerpta Medica, pp 136–139

17. D'Angio GJ, Evans AE (1983) Cyclic low-dose total body radiation for metastatic neuroblastoma. Int J Radiation Oncol Biol Phys 9:1961–1965

18. Delalieux C, Ebonger G, Maurus R et al. (1975) Myoclonic encephalopathy and neuroblastoma. N Engl J Med 292:46–47

19. Evans AE (1980) Natural history of neuroblastoma. In: Evans AE (ed): Advances in neuroblastoma research. Raven, New York, pp 3–12

20. Evans AE, Albo V, D'Angio GJ et al. (1976) Factors influencing survival of children with non-metastatic neuroblastoma. Cancer 38:661–666

21. Evans AE, D'Angio GJ, Randolph J (1971) A proposed staging for children with neuroblastoma. Cancer 27:374–378

22. Evans AE, Heyn RM, Newton WA et al. (1969) Vincristine sulfate and cyclophosphamide for children with metastatic neuroblastoma. JAMA 207:1325–1327

23. Ehrenbard LT, Chaganti RSK (1981) Cancer in the fetal hydantoin syndrome. Lancet 2:97

24. Faerber EN, Carter BL, Jarro RC et al. (1984) Computed tomography of neuroblastic tumors in children. Clin Pediatr 23:17–21

25. Finkelstein JZ, Klemperer MR, Evans AE et al. (1979) Multiagent chemotherapy for children with metastatic neuroblastoma: a report from Children's Cancer Study Group. Med Pediatr Oncol 6:179–188

26. Franklin IM, Pritchard J (1983) Detection of bone marrow invasion by neuroblastoma is improved by sampling at two sites with both aspirates and trephine biopsies. J Clin Pathol (1982) 36:1215–1218

27. Franz CN, Gelber RD, Belli JA et al. (1982) Aggressive treatment of neuroblastoma. In: Raybaud C, Clement R, Lebreuil G, et al. (eds) Pediatric oncology. International Congress Series 570. Excerpta Medica, pp 175–179

28. Friedland GW, Crowe JE (1977) Neuroblastoma and other adrenal neoplasms. In: Parker BR, Castellino RA (eds) Pediatr Oncologic Radiology. CV Mosby, St. Louis, pp 267–300

29. Gasparini M, Bellani FF, Musumeci R et al. (1974) Response and survival of patients with metastatic neuroblastoma after combination chemotherapy with Adriamycin, cyclophosphamide and vincristine. Canc Chem Rep 58:365–370

30. Ghibaudo P, Pastore G, Cordero di Montezemolo L et al. (1983) DTIC, CTX, ADM, e VCR in bambini con neuroblastoma metastatico. Minerva Pediatr 35:139–143

31. Golding SJ, McElwain TJ, Husband JE (1984) The role of computed tomography in the management of children with advanced neuroblastoma. Br J Radiol 57:661–666

32. Graham-Pole J, Coccia P, Lazarus H et al. (1984) High-dose melphalan for the treatment of children with refractory neuroblastoma and Ewing's sarcoma. Am J Pediatr Hematol Oncol 6:17–25

33. Green AA (1983) Neuroblastoma. In: Jaffe N (ed) Solid tumors in childhood. CRC, Boca Roton, Fla. (1981) pp 63–71

34. Green AA, Hayes FA, Hustu HO (1981) Sequential cyclophosphamide and doxorubicin for induction of complete remission in children with disseminated neuroblastoma. Cancer 48:2310–2317

35. Green AA, Hustu HO, Palmer R et al. (1976) Total-body sequential segmental radiation and combination chemotherapy for children with disseminated neuroblastoma. Cancer 38:2250–2257

36. Hann HL, Evans AE, Cohen IJ et al. (1981) Biologic differences between neuroblastoma stages IV-S and IV: measurement of serum ferritin and E-rosette inhibition in 30 children. N Engl J Med 305:425–429

37. Hann HL, Levy HM, Evans AE (1980) Serum ferritin as a guide to therapy in neuroblastoma. Cancer Res 40:1411–1413

38. Hann HL, Stahlhut MN, Evans AE (1985) Serum ferritin as a prognostic indicator in neuroblastoma: biological effects of isoferritin. In: Evans AE, D'Angio GJ, Seeger RC (eds) Advances in neuroblastoma research. Alan R Liss, New York, pp 331–345

39. Hayes FA, Green AA, Casper J et al. (1981) Clinical evaluation of sequentially scheduled cisplatinum and VM-26 in neuroblastoma. Cancer 48:1715–1718

40. Hayes FA, Green A, Huster HO et al. (1983) Surgicopathologic staging of neuroblastoma: prognostic significance of regional lymph node involvement. J Pediatr 102:59–62

41. Hepler AB (1943) Presacral sympathicoblastoma in an infant causing urinary obstruction. J Urol 49:777–784
42. Howman-Giles RB, Gilday DL, Ash JM (1979) Radionuclide skeletal survey in neuroblastoma. Radiology 131:497–502
43. Janetschek G, Weitzel D, Stein W et al. (1984) Prenatal diagnosis of neuroblastoma by sonography. Urol 24:397–402
44. Ishiguro Y, Kato K, Ito T et al. (1984) Enolase isoenzymes as markers for differential diagnosis of neuroblastoma, rhabdomyosarcoma and Wilms' tumor. Gann 75:53–60
45. Johnsonbaugh RE, Cahill R (1975) Screening procedures for neuroblastoma: false negative results. Pediatrics 56:267–270
46. Kauffman RA, Thrall JH, Keyes JW (1978) False negative bone scans in neuroblastoma metastatic to the ends of long bones. Am J Roentgenol 130:131–135
47. Kinney H, Faix R, Brazy J (1980) The fetal alcohol syndrome and neuroblastoma. Pediatrics 66:130–132
48. Knudson AG Jr, Strong LC (1972) Mutation and cancer: neuroblastoma and pheochromocytoma. Am J Hum Genet 24:514–532
49. Koop CE (1968) Neuroblastoma: two year survival and treatment correlation. J Pediatr Surg 3:178–179
50. Kraker J, Hartman O, Voute PA et al. (1982) The effect of high-dose melphalan with autologous bone marrow transplantation in neuroblastoma patients with advanced disease. In: Raybaud C, Clement R, Lebreuil G. et al. (eds) Pediatric oncology. International Congress Series 570. Excerpta Medica, pp 165–167
51. LaBrosse EH (1968) Biochemical diagnosis of neuroblastoma: use of a urine spot test. Proc Am Assoc Cancer Res 9:39
52. Leiken S, Bernstein I, Evans AE et al. (1978) Use of combination Adriamycin and DTIC in children with advanced stage IV neuroblastoma. Cancer Chem Rep 59:1015–1018
53. Leonard AS, Robach SA, Nesbit ME et al. (1972) The VMA test strip: a new tool for mass screening, diagnosis and management of catecholamine-secreting tumors. J Pediatr Surg 7:528–531
54. Mackay B, Masse SR, King OY et al. (1975) Diagnosis of neuroblastoma by electron microscopy of bone marrow aspirates. Pediatrics 56:1045–1049
55. MacManus M (1983) The diagnosis and staging of neuroblastoma. Clin Radiol 34:523–527
56. Marangos PJ (1985) Clinical studies with neuron specific enolase. In: Evans AE, D'Angio GJ, Seeger RC (eds) Advances in neuroblastoma research. AR Liss, New York, pp 285–294
57. Margulis E, Zucker JM, Lemercier N et al. (1982) Intensive multichemotherapy including cis-diamminodichloroplatinum (CDDP) in metastatic neuroblastoma. In: Raybaud C, Clement R, Lebreuil G, et al. (eds) Pediatric oncology, International Congress Series 570, Excerpta Medica, pp 168–174
58. Mendelsohn G, Eggelston JC, Olson JL et al. (1979) Vasoactive intestinal peptide and its relationship to ganglion cell differentation in neuroblastic tumors. Lab Invest 41:144–149
59. Miller RW (1977) Ethnic differences in cancer occurrence: genetic and environmental influences with particular reference to neuroblastoma. In: Mulvihill JJ, Miller RW, Fraumei JF Jr (eds) Genetics of human cancer. Raven, New York
60. Nickerson BG, Hutter JJ (1979) Opsomyoclonus and neuroblastoma. J Clin Pediatr 18:446–448
61. Ninane J, Pritchard J, Malpas J (1981) Chemotherapy of advanced neuroblastoma: does Adriamycin contribute? Arch Dis Child 56:544–548
62. Ninane J, Pritchard J, Morris-Jones PH et al. (1982) Stage II neuroblastoma. Adverse prognostic significance of lymph node involvement. Arch Dis Child 57:438–442
63. Nitschke R, Humphrey B, Sexauer C et al. (1983) Neuroblastoma: therapy for infants with good prognosis. Med Pediatr Oncol 11:154–158
64. Rangecroft L, Lauder I, Wagget J (1978) Spontaneous maturation of stage IV-S neuroblastoma. Arch Dis Child 53:815–817
65. Reynolds CP, Smith RG, Frenkel EP (1981) The diagnostic dilemma of the "small round cell neoplasm." Cancer 48:2088–2094
66. Sawitsky A, Deposito F, Treat C et al. (1970) Vincristine and cyclophosphamide therapy in generalized neuroblastoma. Am J Dis Child 119:308–313
67. Scheibel E, Rechnitzer C, Fahrenkrug J et al. (1982) Vasoactive intestinal polypeptide (VIP) in children with neural crest tumors. Acta Paediatr Scand 71:721–725
68. Schmechel D, Marangos PJ, Brightman M et al. (1978) Brain enolases as specific markers of neuronal and glial cells. Science 199:313–315
69. Schneider KM, Becker JM, Krasna IH (1965) Neonatal neuroblastoma. Pediatrics 36:359–365
70. Seeler RA, Israel JN, Royal JE et al. (1979) Ganglioneuroblastoma and fetal hydantoin-alcohol syndromes. Pediatrics 63:524–527
71. Senelick RC, Bray PF, Lahey ME et al. (1973) Neuroblastoma and myoclonic encephalopathy: two cases and a review of the literature. J Pediatr Surg 8:623
72. Shaw A, Konrad PN (1984) Pediatric surgical oncology: update on Wilms' tumor, neuroblastoma and rhabdomysarcoma. Curr Probl Cancer 8:18–30
73. Shimada H, Chatten J, Newton WA Jr et al. (1984) Histopathologic prognostic factors in neuroblastic tumors: definition of subtypes of ganglio-neuroblastoma and an age-linked classification of neuroblastomas. J National Cancer Inst 73:405–413
74. Shuster JJ, Land VJ, Nitschke R et al. (1983) Phase II study of four-drug chemotherapy for metastatic neuroblastoma. A Pediatric Oncology Group study. Cancer Treat Rep 67:187–188
75. Siegel SE, Laug WE, Hanlow PJ et al. (1980) Patterns of urinary catecholamine excretion in neuroblastoma. In: Evans AE (ed) Advances in neuroblastoma research. Raven, New York, pp 25–32
76. Sitarz A, Finkelstein J, Grossfeld S et al. (1983) An evaluation of the role of surgery in disseminated neuroblastoma: a report from the Children's Cancer Study Group. J Pediatr Surg 18:147–151
77. Starling KA, Sutow WW, Donaldson MH et al. (1974) Drug trials in neuroblastoma: cyclophosphamide alone; vincristine plus cyclophosphamide; 6 mercaptopurine plus 6 methylmercaptopurine riboside; and cytosine arabinoside alone. Cancer Chemother Rep 58:683–668
78. Sty JR, Kun LE, Casper JT (1980) Bone imaging as a diagnostic aid in evaluating neuroblastoma. Am J Pediatr Hematol Oncol 2:115–118
79. Sullivan MP, Nora AH, Kulapongs P et al. (1969) Evaluation of vincristine sulfate and cyclophosphamide chemotherapy for metastatic neuroblastoma. Pediatrics 44:685–694
80. Traggis DG, Filler RM, Druckman H et al. (1977) Prognosis for children with neuroblastoma presenting with paralysis. J Pediatr Surg 12:419–425
81. Treleaven JG, Ugelstad J, Philip T (1984) Removal of neuroblastoma cells from bone marrow with monoclonal antibodies conjugated to magnetic microspheres. Lancet 1:70–73
82. Tsokos M, Linnoila RI, Chandra RS et al. (1984) Neuron-specific enolase in the diagnosis of neuroblastoma and other small round-cell tumors in children. Hum Pathol 15:575–584
83. Ungerleider RS (1981) Working conference on neuroblastoma clinical trials. Cancer Treat Rep 65:719–723

84. Voûte PA, Voss A, Delemarre JFM et al. (1980) The persistent challenge of neuroblastoma. In: Van Eys J, Sullivan MP (eds) Status of the curability of childhood cancer. Raven, New York, pp 145–161
85. Witzleben GL, Landy RA (1975) Disseminated neuroblastoma in a child with von Recklinghausen's disease. Cancer 34:785–790
86. Young JL, Miller RW (1975) Incidence of malignant tumors in U.S. children. J Pediatr 86:254–258
87. Zeltzer PM, Parma AM, Dalton A et al. (1983) Raised neuron-specific enolase in serum of children with metastatic neuroblastoma. Lancet 2:361–363
88. Zucker JM, Mercier JC (1976) Chimiotherapie lourde dans le neuroblastome. Arch Franc Ped 33:555–567
89. Zucker JM, Margulis E (1979) Radiochemotherapy of postoperative minimal residual disease in neuroblastoma. Recent Results Cancer Res 68:423–430

Chapter 12

Metastatic Disease

J. H. Mersey

Introduction

Autopsy series of adrenal pathology reveal a great variety of diseases, many of which are present in a significant proportion of adrenals sampled. The majority of these abnormalities can be described as adrenal masses. These may be of adrenal origin or may be metastatic to the adrenal. Many of these are clinically silent and insignificant, while others may produce hormones which produce distant effects. A third group, those that are metastatic, are usually clinically silent, but may result in adrenal insufficiency. The presence of these adrenal metastases, however, if known may change prognosis or alter therapy. Therefore, the detection and subsequent evaluation of adrenal masses is of great importance.

The problem of the adrenal mass can be divided into two parts. The first is the approach to the incidentally discovered adrenal mass. Those adrenal masses found in conjunction with distant hormonal effects are discussed in other chapters. Often, adrenal enlargement is detected through radiologic evaluation of other suspected disease, in the absence of any related symptomatology. Given the wide range of possibilities, it is important to establish a logical approach to the investigation.

Second is the question of detection of metastases to the adrenal in patients with known cancer. This issue has two parts: (1) screening procedures in patients with known primaries and (2) evaluation of the cause of adrenal enlargement in these patients once an abnormality is found.

In this chapter I will briefly review the pathologic possibilities, then discuss how clinically to detect adrenal enlargement and pathology. I will then proceed to the evaluation of adrenal masses in patients with and without known cancer. Finally I will discuss the incidence of adrenal insufficiency induced by adrenal metastases and methods of detection.

Pathologic Findings

Adrenal pathology is discussed in detail in Chap. 3 and the normal anatomy in Chap. 2. For the purposes of this chapter, adrenal enlargement can be divided into primary and secondary causes. A review of the overall incidence of adrenal tumors has shown that metastatic disease accounts for 70% of adrenal masses [26].

Primary causes are listed in Table 12.1. These include diffuse hyperplasia due to adrenocorticotropic hormone (ACTH) stimulation, from pituitary Cushing's syndrome, ectopic ACTH syndrome, or congenital adrenal hyperplasia. Cortical nodularity without frank adenoma formation occurs in half of all persons over the age of 50 years [48].

Table 12.1 Causes of adrenal enlargement

1. Cortical
   A. Bilateral hyperplasia
      Cushing's disease
      Ectopic ACTH syndrome
      Congenital adrenal hyperplasia
      Idiopathic (primary aldosteronism)
   B. Adenoma
      Functional producing cortisol, aldosterone, androgen,
         estrogen
      Nonfunctional
   C. Cyst
   D. Carcinoma
2. Medullary
   A. Pheochromocytoma
   B. Ganglioneuroma–neuroblastoma
   C. Myelolipoma
3. Metastatic
   A. Medullary, most common (90%)
   B. Sources of metastases
      Lung
      Breast
      Melanoma
      Colon
      Renal cell
      Lymphoma

Adenomas of the adrenal cortex occur in 2%–8% of all autopsies [8]. These are clinically silent for the most part. The incidence of adenomas is higher in elderly obese diabetic patients (30%), women over age 81 years (29%), and patients with hypertension (20%) [48]. Other adrenal tumors include cysts, myelolipomas, ganglioneuromas, and pheochromocytomas. Most of these nonfunctioning adrenal neoplasms are of no clinical significance. Their only importance is in differentiating them from adrenocortical carcinoma and from metastatic adrenal disease. Adrenal carcinoma is discussed in Chap. 9.

Metastatic disease in the adrenal is a very common occurrence. Two large series [2,4] have reported the autopsy incidence of metastases to the adrenal in patients with known malignancy.

Abrams found a 27% incidence of metastases to the adrenal. Bullocks found an incidence of 8.6%. Willis in another series found an incidence of 10% [53]. There is no obvious explanation for the discrepancy in incidence. Abrams' series, which notes the incidence of metastases to most other organs, has a high incidence of metastases in general, as if their patients had more extensive disease.

Thomas [49] and others have observed that adrenal medullary metastases exceed cortical metastases by 10:1 and that more metastases are found in the left adrenal, presumably because of its greater size.

Certain types of malignancy have been found to spread more commonly to the adrenal. These include lung and breast cancers and melanoma. In Abrams' series there was a 35.6% incidence of metastasis to the adrenal from lung cancer. There is no comment about bilaterality in this study. Abrams compared his data with those of previous studies showing a similar incidence. Bullock found a 28.7% incidence for lung cancer. In his series lung cancer was responsible for four times as many adrenal metastases as any other tumor. This incidence of 28%–35% is also similar to that in other series [15]. As will be discussed later, adrenal metastases are more common with small cell cancer than with other lung cancers.

Breast cancer is generally listed as the second most common tumor to be found in the adrenal. In Abrams' series metastases were found in 53.9% of patients with breast cancer. In Bullock's series the incidence was only 12.8%, and in Willis' 20%. De la Monte [10] in a recent series found that 43% had adrenal metastases, and these tended to occur more often in younger patients. There is no description as to how often these were bilateral in any of these studies. In Abrams' series, breast cancer was responsible for more adrenal metastases than lung cancer.

Malignant melanoma may metastasize more frequently to the adrenal than either lung or breast cancer, but because of its lower incidence the total number of cases is smaller. In Bullock's series the incidence was 30%. Abrams' series included no patients with melanoma. Patel found a 35.6% incidence of adrenal spread and de la Monte found 52% adrenal metastases [11,36].

Many other tumors have been described to cause adrenal metastases, but all with a lower frequency. Colon cancer, the next most common visceral malignancy, spread to the adrenals in 3%–13% of cases in the series previously mentioned. Renal cell carcinoma, an uncommon tumor, spreads to the adrenals with a frequency of 18%–24% [5]. These metastases are more often ipsilateral than contralateral, suggesting direct spread, but can occasionally be only contralateral [29,38]. Lymphoma, which often involves the retroperitoneum, has been described to involve the adrenal in about 4% of cases, half of which were bilateral [35]. Stomach and esophageal cancer also metastasize frequently to the adrenal, with at least half of cases showing bilateral involvement [6].

Essentially all other tumor types have been

described to spread to the adrenal, but the frequency of finding such lesions is rare. Nonetheless, if the presence of a primary tumor is known, and adrenal enlargement is found, the possibility of spread to the adrenal must be considered.

Techniques of Evaluation

Techniques of evaluating the adrenal glands without removing them are reviewed in Chaps. 4 and 5. Meschan [26] in his book also has covered this subject in detail. I will discuss here only the data relevant to identifying the presence of adrenal tumors and differentiating intrinsic from extrinsic origins of the tumors.

Many methods have been employed to image the adrenals. These include intravenous pyelography without and with nephrotomography, retroperitoneal air insufflation, plain films of the abdomen, and more recently ultrasound and CT scanning. All but the last two have been abandoned as useful imaging techniques.

Zornoza [54] reviewed 50 cases of adrenal metastases detected by ultrasound, but it is not apparent how many metastases were missed. He did describe bilateral metastases in 10 of 50 patients, which he called the "headlight sign." Sample [41] and Abrams [1] compared ultrasonography with computed tomography in evaluation of the adrenal gland. Sample found the two procedures to be equally effective in identifying adrenal abnormalities, but suggested that CT scanning would be more effective in screening, while ultrasound might be more effective in the thin patient with little retroperitoneal fat, which makes CT imaging more difficult. Abrams et al. found CT to be significantly better, with a sensitivity of 84%, a specificity of 98%, and an accuracy of 90%, versus 79%, 61%, and 70% respectively for ultrasound. Thomas [49] has agreed with Abrams, and explains the discrepancy between the findings of Sample and Abrams by the fact that newer CT scanners have improved imaging and allow for its advantage over ultrasound.

Therefore the consensus is that CT is the imaging technique of choice. Studies dating back to 1978 have shown the ability of CT to demonstrate adrenal masses as small as 1 cm in diameter [22]. Adrenal glands of normal size can be imaged in more than 90% of patients [47]. Karstaedt also concluded that enlargement of adrenal origin could not be differentiated from metastatic disease, a conclusion confirmed by others [39]. Most studies confirm the remarkably good correlation between adrenal disease on CT scan and that found histologically [7,21]. Cedarmark found in one series of 46 studies that CT correctly identified all adrenal metastases that were visible macroscopically at autopsy; CT did fail to identify one pair of adrenals with microscopic metastases. There were no false positives.

Magnetic resonance imaging has been used recently to image the adrenal glands. At present this technique, which is not generally available, has been shown to be as good as, but not better than, current CT scanning [44].

In summary CT scanning will correctly identify the presence of tumors greater than 1 cm more than 90% of the time, but cannot discriminate between primary and metastatic disease. CT scanning can therefore miss small tumors, and can find benign adrenal tumors in patients with known cancer, raising the spectre of metastases which may be in fact be benign adrenal adenomas.

It would be ideal then if pathologic confirmation could be obtained without subjecting patients to surgery unnecessarily to remove benign adenomas or metastases. A recent approach has been to attempt narrow-gauge needle aspiration of the adrenal under CT guidance. The first series reporting this technique [19] described a study in which 14 needle aspirations were attempted in patients with an adrenal mass. As controls a similar biopsy technique was employed on autopsy specimens for evaluation of cytologic specificity. Diagnostic material was obtained in 13 patients. Four patients had primary adrenal neoplasms, two benign, and two malignant. The malignant lesions were diagnosed on the basis of suspicious cells on cytology. Metastatic cancer was correctly diagnosed in eight of nine biopsies. Two patients with fungal infection of the adrenal were accurately diagnosed by aspiration. There were no complications of biopsy; no hemorrhage or pneumothorax was observed. The authors of this study do comment on the difficulty of clearly separating benign from malignant primary tumors of the adrenal. The authors also point out the value of aspiration biopsy in the patient with a primary malignancy elsewhere, since a positive biopsy may well change the therapeutic approach. Gross [17] has agreed with this approach; he performed adrenal biopsies in three patients with malignancies that do not usually involve the adrenal. In each case the biopsy was positive for malignant cells, thereby confirming the presence of metastatic disease, and in each case altering the therapeutic approach from resection to systemic therapy.

Berkman [3] biopsied a series of 16 patients. Fifteen of 16 were successful, the smallest mass being 1.7 cm. Seven had benign adrenal cells and were thought to have adenomas, adrenal hemorrhage, or Cushing's disease. Nine had malignancy elsewhere; only four of these had positive biopsies for malignant cells. The rest had tissue consistent with an adrenal adenoma. No complications occurred. These authors also emphasize the importance of biopsy because an abnormal scan may mislead the clinician about the presence of metastases.

Clearly this procedure is of value and of minimal risk in the hands of experienced physicians. It does, however, require both this experience and a pathologist who can interpret the cytologic findings. This technique will be performed more frequently in the future, but caution must be used before recommending widespread use.

Evaluation of the Adrenal Mass in the Patient Without Known Malignancy

With the advent of CT scanning for evaluation of multiple intraabdominal and retroperitoneal diseases, the discovery of incidental adrenal enlargement has become fairly common. In our clinical experience, many of these masses were removed surgically, with the majority being found to be benign adrenal adenomas. The literature confirms that this was a common experience in many centers. Therefore, to avoid unnecessary surgery, it would be helpful to design an approach to the isolated clinically inapparent mass in order to avoid surgery when possible.

Since CT can demonstrate adrenal masses as small as 1 cm in diameter, and 2%–8% of all patients have adrenal adenomas at autopsy, it is not surprising that CT scanning will identify these adrenal masses. Glazer [14] reported 16 adrenal masses in patients without suspected adrenal disease. These

were gathered over a 2-year period. Size ranged from 1 to 6 cm, with eight being less than 2 cm. Six patients had adrenalectomy or autopsy. Two of the patients had renal cell cancer and epidermoid cancer of the lung, respectively. All pathologic specimens were benign adrenal tissue, five of the six being adenomas, and one a nodular hyperplasia. Based on this information the authors concluded that most small adrenal masses are benign adenomas; also not all adrenal enlargements in patients with cancer represent metastatic disease. Since most adrenal cancers are large on presentation, they suggest follow-up CT scanning in 2-3 months, and adrenal biopsy in patients with cancer elsewhere. They suggest adrenalectomy or biopsy for patients with lesions greater than 3–4 cm.

In another series [27], 22 adrenal masses were found on CT. Four were thought to be cysts or myelolipomas by CT. These were excluded from further evaluation. The rest ranged in size from 1.2 to 5 cm in patients from ages 45 to 73 years. These data are quite consistent with Glazer's. As in Glazer's series there was a left preponderance (12 of 18). Six adrenals were examined pathologically and all were benign adrenal tissue. In five of the patients there was malignancy elsewhere. Two of these had benign biopsies and three had abdominal lymphoma, which responded to chemotherapy, but with no change in adrenal size, therefore suggesting a benign etiology of the adrenal mass. The authors suggest that certain CT criteria help confirm the benign nature of the lesion. These are smooth contour, well-delineated tumor margin, no growth on serial CT over 1 year, and size less than 5 cm. These conclusions are not based on their data, since they had no malignant lesions in this series, but are based on their opinion and quoted literature. Except for size, most other authors would disagree that benign lesions can be separated from malignant ones by CT alone. They suggest a nonoperative approach unless the mass is greater than 5 cm.

Copeland has reviewed this topic recently [8]. He outlines a clinical approach to the problem of the isolated adrenal mass once detected. To begin with patients should be evaluated for the presence of symptoms or physical signs related to biochemical activity of the tumor. These can include medullary tumors such as pheochromocytoma, and cortical tumors. These can result in Cushing's syndrome, primary aldosteronism, or feminizing and masculinizing syndromes. Laboratory evaluation then should include urinary metanephrine for pheochromocytoma, cortisol, 17-hydroxycorticosteroids, 17-ketosteroids, and 17-ketogenic steroids. The reason given for the measurement of ketogenic steroids is that some adrenal carcinomas have been reported to make 17-hydroxy progesterone, which is not measured by ketosteroids, but is by ketogenic steroids. If masculinization or feminization is suspected, then androgens or estrogens should be measured. If hypertension and hypokalemia are present then aldosterone must be measured. See Chap. 7 for details on this evaluation.

Epidemiologic criteria can also be helpful, with most adrenal cancers occurring in older men. More important, however, according to Copeland is the size of the tumor. Adenomas greater than 6 cm are rare. On the other hand most adrenal carcinomas are greater than 6 cm (105 of 114). Without belaboring the obvious, these cancers were smaller at some time, and prognosis is related to size at detection, and so smaller lesions cannot be ignored.

Fine needle aspiration has a limited role in these patients, because of the difficulty in distinguishing benign from malignant adrenal tissue. Review of the incidence of benign and malignant adrenal neoplasms suggests that operating only on tumors greater than 6 cm would result in the finding of adrenal carcinoma in 1 in 60 operations. Operating on all adrenal masses would reveal adrenal carcinoma in 1 of 4000 operations. Copeland therefore recommends follow-up CT scans at 2, 6, and 18 months for lesions less than 6 cm, and immediate surgery for lesions greater than 6 cm. If size changes, then the patient should be reevaluated biochemically and subjected to surgery.

Copeland's approach is logical and comprehensive, but omits one key issue. That is, the incidence of metastatic disease to the adrenal is higher than that of intrinsic disease. Therefore the presence of metastatic cancer must be considered in the approach to the isolated adrenal mass. In Fig. 12.1 is outlined the approach I would use in evaluation of the incidentally discovered adrenal mass. Once a CT scan has been performed and an abnormality is found, evaluation based on size is undertaken. For lesions greater than or equal to 6 cm, hormonal evaluation followed by surgical removal should be performed. If the adrenal abnormality is less than 6 cm, a different approach should be used. Hormonal evaluation, as well as consideration of malignancy elsewhere which has spread to the adrenal, should be done. If the adrenal can be shown to produce excess steroid, it should be removed. If a

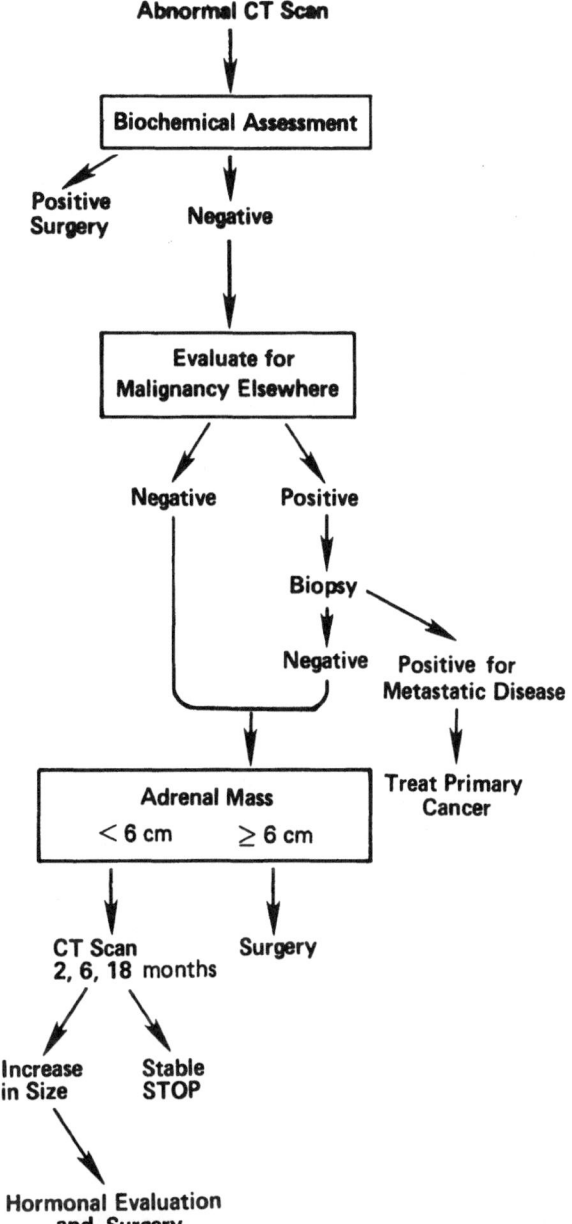

Fig. 12.1. Flow diagram of the evaluation of the isolated adrenal mass. See text for detailed discussion. In brief, if an adrenal mass is detected and biochemical assessment is negative then evaluation for possible metastatic disease to the adrenal should be considered. If negative then the decision for surgery depends on the size. If positive then adrenal biopsy should be performed.

primary cancer is found elsewhere, needle aspiration of the adrenal should be performed to confirm that this adrenal lesion is metastatic. If this workup is negative, serial CT scans should be performed, with a change in size prompting reevaluation and surgery.

Shown in Fig. 12.2 are two examples of CT scans which show adrenal masses. Fig. 12.2a shows the presence of a left adrenal mass discovered in a 45-year-old male who presented with gynecomastia. Endocrine evaluation was carried out as suggested previously. The only abnormality found was an elevated estradiol level. In particular, 17-keto-steroids were always within normal limits. Because the patient had other possible sources of estrogen synthesis, including liver and adipose tissue, we undertook adrenal venous sampling. This demonstrated a step up from the left adrenal vein. The patient underwent adrenalectomy; pathology showed an adrenal adenoma, but the pathologist was unwilling to exclude adrenal carcinoma, based on pathologic criteria.

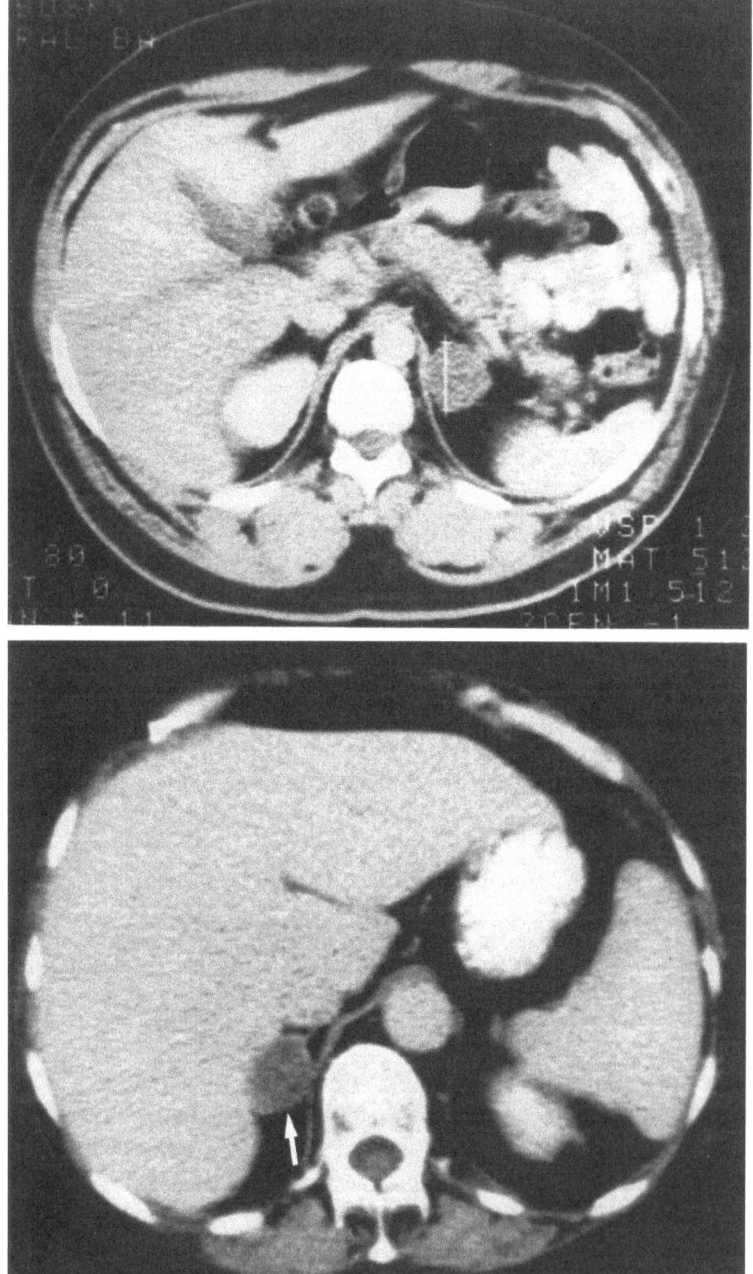

Fig. 12.2. **a** Adrenal mass in a patient with a primary adrenal tumor. Note the 3.5-cm left adrenal mass. **b** Adrenal mass found in an asymptomatic patient with gallbladder disease. Note the 2.5-cm right adrenal mass.

Figure 12.2b shows the CT scan of a patient who underwent CT scanning because of gallbladder disease. In addition to demonstrating the expected finding a 2.5-cm adrenal mass in the right adrenal was found. Biochemical workup was negative, and the patient is being followed by serial CT scans.

Evaluation of the Adrenal in the Oncologic Patient

The assessment of adrenal pathology in the oncologic patient is a two-part issue: first the importance of finding adrenal abnormalities must be considered, and second the necessity of knowing the precise diagnosis of the adrenal abnormality must also be discussed.

As mentioned above, adrenal metastases are found frequently in many types of tumors, particularly, lung, breast and melanoma. These data in the quoted studies do not tell us how often the detection of adrenal masses would change the therapeutic approach. In fact most of these studies predate chemotherapy of cancer. If adrenal metastases are the only ones detected, then this discovery would change therapy from a primary resection to systemic chemotherapy. On the other hand if adrenal enlargement is detected, but is in fact an adrenal adenoma and not metastatic disease, then systemic chemotherapy may be inappropriate when surgery may be curable.

Screening for adrenal metastases has been done in high-risk patients. The highest risk group is patients with small cell cancer of the lung. Dunnick [13] described a series of 45 patients who had abdominal CT scans. Sixteen had metastases detected, four of these in the adrenal. Four also had other retroperitoneal metastases; the study does not say how many had adrenal metastases only. No adrenal biopsies were performed, but two of the adrenal glands decreased in size with chemotherapy. In another series [18] of 50 patients, seven (14%) had adrenal metastases, and in four of these no other metastases were found. Two of four were confirmed pathologically at autopsy. This incidence of 14% is similar to that found in an autopsy study conducted 1 month after surgery for curative therapy [28]. In another study [50] 65 patients underwent abdominal CT. Adrenal enlargement was found in ten (15%) in seven of whom it was

the only abnormality. There was no pathologic confirmation in this study.

Not only may there be false-positive scans, but false-negative ones. Pagani [33] performed a study in 24 patients with small cell carcinoma of the lung and normal adrenal CT scans. The patients then underwent adrenal biopsy by percutaneous CT direction. This was performed bilaterally in 19 patients. Four patients had biopsies positive for small cell carcinoma; in one patient both adrenals were involved. Fourteen of 43 biopsies failed to obtain adequate material for interpretation. Two patients developed pneumothoraces. Therefore there was a 17% false-negative rate for adrenal CT scanning in this study.

Many studies in non-small cell carcinoma of the lung have also been performed. In one study of 110 patients, 11 patients were found to have 16 adrenal tumors. As usual left predominated over right (nine to seven). Five patients had no other evidence of metastatic disease [42]. This finding is more important than in small cell cancer, since curative resection is more likely to be attempted in non-small cell cancer. The question remains, however, of whether the adrenal enlargement is in fact metastatic. Nielsen [30] undertook a similar study in 84 patients with non-small cell cancer, and found abnormal adrenals in 15 patients; in 3 the abnormality was bilateral. Four patients underwent biopsy and all showed metastatic disease. In spite of this the authors suggested that all patients undergo biopsy to exclude a benign adrenal lesion.

In a series of 330 patients with non-small cell lung cancer, Oliver [31] found on CT scanning 32 patients with adrenal masses without other intraabdominal disease. To determine whether or not these adrenal masses were in fact metastatic disease, 25 of the patients underwent needle aspiration. At biopsy only eight of the biopsies were positive for metastatic disease. The rest were consistent with benign adrenal adenomas. The authors concluded that lesions greater than 3 cm were more likely to be metastases, and that all lesions should be biopsied if the presence of metastatic disease would withhold curative surgery.

Pagani [34] in his series on non-small cell lung cancer found a similar incidence of adrenal abnormalities of 12% (20 of 172). Seven of these patients had bilateral disease, with six having only left and eight only right adrenal masses. Fourteen of these 20 had no metastatic disease detected elsewhere, and therefore underwent needle aspiration biopsy.

Thirteen of the 14 had metastatic disease; only one was an adrenal tumor. In addition 32 patients without abnormal adrenal scans underwent biopsy. Four of these (12%) also had positive biopsies. Thus in this study there were few false-positive scans, but a significant number of false-negative ones.

Similar studies have not been done for other types of tumors, except for one study on lymphoma. In this study [35] 173 patients with non-Hodgkin's lymphoma underwent CT scanning. Seven had positive scans, which showed bilateral enlargement in three. All glands showed shrinking with chemotherapy, but no biopsies were done.

Pagani [32] reviewed the incidence of serendipitous findings in 1000 CT scans in patients with cancer and found 37 patients with adrenal abnormalities, 27 of which were unexpected. Ten of these were instrumental in changing therapy in the patient. Nine of these were metastases and one was an adrenal carcinoma.

Based on these data, I would suggest the approach shown in Fig. 12.3. Once a patient is found to have a primary cancer known to metastasize to the adrenal, then abdominal CT should be performed. This is particularly applicable to lung, breast, melanoma, lyphoma, and renal cell carcinomas. If this fails to show adrenal enlargement, no further workup should be done. Adrenal biopsy of nonenlarged glands cannot be supported clinically, even if some studies have shown positive biopsies in normal adrenals. Performing these in all patients is unsupportable because of risk, expense, and low yield.

If CT shows an adrenal mass, and no other metastases have been demonstrated, adrenal biopsy should be performed because of the significant possibility that the adrenal mass is a benign adenoma. The only exception may be if both adrenals show enlargement, which in the absence of Cushing's disease is much more likely to be bilateral metastases (as high as 25% of all patients have bilateral disease). If the biopsy specimen is adequate, then clinical decision making as regards therapy of the malignancy can take place. If biopsy is inadequate or cannot be done, then serial CT scans should be performed at 2, 6, and 12 months.

Adrenal Insufficiency from Adrenal Metastases

As mentioned previously, as many as 25% of patients who have adrenal metastases have bilateral adrenal involvement. These patients may have no worse prognosis in terms of their malignancy (although this has not been evaluated), but obviously run the risk of developing adrenal insufficiency. Most authors have agreed that 90% of adrenal tissue must be destroyed to produce a clinically significant reduction in adrenal secretion. Therefore the presence of bilateral metastases is far from synonymous with an Addisonian state. Nonetheless, clinically apparent adrenal insufficiency is increasingly commonly reported, and represents a real risk.

The diagnosis of adrenal insufficiency may be missed in the presence of widespread metastases because of similarity of symptoms—that is, weight loss, nausea, anorexia, and electrolyte abnormalities. Reviews of adrenal insufficiency secondary

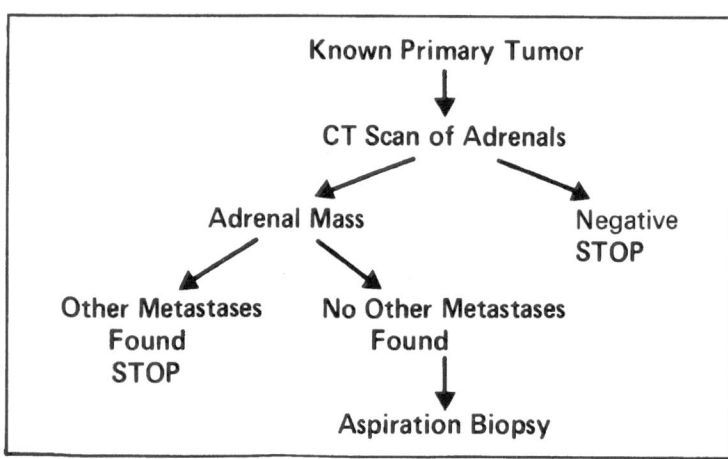

Fig. 12.3. Flow diagram for the evaluation of an adrenal mass in patients with cancer elsewhere. See text for discussion.

to metastatic disease usually discriminate between biochemically confirmed cases and those that could be suspected pre- or postmortem, but were not confirmed. For example, one series reviewed 457 autopsies of patients with colon carcinoma, and 52 were thought to have sufficient adrenal metastases to cause clinically apparent Addison's disease; none of these were confirmed by adrenal testing [6].

The most recent review cites 49 previous cases mentioned in the literature [9]. Two more have been described since [24,37]. Thirty-four patients had some sort of adrenal testing to confirm the diagnosis, but in many of these results are confusing or inadequate for diagnosis. Remarkably, all the confirmed cases have been case reports. There has never been a prospective study to determine the precise prevalence of adrenal failure, even in those patients with bilateral metastases. Review of these many case reports has shown the majority of patients to have metastatic lung cancer [9,20,25,37,40,43,45,46,51,52]. Other tumors described to be responsible include breast [46,51], testis [51], pancreas [40], adrenal [46], renal [16,45], lymphoma [24,45], and transitional cell cancer of the bladder, colon, and melanoma [45]. In short, after lung cancer, many other tumors may be responsible for causing adrenal failure, but no particular tumor is very likely.

Given the likelihood of bilateral adrenal metastases, and the increasing number of reported cases, as well as the increasing duration of survival of patients with metastatic disease, it is important to be aware of the possibility of overt or incipient adrenal insufficiency. No prospective studies have been done, but many authors have proposed that susceptible patients be tested. In our experience and in that of others [12,23] rapid ACTH testing, measuring both cortisol and aldosterone, has been as accurate as more prolonged testing. The procedure that we follow is to administer Cortrosyn (synthetic alpha-1-24-ACTH) $250\,\mu g$ intramuscularly, and to measure cortisol and aldosterone at baseline and 60 min. After 7 years of experience we have always been able to determine whether a patient is normal, Addisonian, or hypopituitary by this test. Results from our study are shown in Table 12.2. For normal volunteers, the minimal morning cortisol level was $7\,\mu g/dl$, with a minimal increment at 60 min of $9\,\mu g/dl$. For patients with adrenal insufficiency the maximal morning cortisol level was $2.4\,\mu g/dl$ and the maximal increment was $0.6\,\mu g/dl$. For hypopituitary patients the maximal morning cortisol level was $4\,\mu g/dl$ and the maximal response $11\,\mu g/dl$. Therefore there was no overlap between normal and abnormal response, but there was overlap between adrenal and pituitary patients in terms of cortisol response. When aldosterone response was included, the separation was complete. Baseline aldosterones were essentially the same, but the minimal increment for hypopituitary patients was 6 ng/dl, and the maximal increment for Addisonian patients was 2.6 ng/dl.

I would propose, therefore, the following approach. If adrenal CT scan reveals bilateral masses, ACTH testing should be performed. If results reveal adrenal insufficiency, the patient should be started on glucocorticoid and mineralocorticoid replacement. This is usually done with cortisone acetate and 9-alpha-fluorocortisone. The dose varies from patient to patient, but is usually 25–37.5 mg/day of cortisone in two doses, and 0.1 mg fluorocortisone. Patients who are ill from their underlying disease will often require larger doses of glucocorticoid and may be better treated with prednisone or other long-acting steroids.

Table 12.2. Rapid ACTH test for diagnosis of adrenal disease

	Cortisol Mean (range) ($\mu g/dl$)	Increment Mean (range) ($\mu g/dl$)	Aldosterone Mean (range) (ng/dl)	Increment Mean (range) (ng/dl)
Normal				
Baseline	12.5 (7–20)		8.5 (0–16)	
60 min	28.7 (23–45)	16.1 (8.5–30.5)	28.0 (15–47)	19.5 (6.1–32.8)
Addison's disease				
Baseline	0.9 (0–2.4)		3.9 (0–12)	
60 min	1.0 (0–3)	0.1 (–0.3–3)	4.5 (0–12)	0.7 (0–2.6)
Hypopituitarism				
Baseline	2.4 (0–4)		4.3 (2–10)	
60 min	9.4 (4–16)	7.0 (3–13)	29.3 (9–70)	25.0 (6–65)

Since the pituitary is also a possible site for lung and breast metastases, the possibility of ACTH deficiency must be considered. The measurement of cortisol and aldosterone in the rapid ACTH test will also allow this diagnosis to be ruled in or out. As the patient is followed clinically, if adrenal masses enlarge, or disease progresses clinically, and the first test showed normal adrenal function, then the patient should be retested. Alternatively as suggested by Seidenwurm, all patients with adrenal masses may be placed on replacement hormones. Either of these approaches will preclude the possibility that adrenal insufficiency will go untreated and worsen the condition of the patient.

Most important is that the physician should be aware of the potential for adrenal failure, and diagnose and treat the patient accordingly.

References

1. Abrams HL, Siegelman SS, Adams DF et al. (1982) Computed tomography vs ultrasound of the adrenal gland: a prospective study. Radiology 143:121–128
2. Abrams HL, Spiro R, Goldstein N (1950) Metastases in carcinoma: analysis of 1000 autopsied cases. Cancer 3:74–85
3. Berkman WA, Bernardino ME, Sewell CW et al. (1984) The computed tomography-guided adrenal biopsy. Cancer 53:2098–2103
4. Bullock WK, Hirst AE (1953) Metastatic carcinoma of the adrenal glands. Am J Med Sci 226:521–524
5. Campbell CM, Middleton RG, Rigby OF (1983) Adrenal metastasis in renal cell carcinoma. Urology 21:403–405
6. Cedarmark BJ, Ohlsin H (1981) Computed tomography in the diagnosis of metastases of the adrenal glands. Surg Gynecol Obstet 152:13–16
7. Cedermark BJ, Blumenson LE, Pickren JW et al. (1977) The significance of metastases to the adrenal gland from carcinoma of the stomach and esophagus. Surg Gynecol Obstet 145:41–48
8. Copeland PM (1983) The incidentally discovered adrenal mass. Ann Intern Med 98:940–945
9. Cowan JD, Kies M, Mulgrew PJ et al. (1984) Addison's disease due to metastatic carcinoma. South Med J 77:796–799
10. de la Monte SM, Hutchins GM, Moore GW (1984) Endocrine organ metastases from breast carcinoma. AJP 114:131–136
11. de la Monte S, Moore G, Hutchins G (1983) Patterned distribution of metastases from malignant melanoma in humans. Cancer Res 43:3427–3433
12. Dluhy RG, Himathongkam T, Greenfield M (1974) Rapid ACTH test with plasma aldosterone levels. Ann Intern Med 80:693–696
13. Dunnick N, Ihde D, Johnston-Early A (1979) Abdominal CT in the evaluation of small cell carcinoma of the lung. AJR 133:1085–1088
14. Glazer H, Weyman P, Sagel S et al. (1982) Nonfunctioning adrenal masses: incidental discovery on computed tomography. AJR 139:81–85
15. Glomset DA (1983) The incidence of metastases of malignant tumors to the adrenals. Am J Cancer 32:57–61
16. Goldenberg Sl, Wright JE, McLoughlin MG (1983) Metastatic renal cell carcinoma: unusual cause of Addison's disease. Urology 23:408–409
17. Gross BH, Goldberg HI, Moss AA et al. (1983) CT demonstration and guided aspiration of unusual adrenal metastases. J Comput Assist Tomogr 7:98–101
18. Harper P, Honang M, Spiro S et al. (1981) Computerized axial tomography in the pretreatment assessment of small-cell carcinoma of the bronchus. Cancer 47:1775–1780
19. Heaston DK, Handel DB, Ashton PR et al. (1982) Narrow gauge needle aspiration of solid adrenal masses. AJR 138:1143–1148
20. Hill GI, Wheeler HB (1965) Adrenal insufficiency due to metastatic carcinoma of the lung. Cancer 18:1467–1473
21. Korobkin M, White EA, Kressel HY et al. (1979) Computed tomography in the diagnosis of adrenal disease. AJR 132:231–238
22. Karstaedt N, Sagel SS, Stanley RJ et al. (1978) Computed tomography of the adrenal gland. Radiology 129:723–730
23. Mersey JH, Goldiner WH, Valente WA et al. (1980) Integrated sampling in testing for adrenal insufficiency. Clin Res 28:626A
24. Mersey J, Bowers B, Jezic D et al. (1986) Adrenal insufficiency secondary to invasion by lymphoma: documentation by CT scan. South Med J 79:71–73
25. Meyer JE, Halperin EC, Levene SR et al. (1983) Adrenal insufficiency secondary to metastatic lung carcinoma: CT aided diagnosis. J Comput Assist Tomogr 7:1107–1108
26. Meschan I, Parker M (1984) Urinary tract. In: I Meschan (ed) Roentgen signs in diagnostic imaging. Saunders, Philadelphia, pp 145–316
27. Mitnick J, Bamik M, Megilow A et al. (1983) Nonfunctioning adrenal adenomas discovered incidentally in computed tomography. Radiology 148:495–499
28. Muggia F, Krezoski S, Hansen K (1974) Cell kinetic studies in patients with small cell carcinoma of the lung. Cancer 34:1683–1690
29. Neal PM, Leach GE, Kaswick JA et al. (1982) Renal cell carcinoma: recognition and treatment of synchronous solitary contralateral adrenal metastasis. J Urol 128:135–136
30. Nielson, Jr ME, Heaston DK, Dunnick NR et al. (1982) Preoperative CT evaluation of adrenal gland in nonsmall-cell bronchogenic carcinoma. AJR 139:317–320
31. Oliver T, Bernardino M, Miller J et al. (1984) Isolated adrenal masses in nonsmall-cell bronchogenic carcinoma. Radiology 153:217–218
32. Pagani JJ, Bernardino M (1982) Incidence and significance of serendipitous CT findings in the oncologic patient. J Comput Assist Tomogr 6:267–275
33. Pagani JJ (1983) Normal adrenal glands in small cell lung carcinoma: CT-guided biopsy. AJR 140:949–951
34. Pagani JJ (1984) Non-small cell lung carcinoma adrenal metastases. Cancer 53:1058–1060
35. Paling MR, Williamson BRJ (1983) Adrenal involvement in non-Hodgkin lymphoma. AJR 141:303–305
36. Patel J, Diddkar M, Pickren J et al. (1978) Metastatic pattern of malignant melanoma. A study of 216 autopsy cases. Am J Surg 135:807–810
37. Payne DK, Levine SN, Franco DP et al. (1984) Adrenal insufficiency due to metastatic lung carcinoma and shown by abdominal CT scan. South Med J 77:1592–1593
38. Previte SR, Willscher MK, Burke CR (1982) Renal cell carcinoma with solitary contralateral adrenal metastasis: experience with 2 cases. J Urol 128:132–134
39. Reynes CJ, Churchill R, Monsada R et al. (1979) Computed tomography of adrenal glands. Radiologic Clinic of North America 17:91–104

40. Rosenthal FD, Davis MK, Burden AC (1978) Malignant disease presenting as Addison's disease. Br Med J 2:1591–1592

41. Sample WF, Sarti DA (1978) Computed tomography and gray scale ultrasonography of the adrenal gland: a comparative study. Radiology 128:377–383

42. Sandler MA, Pearlberg JL, Madrozo BL et al. (1982) Computed tomographic evaluation of the adrenal gland in the preoperative assessment of bronchogenic carcinoma. Radiology 145:733–736

43. Schambelan M, Slaton PE Jr, Murray JF et al. (1969) Adrenal insufficiency and inappropriate secretion of antidiuretic hormone. Arch Intern Med 124:197–201

44. Schultz C, Haaga J, Fletcher B et al. (1984) Magnetic resonance imaging of the adrenal glands: a comparison with computed tomography. AJR 143:1235–1240

45. Seidenwurm DJ, Elmer EB, Kaplan LM et al. (1984) Metastases to the adrenal glands and the development of Addison's disease. Cancer 54:552–557

46. Sheeler LR, Myers JH, Eversman JJ et al. (1983) Adrenal insufficiency secondary to carcinoma metastatic to the adrenal gland. Cancer 52:1312–1316

47. Siekavizza JL, Bernardino ME, Samaan NA (1981) Supra-renal mass and its differential diagnosis. Urology 18:625–632

48. Sommers SC (1985) Adrenal glands. In: John M. Kissane (ed) Anderson's pathology. Mosby, Princeton, pp 1429–1450

49. Thomas JL, Barnes PA, Bernardino ME et al. (1982) Diagnostic approaches to adrenal and renal metastases. Radiol Clin North Am 20:531–544

50. Vas W, Zylak CJ, Mather D et al. (1981) The value of abdominal computed tomography in the pre-treatment assessment of small cell carcinoma of the lung. Radiology 138:417–418

51. Viewig WVR, Reitz RE, Weinstein RL (1973) Addison's disease secondary to metastatic carcinoma: an example of adrenocortical and adrenomedullary insufficiency. Cancer 31:1240–1243

52. Weber CL, Murphy ML (1971) Adrenal hypofunction secondary to adrenocortical destruction by metastatic carcinoma of the lung. J Arkansas Med Soc 68:181–183

53. Willis RA (1948) Pathology of tumors. In: Willis RA (ed). Mosby, St Louis, p 178

54. Zornoza J, Bernardino ME (1980) Bilateral adrenal metastasis "head light" sign. Urology 15:91–92

Chapter 13

Surgical Management

N. Javadpour

Surgical Approaches

The physiologic characteristics of the adrenal glands and their anatomic proximity to the genito-urinary organs have attracted the attention of a number of urologic surgeons. Urologic surgeons are thus familiar with the retroperitoneal structures and some have been trained to manage surgical diseases of the adrenal glands. These glands may be approached by abdominal, lumbar, or combined thoracoabdominal incisions, depending on the nature and location of the pathology and to some extent on the familiarity of the surgeon. For pheo-chromocytomas, transperitoneal approaches are desirable. In the case of a large tumor of either of the adrenal glands, a thoracoabdominal approach will provide good exposure of the diaphragm and upper pole of the kidney. Some surgeons may also use a posterior approach, especially in small adrenal tumors or in bilateral adrenalectomy for breast cancer.

The various approaches are described in more detail below and illustrated in Figs. 13.1–13.3.

Anterior Approach

This approach is usually utilized when bilateral adrenal exploration is undertaken. The incision can be a midline or an upper abdominal transverse incision, with which the liver, pancreas, spleen, stomach, intestines, and other abdominal organs can be evaluated. I usually use a midline incision so that the pelvic organs can also be evaluated. After entering the retroperitoneal area, the colon can be brought back laterally or medially to allow access to the adrenal glands. One may make an incision over the posterior peritoneum from the ligament of Treitz to the ileocecal segment. After ligation of the inferior mesenteric vein, the left renal pedicle and the left suprarenal area may be dissected to expose the left adrenal gland. The right adrenal

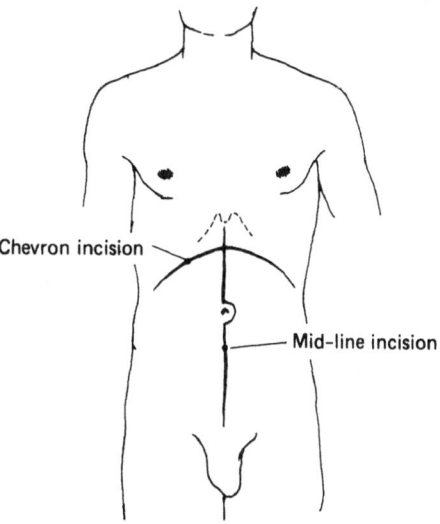

Fig. 13.1. Incisions for transabdominal, transperitoneal simultaneous approaches to both adrenal glands.

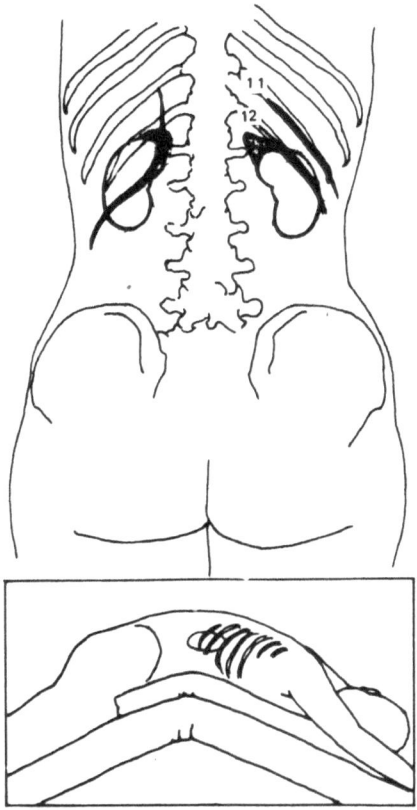

Fig. 13.2. Posterior approach to adrenal glands. Note the position of the table for optimal exposure.

gland may be approached by kocherization of the duodenum and the peritoneal reflection from the anterior surface of the inferior vena cava. This approach is also utilized in the dissection of the retroperitoneal lymph nodes and in addition gives access to the aorta and the lower portion of the urinary tract.

A massive retroperitoneal tumor may be excised safely using this approach, due to excellent control over the great vessels. We have used this approach in a number of cases for an *en bloc* resection of the inferior vena cava surrounded with tumor. Closure of the wound is easy although patients may have ileus for a short period. This can be managed postoperatively by the use of a nasogastric tube for 2–3 days.

Thoracoabdominal Approach

The patient is placed on the operating table with the pelvis flat and the chest rotated about 30° [8]. The arm on the affected side is gently anchored to an ether screen. The kidney rest is elevated to a position under the kidney and the adrenal area. The incision is usually over the tenth rib and after the chest has been opened, the diaphragm is split at its periphery. Then, the adrenal mass and the kidney and the spleen [5] left side will come into view. The mass is dissected from the retroperitoneal area and the tail of the pancreas. The closure is relatively simple and generally a chest tube is inserted and kept in place for 48–72 h. The peritoneum may be opened if an exploration of the intraperitoneal organs is necessary. In the case of a very large retroperitoneal mass, the peritoneal cavity may be opened. This incision lends itself to retroperitoneal exploration for removal of large tumors from the adrenal glands or upper pole of the kidneys.

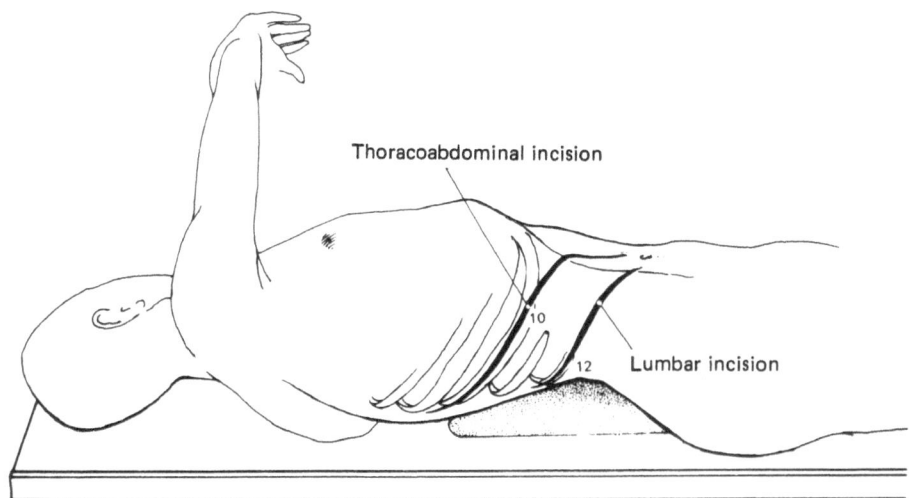

Fig. 13.3. Lateral position including lumbar incision and thoracoabdominal incisions.

Lateral Approach

The lateral flank approach below the ribs or over the 11th or 12th ribs has been used in exposing the kidney and adrenal gland. The disadvantage of this incision is that the abdominal organs and the contralateral adrenal gland can also be exposed. However, if the tumor [1] is small and the lesion unilateral, this exposure is well tolerated.

Combined Sternal and Abdominal Incision

A sternum-splitting midline incision may be made and continued to the abdomen [8]. Alternatively two separate incisions may be made: one on the thoraco-abdominal side, and then, after the primary tumors have been removed to the left and the table tilted to the flat position, a sternum-splitting incision in order to gain access to the upper part of the inferior vena cava and the right atrium. This can be achieved with the patient on cardiopulmonary bypass or without such a bypass. With the assistance of a cardiac surgeon if a cardiopulmonary pump is used, one may remove the tumor from the inferior vena cava without fragments escaping into the right atrium causing pulmonary embolism and possible sudden death.

Surgical Management of Adrenal Diseases

Primary Aldosteronism

The following approaches are used at the University of Maryland and National Institutes of Health in the management of various diseases of the adrenal glands.

Medical treatment of aldosteronism has been tried with spironolactone [3]. This antagonist of aldosterone does not alter the production of this hormone, but works at the level of kidney tubules.

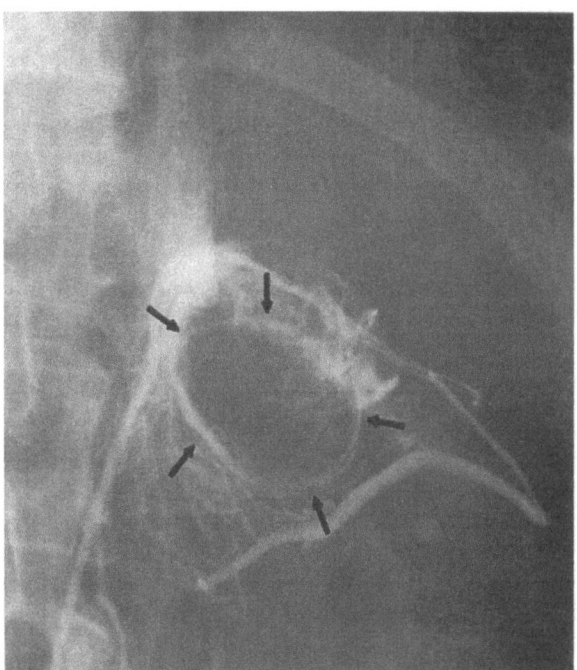

Fig. 13.4. A small adenoma that lateralized on adrenal venography and measurement of adrenal venous aldosterone.

Also, it reduces hypertension, and in selected patients it may be satisfactory as the only therapy.

The advent of accurate localization diagnosis and localization techniques, including the use of computed tomography and venous catheterization (Fig. 13.4) has almost eliminated the need for bilateral exploration of the adrenal glands. Currently, with localization of aldosteronism we use a flank or a posterior approach. Table 13.2 shows a comparison of our current surgical approaches with those used previously. The unilateral approach reduces the postoperative complications.

Table 13.1. Primary aldosteronism: pathology at operation

No. of patients operated on	50
Adrenal pathology found	45
Unilateral adenomas	28
Bilateral multiple adenomas	3
Hyperplasia	9
Adenoma + hyperplasia	4
Atrophy	1

Table 13.2. Primary aldosteronism: surgical approaches at NIH

	No. of cases	Before 1974	After 1974
Anterior abdominal	32	32	—
Thoracoabdominal	1	1	—
Flank	5	—	5
Posterior bilateral	5	5	—
Posterior unilateral	7	—	7

Cushing's Disease

Given the difficulties of diagnosing a pituitary etiology of Cushing's syndrome, and indeed the variable criteria on which such a diagnosis is based, it is not surprising that the incidence of pituitary tumors causing adrenocortical hyperplasia (Cushing's disease) varies between 5% and 20%. Most recently, emphasis on the existence of microadenomas has made previous estimates of the incidence of Cushing's disease erroneously low [4,9,13] (Table 13.3).

Table 13.3. Etiology of Cushing's syndrome in 53 patients who underwent operation at NIH

Adrenal hyperplasia	6
Micronodular hyperplasia	2
Adrenal adenoma	3
Adrenal carcinoma	42

In a series of transsphenoidal microsurgical pituitary explorations for adrenocortical excess, 17 pituitary adenomas were selectively resected, 14 of which were confirmed histologically. Of this total group of 20, normal sella tomography results were obtained in 8 (40%). Sixteen of the 17 undergoing selective tumor removal had their hypercortisolism reversed. This incidence of pituitary adenomas is consistent with autopsy series.

"Normal" plasma ACTH levels can be found in patients with Cushing's disease, but they represent in reality an abnormal response in the presence of hypercortisolism. An elevated peripheral ACTH level does not elucidate a source and may be confused with the ectopic ACTH produced by some tumors. The absence of an obvious neoplasm and the availability of a reliable ACTH assay, selective venous catheterization of the jugular vein, sigmoid sinus, and superior petrosal sinus should be diagnostic.

The surgical approaches depend on the location and type of pathology (Tables 13.1, 13.2).

Adrenal Cancer

Lesions of the adrenal glands are exposed on splitting the diaphragm on a thoracoabdominal approach. If a large unilateral lesion is suspected, the thoracoabdominal approach is preferred. This approach can be combined with a median sternotomy for simultaneous resection of the primary tumor and tumor extending into the supradiaphragmatic portion of the inferior vena cava. Alternatively, for simultaneous resection of the primary lesions and an intrathoracic metastasis, the thoracoabdominal approach through the diaphragm can be used.

A Technique for Resection of Primary Adrenal Carcinoma Extending into the Inferior Vena Cava (IVC) and Right Atrium

The adrenal gland may be exposed through a thoracoabdominal incision resecting the tenth rib. After meticulous dissection of the primary adrenal tumor and the regional lymphatics, attention is focused onto the IVC. Through a sternum-splitting incision, the right atrium, superior vena cava, and the proximal portion of the IVC are identified. The superior vena cava is cannulated and the extracorporeal circulation is initiated using conventional methods of hypothermia. Through a right atriotomy, the superior margin of the tumor can be identified and the atrial extension of the tumor can be removed through this opening. The lower portion of the tumor can be removed through a venotomy in the abdominal portion of the IVC. The atriotomy and venotomy are then closed and the clamp on the IVC distal to the renal veins is removed. Cardiopulmonary bypass is discontinued (Figs. 13.5–13.7).

Pheochromocytoma

The optimal management of patients with pheochromocytoma demands a multidisciplinary approach [2,10,12,16,17]. The radiologic studies recommended include IVP with nephrotomograms, abdominal arteriograms, selective venography, and CT of both adrenal glands. The preoperative localization establishes the surgical approach for excision of these tumors.

The alpha-adrenergic blocking agent phenoxybenzamine is given in a dose of 10–40 mg/day for 10 days to 2 weeks prior to the operation and the dose is titrated to the individual patient's requirement. The efficacy of a particular regimen can be judged by the control of blood pressure, because in some patients other aspects of abnormal catecholamine excess, such as the glucose intolerance and the elevated lipolysis, will not return to normal.

Beta-adrenergic blocking agents (propralonol) can be used in the preoperative or operative period

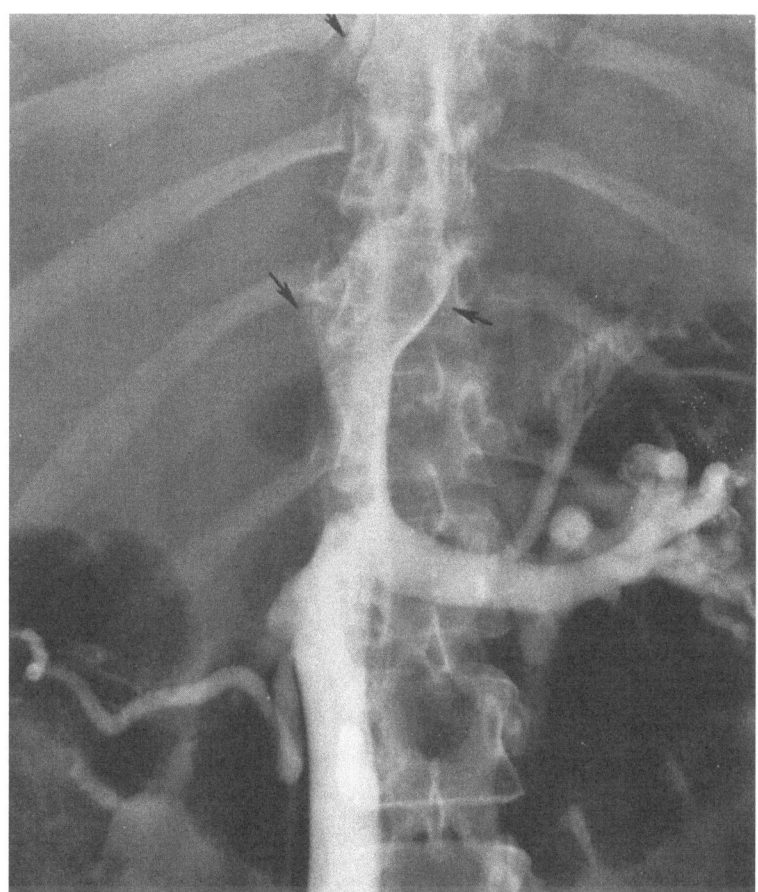

Fig. 13.5. Inferior venacavography of a large adrenal carcinoma. Note the filling defect in the inferior vena cava up to the right atrium (*arrows*).

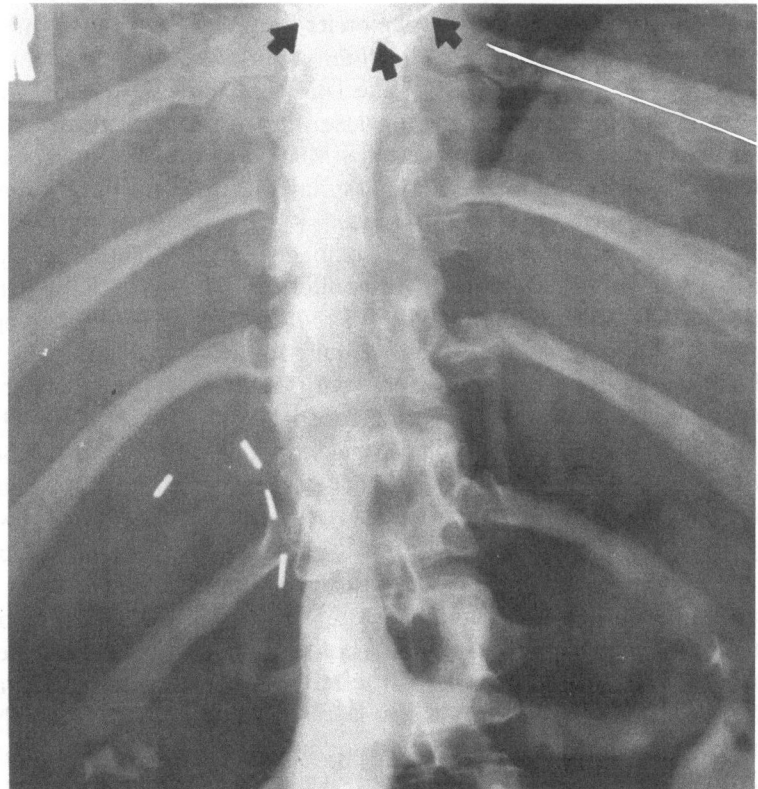

Fig. 13.6. Inferior venacavography of the patient in Fig. 13.5 after the removal of the primary tumor (silver clips) and removal of the tumor thrombus in the vein. Note the loose pursestring suture that was used during the operation in order to prevent pulmonary embolism by tumor fragments (*arrows*). This patient was managed by cardiopulmonary bypass and survived with multiple pulmonary resection.

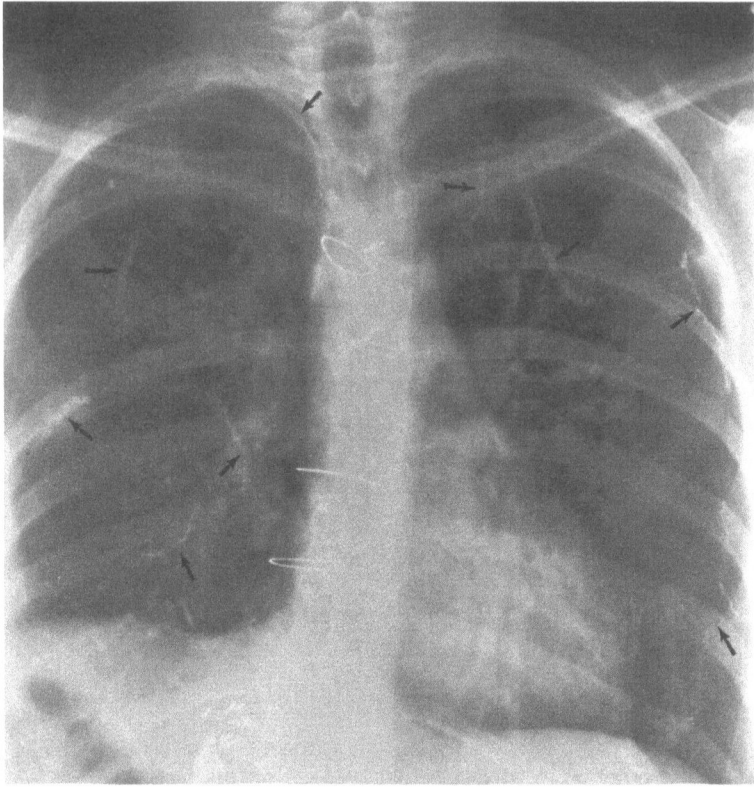

Fig. 13.7. A chest X-ray of the patient in Fig. 13.6 after multiple resections of the pulmonary metastases. (Arrows show the staples for the area of resection.)

especially when patients have myocardial arrhythmia.

An alternative method that we prefer is the use of drugs that decrease catecholamine synthesis, such as alpha-methyl-*para*-tyrosine (AMPT). This agent inhibits tyrosine hydroxylase and thus decreases catecholamine synthesis. AMPT is used in doses ranging from 500 mg to 2 g/day and the dose is titrated to individual tolerance.

The key to successful operative management is extremely careful intraoperative monitoring, particularly at the time of induction. We routinely use arterial pressure monitoring and usually induce a balanced anesthesia, occasionally with Ethrane. Catecholamine-induced arrhythmias can be carefully controlled by the intraoperative use of a beta-blocking agent (propralonol) or lidocaine. Postoperative attention to the large fluid needs of these patients is mandatory.

We have used a midline or a transverse upper abdominal incision for simultaneous bilateral exploration of the adrenal glands; this is an additional reason for bilateral exploration of the adrenal gland. Surgically, the aim is to perform a radical adrenalectomy with removal of all surrounding adjacent fatty tissue and adjacent lymph nodes. On occasion,

in the case of an extensive, invasive tumor, a nephrectomy needs to be performed and most procedures are done through an abdominal approach with the option of entering the chest when appropriate.

The following is an example of the diagnosis and treatment of a metastatic pheochromocytoma. The patient presented with hypertension and was found to have a malignant tumor of the adrenal, which was removed; this was followed by complete resolution of symptoms for approximately 1 year. Then, the patient had recurrence of her symptoms and on angiography was shown to have a vascular lesion in the hilum of the kidney (Fig. 13.8). This was further confirmed by selective venous sampling, which illustrated a marked increase in the release of norepinephrine from the site of the lesion. In addition, markedly elevated levels of norepinephrine were seen in the azygous vein, suggesting the presence of a secondary lesion in the mediastinum (Fig. 13.9). Therapy consisted of complete resection of the locally invasive recurrent lesion followed by removal of the metastases. The patient remained without evidence of tumor approximately 2 years later.

The therapy of choice for malignant pheochromocytoma is resection of the tumor. Blocking

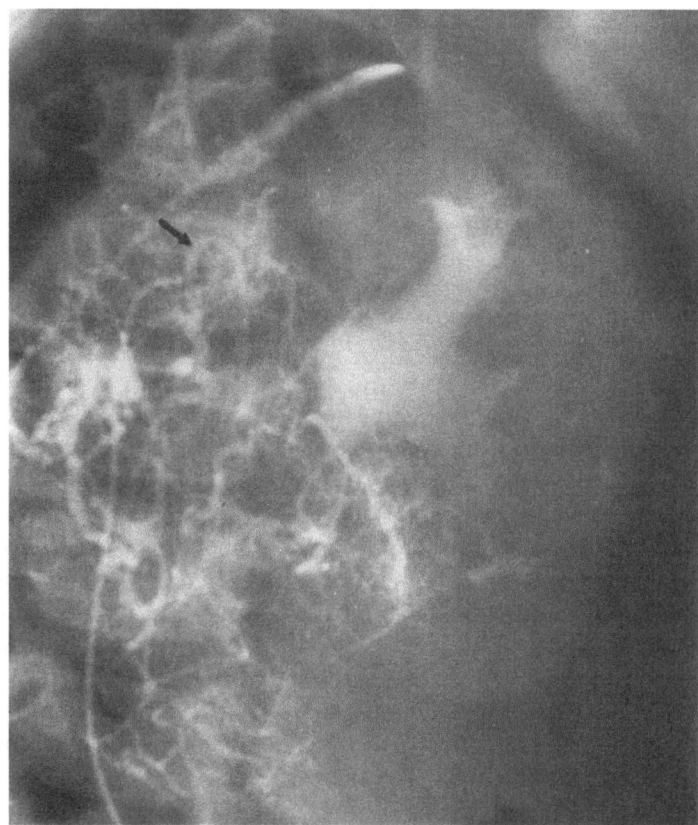

Fig. 13.8. An arteriogram of the recurrence of a left adrenal pheochromocytoma in the hilum of the left kidney. Note the left lumbar artery feeding this recurrent tumor that was not present at the time of the removal of the left adrenal pheochromocytoma.

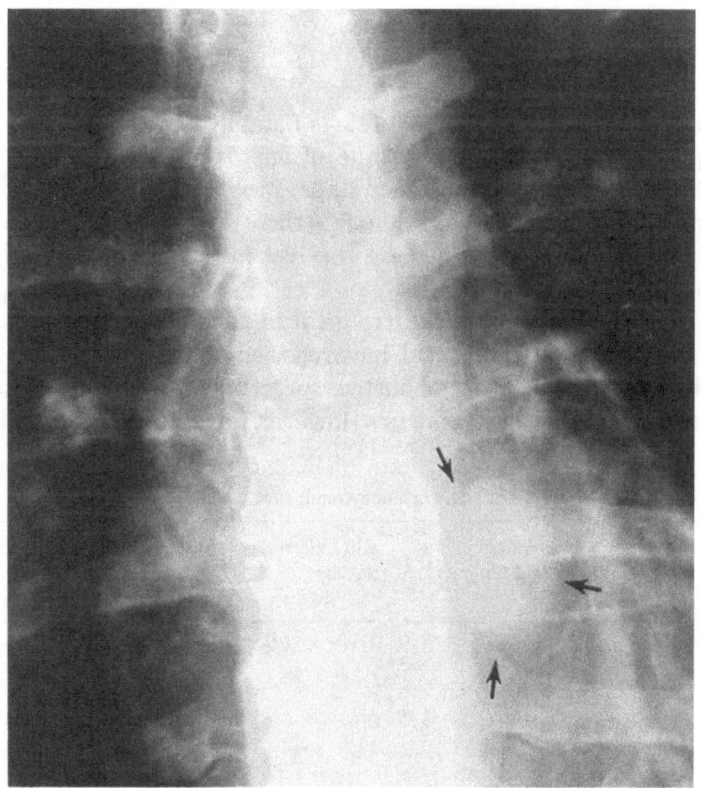

Fig. 13.9. Chest X-ray of the same patient, demonstrating metastasis in the left lung (*arrows*).

Table 13.4. Therapy in 22 patients with malignant pheochromocytoma treated at NIH from 1953 to 1972

Operation alone	6
a-Methyl-*para*-tyrosine (AMPT) alone	2
Surgery plus AMPT	4
Surgery plus propranolol (P)	1
Surgery plus dibenzamine (DBZ)	2
Surgery plus AMPT + P	1
Surgery plus AMPT + DBZ	2
Surgery plus AMPT + AMPP	1
Surgery plus AMPT + AMPP + P + DBZ	1
Surgery plus AMPT + AMPP + DBZ	1
Surgery plus chemotherapy + AMPT + DBZ	1

and synthesis inhibitors may be used for unresectable tumors (Table 13.4). The role of radiation therapy and chemotherapy is not clear at the present time. Patients with disseminated tumors may often benefit symptomatically from tumor debulking, but improvement in survival of the patient with such malignancy is not proven in a control study.

From our limited experience with extraadrenal malignant pheochromocytoma, it appears that the prognosis is worse (Table 13.5), i.e., no 5-year survivors compared with 42% 5-year survivors in patients with adrenal malignant lesions. These figures take no account, however, of the difficulties and delay in the diagnosis.

Neuroblastoma

Complete surgical removal of stage I and II tumors provides a 2-year survival rate of approximately 80%. Its application in other stages has not been proved to be beneficial although there are indications that it may increase survival in selected instances.

Indications for surgical treatment in each stage are less clear. Grosfield et al. have reported a possible beneficial effect of cytoreductive surgery in metastatic neuroblastoma patients. However, their study was not randomized. A prospective randomized study will be needed to evaluate the efficacy of excision in stage III and IV disease. Occasionally, complete resection is possible after chemotherapy and/or irradiation.

The surgical techniques and approaches to the adrenal neoplasms are similar to those for other abdominal tumors such as Wilms' tumor. A midline incision usually lends itself to a careful exploration of the retroperitoneal organs including sympathetic trunks.

The role of radiation therapy remains to be defined. Its use for control of pain due to metastases and for postoperative treatment of stage III residual tumor seems warranted, although the latter is unsupported by properly collected data.

The overall survival rates in neuroblastoma have not improved in relation to those of the other childhood malignancies. Clearly, improved survival will be affected only by an integrated approach to treatment, combining surgical resection, radiation therapy, and prolonged courses of effective chemotherapeutic agents.

References

1. Auda SP, Brennan MF, Gill JR (1980) Evolution of the surgical management of primary aldosteronism. Ann Surg 191:1–7
2. Bergman SM, Sears HF, Javadpour N et al. (1978) Postoperative management of patients with pheochromocytoma. J Urol 120:109
3. Dargo JR, Staten RJ, Lipton A et al (1984) Clinical effect of aminoglutethimide, medical adrenalectomy in treatment of 43 patients with advanced prostatic carcinoma. Cancer 53:1447
4. Schaner EG, Dunnick NR, Doppman JL et al. (1978). Adrenal cortical tumors with low attenuation coefficients: a pitfall in computed tomography diagnosis. J Comput Assist Tomogr 2:11
5. Hajjor RA, Hickey RC, Samaan NA (1975) Adrenal cortical carcinoma. Cancer 35:549

Table 13.5. Malignant pheochromocytoma: survival

Tumor	No. of patients	Alive after 5 years with disease	Alive after 5 years without disease	Dead	Mean survival from diagnosis
Adrenal	16	4/16	3/16	9	6.57 ± 5.3 years Range, 2 months – 16 years
Extraadrenal	6	0/6	0/6	6	1.15 ± 3 years Range, 2 months – 3 years

6. Hunter AM, Kayhoe DE (1968) Adrenal cortical carcinoma: clinical features of 138 patients. Am J Med 41:572

7. Huvos AG, Hajdu SI, Brasfield RD et al. (1970) Adrenal cortical carcinoma: clinicopathologic study of 34 cases. Cancer 25:354

8. Javadpour N, Woltering EA, McIntosh (1978) Technique for resection of primary adrenal carcinoma extending into inferior vena cava and right atrium. Urology 12:626

9. Kullenn F, Couillin P, Girard et al. Late onset of adrenal hyperplasia in hirsutism. N Eng J Med 313:224

10. Mills SR, Doppman JL, Head GI et al. (1978) Transcatheter brush biopsy of intravenous tumor thrombi. Radiology 127:667

11. Punt J, Pritchard J, Pincott JR et al. (1980) Neuroblastoma—a review of 21 cases presenting with spinal cord compression. Cancer 45:3095

12. Rote AR, Flint LD, Ellis FH (1977) Intracaval recurrence of pheochromocytoma extending into right atrium. N Engl J Med 296:1269

13. Sample WF (1978) Adrenal ultrasonography. Radiology 127:461–467

14. Schaner EG, Dunnick NR, Doppmann JL et al. (1978) Adrenal cortical tumors with low attenuation coefficients: a pitfall in computed tomography diagnosis. J Comput Assist Tomogr 2:11

15. Schaner EG, Head GL, Kalman MA et al. (1977) Whole-body computed tomography in the diagnosis of abdominal and thoracic malignancy. Review of 600 cases. Cancer Treat Rep 61:1537

16. Sisson JC, Frager MS, Valk TW et al. (1981) Scintographic localization of pheochromocytoma. N Eng J Med 305:12–17

17. Stewart BH, Bravo EL, Hoaga J et al. (1978) Localization of pheochromocytoma by computed tomography. N Engl J Med 299:460

18. White EA, Schamblen M, Rost ER et al. (1980) Use of computed tomography in diagnosing the cause of primary aldosteronism. N Engl J Med 303: 1503

Subject Index